To my ,
Larry Faulkner
with my best regards
Michael Anundh

BROWN-SÉQUARD

Brown-Séquard

An Improbable Genius Who Transformed Medicine

Michael J. Aminoff, MD, DSc, FRCP
Professor of Neurology
School of Medicine
University of California
San Francisco, California

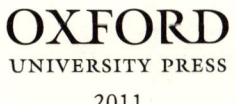

2011

OXFORD
UNIVERSITY PRESS

Oxford University Press, Inc., publishes works that further
Oxford University's objective of excellence
in research, scholarship, and education.

Oxford   New York
Auckland   Cape Town   Dar es Salaam   Hong Kong   Karachi
Kuala Lumpur   Madrid   Melbourne   Mexico City   Nairobi
New Delhi   Shanghai   Taipei   Toronto

With offices in
Argentina   Austria   Brazil   Chile   Czech Republic   France   Greece
Guatemala   Hungary   Italy   Japan   Poland   Portugal   Singapore
South Korea   Switzerland   Thailand   Turkey   Ukraine   Vietnam

Copyright © 2011 by Michael J. Aminoff.

Published by Oxford University Press, Inc.
198 Madison Avenue, New York, New York 10016

www.oup.com

Oxford is a registered trademark of Oxford University Press

All rights reserved. No part of this publication may be reproduced,
stored in a retrieval system, or transmitted, in any form or by any means,
electronic, mechanical, photocopying, recording, or otherwise,
without the prior permission of Oxford University Press.

Library of Congress Cataloging-in-Publication Data

Aminoff, Michael J. (Michael Jeffrey)
   Brown-Séquard : an improbable genius who transformed
medicine / Michael J. Aminoff.
      p. ; cm.
   Includes bibliographical references and index.
   ISBN 978-0-19-974263-9 (alk. paper)
1. Brown-Séquard, Charles-Edouard, 1817–1894.   2. Physicians—France—Biography.
3. Physiologists—France—Biography.   4. Neurologists—France—Biography.   I. Title.
   [DNLM: 1. Brown-Séquard, Charles-Edouard, 1817–1894.   2. Neurology—Great Britain—
Biography.   3. Neurology—Mauritius—Biography.   4. Neurology—Paris—Biography.
5. History, 19th Century—Great Britain.   6. History, 19th Century—Mauritius.   7. History,
19th Century—Paris.   8. Neurology—history—Great Britain.   9. Neurology—history—
Mauritius.   10. Neurology—history—Paris. WZ 100 B881a 2011]
R507.B7.A83 2011
610.92–dc22   [B]   2010013439

This book is dedicated to my father, Abraham S. Aminoff, who died in 1994. He is remembered with love, respect, and admiration. It is also dedicated to Jan, my wife and companion for more than thirty-four years, and to our three children—Alexandra, Jonathan, and Anthony—who have given me much happiness and of whom I am so proud.

Preface

THE FACE OF medicine was changed forever by the experimental observations of Charles Edouard Brown-Séquard, a man whose name came to be known widely throughout the centers of learning in the Old World and the New in the latter half of the nineteenth century. Without benefit of family connections or personal wealth, the young Mauritian, who studied medicine in Paris, led an improbable life as an experimenter and academic clinician. He rose to the very top of his chosen profession in England, France, and the United States, but then destroyed his reputation by experiments that were widely misinterpreted and misunderstood by the public and many of his professional colleagues, even as they led to a new understanding of biology, a new system of medicine, and new treatments for ancient diseases.

Historians of modern medicine encounter the name of Brown-Séquard in many different contexts, but most people have never heard of him, and he is familiar to physicians only because of the spinal cord disorder named after him. His multifaceted contributions to the biomedical sciences and to clinical medicine have been forgotten or, perhaps, were never truly appreciated. It is therefore worth mentioning just some of them here, so that the reader can begin to see the breadth of his achievements.

Brown-Séquard was the first to show that the adrenal glands, previously regarded as vestigial structures, are essential to life. His work revealed that the nervous system controlled the caliber of blood vessels and enabled blood flow to be directed to different regions of the body as needed. He showed that acute damage to the brain affected the function of the lungs, a disorder (neurogenic pulmonary edema) that may have a fatal outcome. It was many years before the phenomenon was rediscovered by others, and not until one hundred years after his original observations that successful attempts were made to treat it, based on mechanisms that he had suggested. By irrigating parts of a dead body with fresh or oxygenated blood, he was able to keep them alive for longer, and this work paved the way for the subsequent development of cardiopulmonary bypass and various transplant procedures. His studies on the hibernating behavior of a small tropical mammal are said to have pointed to the eventual use of hypothermia in patients undergoing heart surgery. His conception of the functional processes that regulate how the brain functions and how—through the nervous system and various chemical (hormonal) mechanisms—the organism is able to function as a seamlessly integrated unit are now generally accepted, but were not well received when first he made his views known. He did not accept the concept, emerging in the latter half of the nineteenth century, that specific functions were localized to anatomically distinct regions of the brain. Instead, he believed that functionally specialized networks of nerve cells were distributed throughout different brain regions, a view that has only recently reemerged, a century later, and is not without merit. His views on the basis of sleep were widely accepted for years although they are remembered no longer. His work on rigor mortis—more than one hundred and fifty years ago—still has major implications for forensic pathologists trying to establish the time of death of their unfortunate subjects. Brown-Séquard's studies on the cause of bed sores and on the eyes and ears—long forgotten—led to important clinical or scientific advances. But it was his work on the central pathways mediating pain sensation that brought him recognition and reward, and his conclusions still serve as a cornerstone of modern teaching in neurobiology. Interestingly, he subsequently revised his beliefs to suggest that dynamic mechanisms within the spinal cord account, at least in part, for the alterations in sensation that result from spinal cord lesions, and only recently—more than one hundred years later—have neuroscientists come round to a point of view not far removed from that which he described just a few months before he died.

In the last years of his life Brown-Séquard faced ruin, both financial and professional, by his work on organ extracts. It began when he injected himself with the mashed-up testicles of various animals and reported improvement in his general condition. He had come to believe that the testicles manufacture a substance that passes into the blood and affects other parts of the body, and that the changes that develop in the elderly relate at least in part to a decline in function of the genital glands. His report caused a sensation and an uproar. It led to disbelief and outrage, but held the attention of the public by its focus on sex, aging, rejuvenation, and the seemingly bizarre use of extracts of animal testicles. The work led directly to a new therapeutic method—hormone replacement therapy—that initially involved the administration of extracts of organs, selected on the basis of the disease to be treated, to restore to the blood substances that he thought were lacking.

A number of biographical essays that briefly catalogue the main events and achievements of Brown-Séquard's life have been published in scholarly journals over the years. These are generally based on secondary sources, however, and—to my knowledge—there have been only two full-length English-language biographies of Brown-Séquard, one by J.M.D. Olmsted and the other by myself. Both of those books, which were written for a somewhat specialized audience, have long been out of print and command unreasonable sums on the few occasions that copies become available from various web-based book outlets. The present volume is intended to be an easily accessible biography that brings the life and work of Brown-Séquard to a wider audience than my earlier monograph, and it is written from a somewhat different perspective, even as it draws from and builds on that earlier work. Indeed, I hope it will appeal not only to neurologists, neurosurgeons, and neuroscientists but also to experimental and clinical endocrinologists, general physicians and surgeons, those interested in the history of medicine and science, and a segment of the lay public. More general information is provided than in my earlier work, including details of important contemporaries, institutions, concepts of disease, beliefs, and customs, and new archival material, especially from Paris and the United States, is included.

To write about such a colorful man—who for a time was the popular face of science—was daunting, if only because original information concerning him is to be found on both sides of the English Channel, in the New World as well as the Old, and in the distant land of Mauritius, his birthplace. There remain gaps in the account of his private life, but I suspect that little is lost, for his life was his work. The sheer volume of work put out by this prodigious and enthusiastic investigator, whose interests spanned so many fields, and the vagaries and eccentricities of his private life, also made it challenging to document his life. He had three wives, fathered three children, and founded three journals, and he was a founder physician of the leading neurological hospital in England, the first professor of neurology in the world, and the holder of chairs at Harvard College, the Collège de France, and other prestigious institutions. He was offered several other chairs throughout his remarkable career, and was an elected member of the three leading scientific societies in the world, namely the Royal Society (England), the National Academy of Sciences (USA), and the Académie des Sciences (France). He spent some six years of his restless life at sea, and his larger-than-life but flawed personality was associated with a private life as turbulent and troubled as his professional life was erratic. He managed to bring on himself the enmity of the church, the antivivisectionists, and much of the medical profession. A man of ideas—indeed, a visionary of science, as I have labeled him elsewhere—he has always been an easy target for professional critics because some of his ideas have failed to stand the test of time. Nevertheless, many of his ideas, important ones, were correct, even though—in some cases—they were based on vague suppositions and supported by incomplete experimental studies. Although they influenced the subsequent course of events, leaving a lasting impression on the face of medicine, Brown-Séquard has never received proper credit as their originator, coming instead to be marginalized. I have tried to examine some of the reasons for this neglect in the pages that follow.

In discussing Brown-Séquard's scientific contributions, I have endeavored to do so in terms free of medical jargon and have included a glossary of any technical terms that had to be used in the text. I have placed his contributions in the context of the times, but have also discussed subsequent developments in the field to show their relevance to modern concepts. I hope that this has helped the general reader to appreciate the clinical and scientific issues under discussion. Although their scientific validity can be questioned, I have included his somewhat sensational experiments on himself because of their profound implications and because of the advances to which they led.

I have been led to an appreciation of Brown-Séquard by a long career as a clinical neurologist and neurophysiologist, and have come to admire his versatility and foresight even if I have at times come to wonder about the oddities of his life. Today, he should rank as one of the great clinician-scientists of his generation, an unhappy genius who had profound insight and intuition into the mechanisms that allow living organisms to function as an integrated whole.

I have derived enormous pleasure in studying the life and works of Brown-Séquard, even as I have marveled at the extent of his achievements, have been engrossed by the concepts that he advanced, and have wondered at the wild swings in his fortunes over the years. Many of the issues with which he struggled still baffle us, and I hope that readers will find challenging the sometimes wild imaginings of this captain of science.

Michael J. Aminoff
San Francisco, 2010

Acknowledgments

I RECEIVED HELP FROM many people in preparing this book, and welcome the opportunity to express my gratitude to them. I was first introduced to the curious life of Brown-Séquard while working as an intern on the clinical service of the eminent British neurologist, William Gooddy, in the mid-1960s. Dr. Gooddy was a cultured man of enormous charm, and he easily infected me with his enthusiasm and admiration for Brown-Séquard and his achievements. He had traced the surviving members of Brown-Séquard's family, who still had some of his papers, correspondence, and clinical and scientific notes, and these were subsequently purchased by the Royal College of Physicians of London and placed in their archives.

Mr. Geoffrey Davenport, then librarian at the College, and his assistant Ms. Terry Picton, were most generous, not only in facilitating my access to this archival material but in photocopying the entire collection for me to study at my leisure in California. I have referenced this archival material in the bibliography of various chapters by manuscript number, indicating the source simply as "Archives, Royal College of Physicians, London."

I am most appreciative for the assistance that I received from the staff of the library at the University of California, San Francisco, and especially from Ms. Azar Khatibi and Mr. Josue Hurtado, as well as from the staff at the Lane Medical Library at Stanford University Medical Center, the Francis A. Countway Library of Medicine in Boston, and the archives of the Académie des Sciences in Paris. Numerous archivists and librarians at other institutions found time to delve into their records on my behalf with regard to specific queries, and I have acknowledged their assistance in the footnotes to the text. I am pleased also to thank Mr. Timothy Underwood and Ms. Sarah Corr at the University of California, San Francisco, for their help.

Working on this book has afforded me great pleasure, not least because of the many discussions I had over the years with friends such as Professors Douglas S. Goodin and Richard K. Olney at the University of California, San Francisco, on various aspects of Brown-Séquard's experimental work, as well as with friends and colleagues at many other universities and medical schools in this country and abroad. My three children each read portions of the manuscript and offered suggestions for improvement, and I am grateful to them for their assistance. Alexandra is a physician who is specializing in pediatrics, Jonathan is an attorney who works as a deputy Federal Public Defender, and Anthony is a law student. They were thus able to comment on the manuscript from different perspectives than my own, which was particularly helpful. I thank them also for the patience with which they listened as I recounted over the dinner table what I hope were amusing vignettes about Brown-Séquard and his contemporaries. I also thank my wife, Jan, for ensuring that I had the time to work undisturbed on this book and for her love and support.

I am grateful to those who helped me with the artwork for this book. The illustrative material was derived from various sources, as indicated by the credit line that appears in the legends to the figures in the plates. Ms. Kathy Jee made up the diagrams of the anatomy and physiology of the spinal cord that appear in the text, and I greatly appreciate her help. I am also grateful to Mr. Max Morath, the entertainer and an authority on ragtime, for a copy of his production notes and his recording of the song "Brown-Séquard's Elixir" by Winchell Forbes, which became popular in American music halls soon after Brown-Séquard reported on his work with testicular extracts.

Mr. Craig A. Panner, my editor at the Oxford University Press, never failed to offer me advice, encouragement, and assistance in seeing this volume through to publication, and I greatly appreciated his help and value his continuing friendship. I am also grateful to Ms. Karen Harmon, Ms. Joann Woy, Mr. Viswanath Prasanna, and the production team who guided this book through the publication process with patience, skill, and understanding.

Contents

Chapter 1 The Death of a Professor 3

Chapter 2 At Home in Mauritius 11

Chapter 3 A Medical Student in Paris 23

Chapter 4 Great Expectations 45

Chapter 5 The Physics of the Circulation: Why We Don't Faint on Standing, and Why We Get Bedsores on Lying Still for Too Long 65

Chapter 6 Fame in the Making 81

Chapter 7 Fame and Fortune in Britain: A Piece of Cake 97

Chapter 8 Broken Dreams and Promises 121

Chapter 9 Musical Chairs 137

Chapter 10 Thoughts About the Brain 157

Chapter 11 The Disease of Devils and Demons 183

Chapter 12 The Magnificent Maverick 197

Chapter 13 A New System of Medicine 235

Chapter 14 Scenes from the World of a Scientist 261

Chapter 15 A Backward Glance and a Reckoning 283

General Biographical References 289

Appendix: The Scientific Works of Brown-Séquard 291

Glossary 335

Index 343

BROWN-SÉQUARD

1

The Death of a Professor

It was April 2, 1894. Monsieur Loewy, president of the Académie des Sciences in Paris, announced to the assembled members that Charles Edouard Brown-Séquard had died a few hours earlier. He read out a telegram of condolence from the president of the section of physiology of the International Medical Congress then meeting in Rome, commented briefly on the life and accomplishments of the elderly physician and physiologist who had been professor of medicine at the Collège de France, and—after five minutes—brought the meeting to an end as a sign of mourning and respect.[1] The academicians, having heard rumors of his death, had come in great number to the meeting to show their respect for an illustrious colleague, and they now gathered in the corridors to talk and remember him.

Brown-Séquard's death—along with that of many other grandees of history—was part of the fabric of a turbulent year, filled with many distractions. Anarchists tried to blow up the Royal Observatory in Greenwich; the First Sino-Japanese war broke out; there was revolution in Sicily and civil unrest in the United States, with strikes and marches by the unemployed on Washington and riots in Cleveland; and President Carnot of France was assassinated and Captain Dreyfus arrested for espionage in a case that was to challenge the very underpinnings of the French Republic. Nevertheless, Brown-Séquard's death was widely noted in the lay press as well as in the scientific periodicals. Obituaries were published in the leading dailies and weeklies of the time, not only in Paris, London, and New York, but in Budapest, Vienna, and St. Petersburg, and in the obscure local newspapers of other towns and provinces in the major countries of Europe, as well as in his distant birthplace of Mauritius. All of Europe seemed to have been taken by surprise and to miss him. The entire academic world seemed to mourn him.[2]

The aging Brown-Séquard had, in fact, been ill for at least a year with phlebitis of the right leg, and he had also been depressed by the death of his third wife, Emma, in January 1894, as they wintered in Nice.[3] Indeed, he felt lost without her. Perhaps he should have stayed in the warmth of the south of France, as his friends and collaborators had urged, but he felt the need to return to the metropolitan bustle of the capital and to his second-floor apartment at 19 rue François Premier, and it was there that he died of "cerebral congestion" at 11:30 P.M. on April 1, under the care of his devoted physician, Eugene Dupuy, another Mauritian, who had worked under him as a young medical student and dedicated his doctoral thesis to the older man who had come to regard him as a son:

> To my illustrious Master, to him who gave me without reservation the treasures of his heart and mind, C. E. Brown-Séquard.[4]

Brown-Séquard himself described his last illness in a letter to Dr. Waterhouse, a friend to whom he was related by marriage,[5] and an account by Dr. Dupuy provides further information,[6] as is described in detail in Chapter 12. At his request, there was no state funeral, no pomp or speeches, no wreaths or symbols on the coffin. He had requested that no religious rites be performed, but a private and simple service was nevertheless held at his home, with an Anglican clergyman officiating and giving a brief eulogy. A magnificent wreath of lilacs, camellias, and roses addressed "To Brown-Séquard, [from] the island of Mauritius" was delivered to his home,[7,8] and there were flowers from others, despite his wishes. His body was then conveyed to the cemetery of Montparnasse, where it was interred in the presence of representatives of the Académie des Sciences, the Institut de France, the Collège de France, the Société de Biologie, the governments of France and the island of Mauritius, and his friends and collaborators. The pall bearers were Loewy[A] and Bertrand (president and permanent secretary, respectively, of the Académie des Sciences), Boissier (administrator of the Collège de France), Dumontpallier (secretary of the Société de Biologie),[B] the sculptor Prosper d'Epinay (representing

---

[A] Maurice Loewy (1833–1907), astronomer and director of the Paris Observatory, has a crater on the moon named after him.

[B] Alphonse Dumontpallier (1827–1899), French physician, interested in hypnotism and suggestion.

Mauritius),[C] and Etienne-Jules Marey[D] (another of the professors at the Collège).[7-9]

Time has not been kind to the memory of Brown-Séquard. His legacy is all but forgotten, save for a neurological disorder named after him. Ironically, he revised his view of this disorder in his later years in favor of a concept of sensation and sensory loss so modern and far-reaching in its implications that, despite its importance, it is poorly understood even by modern neuroscientists. That he is the father of modern experimental endocrinology, the originator of hormone replacement therapy, one of the founding fathers of neurology (the study of the nervous system in health and disease), a pioneer in transplant surgery, the discoverer of the nerves that regulate the caliber of blood vessels and thereby influence the "physics of the circulation,"[10] a champion of translational medicine, and a visionary whose ideas spawned a new system of medicine is quietly forgotten or, perhaps, never received the wide recognition that it merited. That he stimulated research and scientific investigation, and a scientific approach to clinical medicine wherever he worked or visited—whether in London, Paris, Boston, New York, Richmond (Virginia), Glasgow, Geneva—and generated an enthusiasm for pure science that he passed on to all with whom he came into contact has rarely been acknowledged, although a number of his contemporaries have attributed their subsequent success to his example.

Brown-Séquard was an eccentric whose background and lifestyle doubtless contributed to his decline into obscurity. He was a colonial, without connections or influence, who reached out to the academic world and achieved great stature but remained always an outsider. Contemptuous of money, he could not be induced by unrestrained offers to take on responsibilities that had no appeal or for which he felt unqualified. He refused to profit from the organotherapy that he developed, instead making his organ extracts available freely to physicians requesting them and publishing the technical details of his approach so that others could follow the *methode séquardienne* (and personally profited by it). He rejected fashionable medical practices in the Old World and

---

[C] Prosper d'Epinay (1836–1914), son of a Mauritian politician, was a well-known sculptor, among whose subjects were King Edward VII, Queen Alexandra, other royalty, and many illustrious personalities of the age. He lived in London, Paris, Rome, and Mauritius. Many famous museums, including the Hermitage, display his works.

[D] Etienne-Jules Marey (1830–1904), scientist renown for the development of measurement devices for physiological studies and a pioneer in the developing field of cinematography. He was interested in movement and, among his other achievements, showed photographically that a galloping horse has all four hooves off the ground at once.

the New, preferring to devote himself to more academic pursuits, and at several points became almost destitute in consequence.

Convinced that the advance of medicine depended on experimental studies in animals, he embraced this approach in his own laboratory and brought on himself the wrath of the antivivisectionists, who attacked him both physically and in print. The obituary published in *The Echo* of London noted that he "had earned the infamous fame of being the greatest torturer of animals next to Pasteur himself" and that he had shown "to what a bottomless abyss of selfishness vivisectors and their patrons may descend."[11] And *Le Tintamarre* of Paris gleefully seized the opportunity to publish a poem, "The Revenge of the Guinea Pig."[12] Brown-Séquard's later work on organotherapy was also a provocation to religious groups, which showed him little charity in response. Moreover, his love of the scientific method, with its emphasis on measurement and quantification, seemed sometimes to lead him to almost absurd activities, such as counting the number of gray hairs in his beard or measuring the force of his urinary stream. He did not hesitate to dismiss or oppose scientific doctrines with all his scientific authority when they failed to satisfy him, regardless of their general acceptance by his peers. He did so without the sensitivity, grace, and easy charm that characterize the natural leader. Restless, moody, and uneasy, he is popularly supposed to have crossed the Atlantic some sixty times, spending more than six years of his life at sea. This failure to put down roots or to build a school of disciples to follow in his path, coupled with his diverse rather than focused interests and the scorn generated by his work or style in various segments of the population, opened the gateway to his subsequent obscurity.

Only a few plaques or memorials attest to his substantial achievements—streets named after him in Paris and Nice, a bust, hospital and streets in Mauritius, a postage stamp, a medal even—but his many published articles and books provide a guide to the trail of ideas followed by this eccentric man of science. Many of these ideas retain a freshness and startling originality more than a century after they were formulated, generating exciting new thoughts and possibilities that vindicate Winston Churchill's famous belief that "the farther back you can look, the farther forward you are likely to see." Sadly, however, Brown-Séquard died before many of his ideas and insights could be validated by the disciplined and meticulous experimentation that characterizes the scientific method, a method that he himself sometimes appeared to forego.

Although Brown-Séquard dwarfed many of his colleagues in the originality of his ideas, he flouted the rituals of scientific discovery, and his ideas sometimes superseded reasoned judgment, leading to unrealistic expectations by the general public and chilling disenchantment by the scientific and academic communities, which suspected that much of his work was based on the shifting sands of self-delusion. Furthermore, as his obituarist in the *New York Herald* remarked, his work on organotherapy, in which mashed up testicles and other organ extracts were used to treat human aging and disease, "had to make headway against a great amount of ridicule from the incredulous, misunderstanding from the indifferent, and determined opposition from the haters of innovation."[13]

And yet, he was indeed one of the most extraordinary men of his time, an experimentalist of restless energy, a scientist driven by a compelling urge to understand the physiology—the function—of living organisms. It is ironic, sad even, that the young man who established his reputation through an ability to look with fresh eyes at established beliefs and show their fallacious underpinnings eventually was himself to follow a path that was a shortcut to ridicule and exposed him to the satirists and cartoonists of the popular press.

Even at his death, a few of these journalists could not resist a final opportunity to amuse themselves at the expense of Brown-Séquard's organotherapy, for despite the master's carefully worded communications, others had made injudicious claims for an "elixir of life" that delayed aging. Thus, the now mercifully forgotten Tristan Bernard, in *Le Journal* of 4 April 1894, took the opportunity to describe at length the "arrival of Brown-Séquard in paradise" to the apparent consternation of both St. Peter and God.[14] The Almighty's initial reaction was to greet the scientist with the reproving comment: "Ah! Ah! It is Monsieur Brown-Séquard. It is you, monsieur, who believes that we already have too many clients in paradise and finds the need to prolong the lives of men, giving chaste old men in their sixties the desire and power to depart from the path of virtue ..." Others were kinder in their reaction to the novel therapeutic approach. His obituarist in *Nature*,[15] the leading English-language journal of science, remarked that "Dreams allowed to a poet are forbidden to the philosopher, and time will alone tell whether there be any germ of reason in Brown-Séquard's investigations; if not, they may be forgotten and forgiven." And in *The Lancet*,[16] the implications of his controversial work were spelled out clearly: "It is to be feared, however, that all the evidence goes to show that the sanguine hopes of its single-minded inventor [that testicular extracts might affect the function of many parts of the body] were based upon insufficient evidence, yet in view of the recent developments of therapeutics by means of animal extracts the introduction of this fluid at the particular time at which it was brought forward is not without a considerable degree of significance." Indeed, *The Lancet's* correspondent, in a separate article, wrote that "It is no exaggeration to say that ... Dr Brown-Séquard has invented a new system of medicine which has a great future before it."[17]

Brown-Séquard is a man worthy of recognition as a visionary of science. Indeed, at his death, three great nations claimed him as one of their own, including Britain (for he was a British subject by birth), France (as he became a naturalized citizen of the Republic), and the United States (because he was fathered by an American sea captain). This eccentric, colorful, and peripatetic professor, with his intuitive vision of the integrative mechanisms that maintain the organism—namely, the nervous and the endocrine/hormonal (chemical) systems—has had a tremendous impact on clinical and academic medicine. Henry Bowditch,[E] dean of Harvard Medical School, in reading a memoir on Brown-Séquard to the U.S. National Academy of Sciences in 1897, concluded of him that "if his reasoning power had equaled his power of observation he [Brown-Séquard] might have done for physiology what Newton did for physics."[18] In fact, the advances that have occurred in the biomedical sciences in the years since Brown-Séquard's death have provided increasing support for many of the concepts to which his reasoning—faulty or otherwise—led him, but which met with such fierce opposition from the establishment of his day.

References and Source Notes

1. Anonymous. Académie des Sciences. Séance du 2 Avril. *Le Journal des Debats*, 3 April 1894.
2. Anonymous. Nouvelles de l'étranger. France. *La Gazette de Lausanne*, 3 April 1894.
3. Ville de Nice. Extrait du Registre des Actes de Décès, tenu à la Mairie de Nice pour l'année 1894.
4. Rouget FA. *Brown-Séquard et Son Oeuvre. Esquisse Biographique* (pp. 83–85). Ile Maurice: General Printing and Stationery Co., 1930.
5. Brown-Séquard CE. Extracts from letters written to Dr. W.D. Waterhouse. *Lancet* 1; 977, 1894.
6. Ogle JW. Further remarks on Dr. Brown-Séquard's last illness. *Lancet* 1; 1391, 1894.
7. Anonymous. Obsèques de M. Brown-Séquard. *La Presse*, 5 April 1894.
8. Anonymous. Obsèques du Docteur Brown-Séquard. *Le Gaulois*, 5 April 1894.
9. Anonymous. Les obsèques de M. Brown-Séquard. *Le Figaro*, 5 April 1894.
10. Annotations. Great Mauritians. *Lancet*, 2; 491, 1919.
11. Anonymous. *The Echo (London)*, 3 April 1894.
12. Pichenette. La revanche du cobaye. *Le Tintamarre (Paris)*, 7 April 1894.
13. Anonymous. Dr Brown-Séquard dead. The great physician and scientist succombs [sic] to congestion of the brain. His life and work. *New York Herald*, 3 April 1894.

[E] Henry Bowditch (1840–1911), medical researcher, educator, and dean for ten years of Harvard Medical School, was one of the founders of the American Physiological Society and a vigorous defender of freedom for animal research. See also Chapter 8.

14. Tristan Bernard. Arrivée de Brown-Séquard au paradis. *Le Journal*, 4 April 1894.
15. Anonymous. Obituary: Charles Edouard Brown-Séquard. *Nature*, 49; 556–557, 1894.
16. Anonymous. Obituary: Professor Brown-Séquard. *Lancet*, 1; 975–977, 1894.
17. Anonymous. Death of Professor Brown-Séquard. *Lancet*, 1; 906–907, 1894.
18. Bowditch HP. Memoir of Charles Edouard Brown-Séquard, 1817–1894. *Biographical Memoirs Natl Acad Sci USA* (pp. 93–97). Read before the National Academy, April 1897.

At Home in Mauritius

BROWN-SÉQUARD'S MEDICAL and scientific career had an unsteady beginning. It was November 1838, when the intense young Mauritian enrolled as a student in the Faculty of Medicine in Paris. The study of medicine was his second choice, for he had a passion for literature, had tried his hand at numerous plays, poems, and philosophical vignettes,[1] and had come to the metropolis with hopes of following a literary career. His aspirations were perhaps somewhat foolhardy, as he needed to support both himself and his mother, and he was therefore advised against pursuing them by the several literary persons from whom he sought guidance, including the illustrious Charles Nodier,[A] to whom he had an introduction and to whom he entrusted his best offerings.[1] He may have seemed talented to his friends back home, but the sophisticated Parisians were apparently not impressed. Discouraged and disillusioned, he burned all the manuscripts he had at hand, leaving only the few that remained in distant Mauritius or lay forgotten in some drawer. In his own words, he sacrificed the hopes nurtured over several years solely for the sake of his mother.[1] If this was indeed the case, it would seem that his aspirations were built on the quicksand of indulgent fantasy, and it is more likely that he simply chose for his future the surer path of a profession than the haphazard trail of a literary career as a means of rising to a higher social class and of

---

[A] Charles Nodier (1780–1844), a poet, novelist, bibliophile, and member of the Académie française, influenced many writers of the period, including Victor Hugo, Alexandre Dumas (père), Prosper Mérimée, Alfred de Musset, and Sainte-Beuve. He was also director of the Bibliothèque de l'Arsenal in Paris.

ensuring his future financial stability. It is less clear why he chose a career in medicine rather than some other profession, for at the time many viewed a medical career as inferior to one in law or holy orders, or even the army, and it often provided less financial reward or time for leisurely relaxation. The choice was not related to family tradition or to the influence of some dominant figure encountered in early childhood, and up until this time, he seemed to have shown no particular interest in medicine.

Paris in the first half of the nineteenth century was quite unlike the modern capital of France, despite the efforts of Napoleon Bonaparte, who built various monuments, the arcades of the rue de Rivoli, and the Arc du Carrousel and Arc de Triomphe, and who even improved the sewer system. Its cramped and malodorous slums and crooked alleyways, a reminder of the city's medieval past, were not replaced with sweeping boulevards and wide avenues (which were more difficult to barricade), lined by trees and imposing buildings, until the latter half of the century. The population of Paris was only 714,000 in 1817, the year of Brown-Séquard's birth, and around 900,000 when he enrolled as a student; by the early 1860s, however, it exceeded 1.5 million. The first railway line was opened in Paris in 1837, and the subsequent physical expansion of the city reflected its increasing importance as a commercial, industrial, and cultural center

The city must have seemed bleak in November to the young man who had come from an exotic, far-off island in the Indian Ocean, but he was at least familiar with its language and culture. Mauritius had, after all, been French until the end of the Napoleonic war.

Mauritius is unknown to many people except perhaps as a tourist resort, the source of certain rare stamps—the penny-red and twopenny-blue of 1847—that command vast sums in the auction rooms of the world,[2] or the home of the dodo immortalized in Lewis Carroll's *Alice In Wonderland*. This pigeon-like bird, supposedly obese (although this has recently been questioned and its weight related to seasonal variation in its size), was unable to fly, nested on the ground, and survived the arrival of humans on the island by less than two hundred years, serving as a source of food for the colonists and their domestic animals.[3] One of these luckless animals was preserved after death and kept in the Ashmolean Museum at Oxford, but in 1755 it was thrown on a bonfire because it looked so poorly, and only its head and one leg could be rescued when the new curator made a timely appearance.

Midway between the Cape of Good Hope and India, about a thousand miles from Durban and Mombasa, the volcanic island that is Mauritius rises from the Indian Ocean, ringed by shoals of coral reefs.[2-5] It is small, just over 700 square miles in area, has a tropical climate with high humidity, and—especially in February—is prone to cyclones. Nevertheless, during the nineteenth century, its location made it an important base in times of war and a major commercial center in times of peace. Charles Darwin visited it in 1836 on *H.M.S. Beagle* and found that

> The island equalled the expectations raised by the many well-known descriptions of its beautiful scenery. The sloping plain of the Pamplemousses, interspersed with houses, and coloured by the large fields of sugar-cane of a bright green, composed the foreground. The brilliancy of the green was the more remarkable because it is a colour which generally is conspicuous only from a very short distance. Towards the centre of the island groups of wooded mountains rose out of this highly cultivated plain; their summits, as so commonly happens with ancient volcanic rocks, being jagged into the sharpest points. Masses of white clouds were collected around these pinnacles, as if for the sake of pleasing the stranger's eye. The whole island, with its sloping border and central mountains, was adorned with an air of perfect elegance: the scenery, if I may use such an expression, appeared to the sight harmonious.[6]

Originally discovered by the Portuguese Captain Domingos Fernández in 1505 and called Ilha do Cerne (Island of the Swan),[B] it was rediscovered in 1513 by his compatriot Pedro de Mascarenhas, and is one of the Mascarene Islands. A Dutch expedition under Admiral Wybrandt van Warwyck took formal but only brief possession of it in September 1598, naming it after Prince Maurice van Naussau, Stadthouder of the Netherlands. Over the following years, the Dutch occasionally called at the island for food and shelter, but it was not until 1637 that it was formally occupied by the Dutch East India Company (Vereenigde Oostindische Compagnie) and became a penal settlement. During the seventy-five years of their rule, the Dutch left Mauritius three times, finally abandoning it in 1712, when they moved to the Cape in the hope of finding an easier livelihood.[7] Three years later, Captain Guillaume Dufresne and the French Compagnie des Indes took possession, renaming it L'Isle de France; but the colonists—from Brittany and the island of Reunion—and the Swiss mercenaries who accompanied them grew so restless with the shortage of women that the Compagnie was forced to ship out *filles de joie* from western France to appease them and lure future settlers to the colony.

[B] It is unclear why this name was chosen, but suggestions include that it relates to the shape of the island, the large birds found on the island, or the name of the ship bearing its discoverer.

Not until 1734, when Bertrand François Mahe de Labourdonnais[C] was appointed Governor-General, did the island begin to develop commercial significance as an agricultural colony and strategic importance as a naval base. With the liquidation of the Compagnie des Indes in 1767, Mauritius became a French Crown Colony and remained so until the French Revolution.[7,8] In 1785, it became the seat of government of all French possessions east of the Cape, and its capital city, Port Louis, became renowned for its extravagant social life with its dancing parties, hunting, drinking, gambling, and scandals, as well as for the fraud and corruption that characterized its administration.

The revolutionary ferment of metropolitan France, when finally it spread to the island, had a comic aspect compared with the upheavals in Paris, and was probably muted by the warmth of the sun as well as by an outbreak of smallpox. In an atmosphere of excitement and gaiety, revolutionary placards were posted in prominent places, clubs modeled on their Parisian prototypes were started in Port Louis—these included the Chaumière, an imitation of the Jacobin Club that had branches in the various towns of the island—and a Colonial Assembly was established.[4,9] In the church of St. Louis, a solemn Mass was sung for the soul of the assassinated Jacobin leader, Jean-Paul Marat, with great pomp and splendor; so shaken were the foundations by repeated salvos from saluting cannons that the church has been regarded as unsafe for public assembly ever since.[7] The members of the Chaumière Club, who initially were satisfied by talk of liberty and equality and by the planting of trees and the wearing of red caps, suddenly decided in mid-1794 to become more active in politics.[9] The governor-general was persuaded to bring to trial three officials accused of corresponding with the English, and the Club set up a guillotine in the public square. The wily governor, however, managed to delay things with great skill until the revolutionary excitement had diminished and the Reign of Terror in France had ceased; the Chaumière Club was then closed, the prisoners released, and the guillotine destroyed after it had severed only the head of an unlucky goat. Other high-points of the period included the collapse of a platform on which the leaders of the local revolution had gathered, and the demise of Macnamara, the Irish commander of the local

---

[C] Bertrand François Mahe de Labourdonnais (1699–1753), as governor-general of the Mascarene Islands (1735–1746), transformed Mauritius, constructing roads, houses, warehouses, fortresses, and barracks, and establishing a ship-building industry. In 1746, with England and France at war, he led an expedition to India, defeated a British squadron, and captured Madras (now Chennai) but was subsequently accused of accepting a bribe to preserve the city. Replaced as governor of Mauritius, he returned to France but was imprisoned in the Bastille on false charges. Although eventually exonerated, he died a broken man, aged 54. His statue stands in Port Louis, and the town of Mahebourg is named after him.

French naval forces, who was arrested and murdered by a mob after an attempted escape led to "an unfortunate misunderstanding."[7]

The more extreme decrees of the National Convention were muted by the wisdom and good sense of the leading local officials.[9] The governor-general, reassured by the distance between the island and mainland France, issued two important decrees. One stated that all resolutions of the Colonial Assembly that received his assent had the force of law, and the other required that laws passed in France had to be submitted to the Colonial Assembly, which would have the power of approving or delaying their application to the colony.[9] Order was therefore maintained on the island despite the ferment.

In 1794, the government in Paris decreed that all slaves were to be given their freedom, but offered no compensation to their luckless owners, who thereupon lost much of their enthusiasm for the ideals of the Revolution. When agents of the Directoire, clad in splendid orange cloaks, arrived from France to enforce these laws, they were promptly deported by the Mauritians, who had already heard of the massacre of white settlers that had followed emancipation in the Antilles. The island, despite such almost treasonable civil disobedience, remained loyal to France and served also as a base for corsairs who, encouraged by the French authorities, threatened to disrupt commercial shipping of all nationalities, but especially the British. Between 1797 and 1801, the island was organized as a *département* of France, but with a colonial assembly that divided the colony into eight cantons. Between 1803 and 1810, it became part of the French colony of Indes Orientales, which included various French territories in the area. Over these years, pirate loot poured into Port Louis (renamed Port Napoleon), attracting American traders who were able to get better terms there than in India, until President Thomas Jefferson put a stop to such American involvement in 1807.[2] Nevertheless, trade with America was important for both countries, and Mauritius promoted it by providing the necessary warehousing and supply facilities. An American ship with a cargo of American and West Indian goods, for example, would arrive in Mauritius after perhaps stopping in Cape Town and then, if the prices were right, often trade its remaining cargo for coffee, pepper, and tea. The alternative was to sail on to Bombay, where its cargo could be exchanged for cotton and other goods that—in turn—might be sold elsewhere in Asia for a tidy sum before the return voyage to Cape Town and then to the United States with local goods.

In 1809, five Indiamen were captured by privateers and others, and the losses of the British East India Company in that year amounted to thirteen ships captured or shipwrecked. These events, fears that the French would use Mauritius as a base for attacking India itself, and concerns that trade in India could be hurt by trading in Mauritius eventually led the British to mount an assault on the island. In December 1810, sixteen thousand men landed to find themselves opposed by a much smaller local force. The French surrendered after a campaign that lasted no more than four days and cost the British less than one hundred and fifty casualties.[4] The surrender clauses guaranteed the maintenance of local laws, languages, and customs. By the Treaty of Paris, signed in 1814, the island was ceded to Britain "in full right and sovereignty," but it retained its French culture, language, the Napoleonic code, and Catholic beliefs. As Charles Darwin commented when he visited Mauritius some years later:

> Although the island has been so many years under the English government, the general character of the place is quite French: Englishmen speak to their servants in French; indeed I should think that Calais or Boulogne was much more Anglified [than Port Louis].[6]

Under Britain, the island prospered, with the export of sugar leading to economic growth. Thus, an economy based on trade was gradually replaced by one dependent on sugar cane. The population of Mauritius consisted of Europeans, half-castes, and black slaves. In 1807, there were 6,489 Caucasians and 65,367 black slaves, and in 1817—the year of Brown-Séquard's birth—there were 7,385 whites, 10,979 "free colored" persons (manumitted slaves and those of color who had come to the colony of their own accord or to work under contract, such as carpenters, masons, and other artisans), and 79,493 slaves of various races,[10–12] who were needed for work on the sugar plantations and as domestic servants. The first slaves were probably from Madagascar, but they later were brought to Mauritius from both the west and east coasts of Africa, Indonesia, Malaysia, and elsewhere. Mortality among the slave population was high because of their harsh treatment and primitive living conditions, and because of the frequent outbreaks of cholera that occurred on the island. Britain had abolished the oceanic slave trade in 1807, but slavery remained an essential ingredient of Mauritian life for the next quarter-century, and slaves continued to be transported there illegally to fill this need.

By 1835, the population had reached one hundred thousand, of whom only 10 percent were white whereas 75 percent were black slaves from Africa and Madagascar. In that year, slavery was finally abolished after much civil unrest and after payment of two million pounds sterling in compensation to former slave owners,[8] based on an 1833 Act of Parliament that abolished slavery throughout the British colonies.[D] The former slaves were required to remain

---

[D] The Slavery Abolition Bill of 1833 was passed by both Houses of Parliament and received the Royal Assent from King William IV. It called "for the abolition of slavery throughout the

as apprentices with their previous owners for several years, working for six days per week without pay but with meals provided, to acquire good work habits and to allow for a gradual change-over to a new system of working the plantations. The immigration of coolie laborers from India was subsequently encouraged by the government to provide a solution to the resulting shortage of workers, but led to many abuses.

Because of its cultural link with France, the island was able to offer its inhabitants many of the social amenities that were readily taken for granted in Europe but which generally were so lacking in the Old World's distant colonies. The capital city of Port Louis, on the northwest side of the island, is at the head of a splendid harbor protected by military forts. It has been described as resembling "an amphitheatre, being situated in a valley, opening to the sea on one side, and on the other surrounded by a grand range of mountains, whose declivities are diversified with rugged and broken precipices."[13] Goats and monkeys inhabit the surrounding hills, where many of the exotic trees and shrubs yield edible fruits. Even in the early nineteenth century, Port Louis was a thriving metropolis, with its schools, theaters, dance-halls, cathedrals, churches, government buildings, town hall, barracks, shops, bazaars, and broad thoroughfares shaded by grand trees. A visitor at that time found that much cordiality and mutual and unaffected kindness existed in the local society.

> The visiting hour was about eight o'clock in the evening, and you take your leave at ten, unless invited to stay for supper. The supposed reigning vice is gallantry. And both sexes are passionately fond of dancing, an exercise in which they excel. The men are well made, and the number of elegant females is surprising; they are remarkably handsome, have a great deal of wit and vivacity, and are very engaging in their manners.[13]

Charles Edouard Brown (or Brown-Séquard as he was to become) was born in Port Louis at 11 A.M. on April 8, 1817,[14] the same year as Thoreau and Tolstoy, and the year that James Monroe succeeded Madison as president of the United States. In England, the Prince of Wales served as regent for his insane father, George III. The unification of the states comprising the Italian peninsula and of the German states was still a dream. It was the year that Parkinson's disease was first described (by James Parkinson, an English physician), two years

---

British colonies, for promoting the industry of the manumitted slaves, and for compensating the persons hitherto entitled to the services of such slaves." It came into effect in Mauritius in February 1835.

before the invention of the stethoscope, eight years before the opening of the world's first railway line, and nine before the first steam crossing of the Atlantic. The first practical electrical telegraph was yet to be invented by Morse, and the revolver by Samuel Colt.

The little boy's father, Charles Edward Brown, a merchant sea captain born in Philadelphia on October 29, 1784, to parents of Irish origin, was not present at his birth and would never set eyes on the lad. He had been lost at sea several weeks earlier, probably while returning from India, where he had gone to pick up a cargo of rice to relieve a shortage of food in Mauritius. It has been said that the ship was lost in a storm or taken by the pirates who infested the waters of the Bay of Bengal; one fanciful account has it that Brown was captured within sight of his father-in-law's hilltop villa and had to walk the plank.[15,16] The true story will probably never be told, and little is known of the man save that he reportedly served when young in the United States Navy as a midshipman.[E] However, a letter sent to him from Henry Feltus, an uncle by marriage, expatriate Irishman, and the rector of St. Stephen's Church in New York City (then a rapidly growing town of 120,000 souls), indicates that the family still communicated with relatives in Dublin and owned property there.[17] One story, recorded in a genealogical account of the Feltus family, has it that the sister of Dr. Feltus married a Montreal merchant named Brown and by him became the mother of Brown-Séquard[18]; this is incorrect, although Brown-Séquard's father, Captain Edward Brown, was indeed connected by marital ties with Miss Feltus.

As for the infant's mother, Henriette Perrine Charlotte Séquard was born of French (Provençal) parents in Port Louis in August 1788, while the island still belonged to France. She was the only one of three children to survive infancy. Charlotte's father, Pierre Paul Séquard, was originally from Marseilles and had arrived in Mauritius in 1783, to seek his fortune. Four years later, he married Marie-Jeanne Geneviève Elisabeth Nativel from the neighboring island of Reunion, but he was widowed in 1792 and never remarried. Pierre did quite well in commerce but was ruined by a fire[4] and later entered government service.

Charlotte's marriage contract to Brown,[19] dated July 22, 1813, indicates that she brought to the union property generously assessed at twelve hundred piastres (equivalent to twelve hundred American dollars), as well as three

---

[E] I could find no record of service for Charles Edward Brown as a midshipman in the U.S. Navy.

slaves with a combined worth of four hundred and fifty piastres.[F] Nevertheless, she was left in difficult circumstances by the loss of her husband within four years, in 1817. The name of her widowed father appears as witness on the baby's birth certificate.[14] He helped her bring up the child as best he could, but the resilient young Charlotte had nevertheless to struggle to make ends meet. Indeed, she took on work of the same type as that favored by many free black women[20]: she worked as a seamstress, selling some of her embroidery with the help of an ageing black woman, a one-time slave, and may also have let lodgings to British officers and others wishing to break the long voyage between England and the Indian subcontinent.[16] Perhaps in consequence, unsubstantiated rumor has it that she was herself either black or part black. Looking back on their life together some years later, the boy—now grown to manhood—wrote of his mother's devotion in a letter to the woman who was to become his first wife, "her love for me gave her the strength and she succeeded in making enough money to give me as good an education as possible in a country such as mine, and to accompany me to France and there to enable me to study medicine."[1]

The young Brown inherited his father's wanderlust and his mother's self-discipline. He grew up in Port Louis,[G] which in the late 1820s was said to be a city of laughter and gaiety, with broad thoroughfares, leafy promenades, schools, libraries, a theater, bands performing in the Champs de Mars, and an active social calendar. The houses were generally made of wood, no more than two storeys in height, painted, and well maintained; many were furnished with French style and elegance,[13] and had adjoining gardens with fine trees, palms, and plants. The streets were laid out at right angles, the footpaths were paved with basaltic stone, and many of the grander avenues were lined with

---

[F] In the past, the piastre (or piaster) was used as currency in many regions, such as French Indochina and the Ottoman Empire, and in countries that emerged in the near east after World War I. It was the original French word for the American dollar. It is still used in Mauritius for certain purposes (such as in auctions) and is the equivalent of two rupees. The piastre was originally equal to a silver dollar. According to Mr. Tim DeWolf, manager of the research library at the Federal Reserve Bank of San Francisco, to whom I am grateful, this was probably the exchange rate in 1813 although there is some uncertainty about this. He also pointed out to me the difficulty in trying to express currency in terms of present-day values, as any computation depends on which of several different measures (such as the consumer price index, gross domestic product, or unskilled wage rate) is used. Accordingly, I have made no attempt in this or subsequent chapters to convert any currency to present-day values.

[G] There is some uncertainty as to the exact location of the house where he was born and brought up, in part because of a fire that destroyed much of the city. Some years after Brown-Séquard's death, it was hoped to place a plaque on the building, but the project was abandoned for this reason.

colorful acacias, tamarinds, and other trees. He spoke French both at home and at school—the Pensionnat Singery, a secondary school for boys—and did not learn English until his first visit to North America when he was in his fourth decade. Little is known of his childhood except that, when he was 15, he began to work in one of the large bazaars that served as a focal point of life in many colonial towns, a sort of emporium or general store selling essential commodities, foodstuffs, books, periodicals, and trinkets, but which also served as a coffee-house or meeting place. There, one could join with friends to argue and gossip or be entertained with music, stories, or poetry readings.

With youthful self-confidence and with dreams of success in that elegant city that beckons French-speaking peoples from all points of the compass, at the age of twenty he persuaded his mother that the time was right for them to journey to Paris. Their carefully hoarded savings, and the generous help of friends, enabled them to get passage on a boat sailing for Nantes, the capital city of Brittany. At that time, Nantes was a great seaport with cobbled streets, busy quays, a Gothic cathedral, and fine houses, situated prosperously where the Loire, Erdre, and Sèvre rivers converge on the Atlantic Ocean. The voyage itself took eleven months, with the boat becalmed for two months at the equator. Thus it was that, in April 1838, mother and son arrived in Paris and rented accommodations. During the early months in Paris, Brown worked hard to obtain the baccalaureate in letters and in science, and was especially close to his mother. In a letter to a friend in Mauritius, dated December 1838, his mother pointed out that Brown did not know any of the frivolity and pleasures of the metropolis and never went out except to study,[21] which she felt was not good for him; however, he seemed to want to learn everything at once. To spare her anxiety and himself embarrassment if he should fail, he hid the dates of his examinations from her but, with his excellent memory for facts and figures, he passed his baccalaureate in letters toward the end of 1838,[15] and in science within a further few months. Charlotte watched devotedly over him. Their rented apartment was on the rue Férou, near the Luxembourg Gardens, where she took in up to three lodgers, typically Mauritians who were studying in Paris, and busied herself with all the housekeeping, shopping, and cooking that was required to maintain the establishment and provide for their daily needs; even at night, she worked hard with a sewing needle while sitting next to her son, to ensure that their needs were met.[22] She was justifiably proud of his achievements, particularly when the young man—his literary ambitions cast aside—enrolled as a medical student in the Paris Faculty of Medicine.

References and Source Notes

1. Brown-Séquard CE. Autobiographic details provided in a letter dated 17 December 1852, and addressed to Lady Blanche [Ellen Fletcher] who was to become his first wife. MS 977/1. Archives, Royal College of Physicians, London.
2. Wright C. *Mauritius*. Newton Abbot, UK: David & Charles, 1974.
3. Staub F. Dodo and solitaires, myths and reality. *Proc R Soc Arts Sci Mauritius*, 6:89–122, 1996.
4. Hollingworth D. *They came to Mauritius: Portraits of the eighteenth and nineteenth centuries*. London: Oxford University Press, 1965.
5. Toussaint A. *History of the Indian Ocean*. Chicago: University of Chicago Press, 1966.
6. Darwin C. *Journal of researches into the natural history and geology of the countries visited during the voyage of H.M.S. Beagle round the world* (Chapter 21, p. 483). London: John Murray, 1876.
7. Malim M. *Island of the Swan. Mauritius* (pp. 10–13). London: Longmans, Green & Co., 1952.
8. Barnwell PJ, Toussaint A. *A short history of Mauritius* (pp. 152–153, 255). London: Longmans, Green & Co. (for the Government of Mauritius), 1949.
9. Stephens HM. *A history of the French Revolution* (Vol. 2, pp. 486–489). New York: Scribner's Sons, 1891.
10. Martin RM. *History of the colonies of the British Empire in the West Indies, South America, North America, Asia, Austral-Asia, Africa, and Europe ... from the official records of the Colonial Office* (pp. 497–519). London: WH Allen, 1843.
11. Valentine B. *The dark soul of the people: Slaves in Mauritius, 1835*. Thesis submitted for B.A. (Hons.) degree, Rhodes University, 2000. Accessed online on 1 May 2008, at http://www.nrf.ac.za/SADA/CodebookPDF/S0102.pdf.
12. Barker AJ. *The conflict between economic expansion and humanitarian reform under British rule* (pp. 53, 168). London: MacMillan, 1996.
13. An officer who served on the expedition. [Carmichael D ?] *Account of the conquest of Mauritius with some notices on the history, soil, products, defences, and the political importance of this island*. London: Printed for T. Egerton, Military Library, Whitehall, 1811.
14. Extract from the *Registers of the Acts of the Civil Status of the Population of the Town of Port Louis in the Island of Mauritius in the year 1817*. Folio I55. MS 987/9. Archives, Royal College of Physicians, London.
15. Anonymous. Obituary [of Brown-Séquard]. *The Daily News (London)*, 3 April 1894.
16. Anonymous. Brown-Séquard: The story of his life. *The Tribune (New York)*, 22 April 1894.
17. Letter from Canon H. Feltus to Captain Brown, father of Brown-Séquard, dated 1 May 1816. MS 981/145. Archives, Royal College of Physicians, London.
18. Feltus GH. *The Feltus family book, containing a biographical sketch of The Rev. Henry James Feltus, D. D., Late Rector of St. Stephens, New York City. Together with a genealogy of all descendants to date* (p. VI). New York City: Privately printed, 1917.
19. Marriage contract between Edward Brown and Henriette Charlotte Perrine Séquard. MS 999/75. Archives, Royal College of Physicians, London.
20. Allen RB. *Slaves, freedmen, and indentured laborers in colonial Mauritius*. Cambridge: Cambridge University Press, 1999.
21. Brown, Charlotte (née Séquard). Letter to Augustine Maisonneuve dated 9 December 1838. MS 975/1. Archives, Royal College of Physicians, London.
22. Brown, Charlotte (née Séquard). Letter to Augustine Maisonneuve dated 21 April 1840. MS 975/3. Archives, Royal College of Physicians, London.

3

A Medical Student in Paris

THERE CAN BE little doubt that the education that Brown-Séquard received in Paris was a major determinant of his subsequent success both as a physician and scientist. Medical education in France had undergone a radical change after the Revolution of 1789, when there was a desperate need for trained doctors. The Faculty of Medicine of Paris, founded in 1253, was renown in pre-revolutionary France because of its reputation and antiquity. Up to the end of the eighteenth century, however, one of the main failings in medical instruction at the universities was a lack of bedside teaching. The traditions and inadequacies of more than 500 years came to an end with the law of the Legislative Assembly, in August 1792, and the decree of the National Convention[A] on 15 September 1793, which abolished the faculties of Theology, Medicine, Arts, and Law in the Republic.[1] In 1790, the anatomist Felix Vicq d'Azyr[B] had put forward a plan to reorganize medical teaching.[1] The plan

---

[A] During the French Revolution, the National Convention governed France for three years (1792–1795), during which it made major changes to many aspects of public life.

[B] Vicq d'Azyr (1748–1794), French physician and anatomist. Various anatomical tracts (pathways) in the brain are named after him. He created a classic anatomical folio of the brain and named many of the gyri (the convolutions or folds seen on the surface of the brain). Among his patients was Marie Antoinette. Vicq d'Azyr described new ways of dealing with human and animal epidemics, and was a pioneer in public hygiene and preventive medicine. An interesting account of him is provided in Parent A, Felix Vicq d'Azyr: Anatomy, medicine and revolution. *Can J Neurol Sci*, 34:30–37, 2007.

was subsequently advanced by Antoine de Fourcroy,[C] a Jacobin[D] and one of the great reformers of the period, and submitted to the Convention on 27 November 1794, with the intent that learning should occur through clinical observation of patients rather than just from books.[1] Fourcroy reminded the authorities of the drawbacks of the existing system: "Those who have learned their art are confused with those who have no ideas. The life of the citizens is in the hands of greedy as well as ignorant men .... No proof of knowledge is required."

The Convention moved to establish new teaching institutions in the young republic. Schools of health (so called, instead of schools of medicine, to emphasize the integration of medicine and surgery) were set up in Paris, Montpellier, and Strasbourg in place of the old faculties, and medical education was reorganized to encourage future clinicians to gain practical experience, rather than relying on theoretical knowledge gleaned from books.[1–3] The previous separation of medicine and surgery was ended. Courses were made more practical, and doctoral degrees were awarded only after four years of study, compulsory examinations, and the preparation and defense of a thesis in French or Latin. In Paris, courses were established in the hospitals, clinical cases were grouped together for teaching purposes, and students became more involved in patient care and keeping accurate medical records.[3] Novel approaches to clinical diagnosis and an emphasis on pathological anatomy provided greater breadth to medical education.[4] However, the relationship between the school and the hospitals and clinics was problematic, for the school had no control over the clinics or the teaching that occurred there. Moreover, the sheer number of students limited access to bedside teaching, and clinical lectures, demonstrations, and conferences therefore became an important aspect of medical education in France.

The schools of health were integrated into the university system in 1806, and were renamed Faculties of Medicine in 1808. After the Revolution and during the first Empire (1804–1814), the study of medicine was made more

---

[C] Antoine François, Comte de Fourcroy (1755–1809), French chemist who studied medicine on the advice of Felix Vicq d'Azyr. In 1784, he became lecturer in chemistry at the college of the Jardin du Roi, where his lectures were popular. He was a member of the committees for public instruction and public safety, and later, under Napoleon, director-general of instruction, so that he had a leading role in organizing the educational system of France. He was also involved in the introduction of the metric system. His *Philosophy of Chemistry* is perhaps his best-known publication, but he was also editor of a periodical, *Le Médecin Eclairé*. Fourcroy died in 1809, after being created a count of the French empire.

[D] The radical Jacobin Club was a powerful political organization that played a major role in the Reign of Terror (1793–1794) organized by Robespierre and the Committee of Public Safety during the French Revolution, when opponents of the state were sent to the guillotine.

open to all, perhaps because of the need for medical practitioners in both the civil population and armed forces. Courses of instruction were initially free, and there were no heavy expenses entailed in obtaining a medical degree other than the cost of board and lodging for students living away from home.

The medical curriculum in the first half of the nineteenth century emphasized primarily clinical teaching. As Armand Trousseau, one of the most eminent clinician-teachers of the era commented in the introduction to his *Clinical Lectures at the Hôtel-Dieu* (1857):

> The small amount of time that you dedicate to medicine makes it very difficult for you to study auxiliary sciences. You must have a sufficient notion of chemistry and physics to be able to understand the application of these sciences to medicine. But I should profoundly deplore the time that you might lose in order to acquire a more extended knowledge of chemistry .... Gentlemen, let us have a little less science, and a little more art.[5]

By an official decree in 1841, every medical student was required to attend hospital clinic for at least a year, either as a medical student or extern, beginning in the third year. The *externat* and *internat*, a characteristic feature of the French hospital system, was established during the early nineteenth century.[1] The habit of employing external apprentices and internal assistants (who boarded at the hospital) had existed earlier, but the system was reorganized under the Consulate in 1802. Students were divided into externs and interns, based upon competitive examinations (*concours*) that were administered by the hospitals, rather than by the university, and took place in November. Students commenced their duties in the following January. Selection for these prestigious but optional appointments was not based on talent alone, however, as patronage was also important—examiners were often approached by colleagues in support of particular candidates. During the time that Brown-Séquard was a student, only about one-quarter of the student population became interns or externs and therefore got the best out of the French system. The externs and interns were both students and colleagues of more senior and experienced physicians. Interns were paid, but externs received little compensation (300 francs annually to be divided among all the externs on a service). Typically, each medical service was under the direction of a senior physician and included an intern and three or four externs. Interns were in charge of patients, monitored their treatment, assisted during surgery, and undertook autopsies. They accompanied their chief on his morning rounds, made rounds in the later part of the day, and took calls at night, acting as the physician or surgeon in charge. The externs, appointed for three years after they had completed two years of their medical training, were responsible for minor surgical tasks and for maintaining the patients' records, but they also had spare time for other work or studies. The *concours* for the *externat* involved both written and oral examinations; the latter requiring a five-minute description of some subject in descriptive anatomy and another of some elementary subject in pathology or minor surgery before four senior physicians and three surgeons.[6]

Paris in the 1840s had become perhaps the premier place in Europe to obtain a clinical medical education.[7] The medical students there started clinical work from the first year of their studies, working on the wards for much of the morning and attending lectures later in the day. Furthermore, the physicians with whom they came into contact generally had a remarkable cultural background, in part because of the French educational system, with its emphasis on the classics. It is said that the great Trousseau once quoted some verses of Virgil and when a young student from Toulouse completed his quotation without hesitation or error the young man's career was made—Trousseau helped the student, Georges Dieulafoy,[E] in his studies and promoted his career, so that he eventually became one of the most brilliant of the clinical professors in Paris.[7]

By the middle of the nineteenth century, the excellence of its clinical school began to overshadow the more limited influence of the Faculty of Sciences and thereby hinder further progress in the French medical and educational system.[2] Trousseau's exhortation for "a little less science, and a little more art"[5] reflected a developing problem. In the France of that time, the study of physiology—of function in living organisms—had become more experimentally based and had led to significant advances in the field. Unfortunately, only modest support was available from official sources, so that courses were held privately or at institutions such as the Collège de France, which were distinct from the school of medicine, and only rarely were medical students able to benefit from them. Furthermore, as the century advanced, the French medical schools seemed reluctant to encourage their faculty or students in the pursuit of fundamental research or acquisition of new knowledge. Thus, the French system began to have difficulty in keeping up with developments in the medical sciences, and many of the outstanding French scientists of the era did not—or chose not to—become professors in French medical schools, but were

---

[E] Georges Dieulafoy (1839–1911), French physician, was an outstanding clinician whose good looks and theatrical talents made him a brilliant lecturer. One of his major interests was in the complications of appendicitis (Dieulafoy's triad of hypersensitivity of the skin, localized tenderness, and focal contraction or guarding on palpation of the abdominal wall musculature overlying the appendix is well known to general surgeons), and he also described a blood-vessel abnormality in the stomach that can present with bleeding.

based at professional schools such as the École Normale Supérieure[F] or the Collège de France.[2] Indeed, Brown (or Brown-Séquard, the name by which he soon became known and by which he will be referred to hereafter) and Claude Bernard—the eminent physiologist and his rival in France—were to become professors at this latter institution, which was founded in Paris in 1530 by François I as the Collège Royale. Particularly during the nineteenth century, the Collège de France played an important part in teaching and medical research. Nevertheless, the influence of French medicine on the development of experimental physiology was significant. The clinical, especially surgical, background of many of the early experimentalists, such as François Magendie (p. 39), helped them to obtain material support, and their operative skills and practical knowledge allowed them to seek solutions to problems that came to their awareness because of their background knowledge. Furthermore, there was often close cooperation between clinicians and experimentalists.[4] In the period from 1830 to the middle of the century, by contrast, British and American medical schools attached less importance to physiological research than was the case in France, and such research tended to be subordinated to moral or theological ends.[4]

Brown-Séquard As a Medical Student

Medicine must have been a depressing career at a time when therapeutic options were limited, consultation often occurred too late to be of any practical benefit, clinical work required exposure to illness and therefore some personal risk, and practice typically involved exposure to the vulnerable underbelly of civilized society, with pain, poverty, and pestilence as constant companions. Success depended not only on talent but also on the social stature of patients and on recognition by one's colleagues, and thus required a certain grace, charm, self-confidence, and wit that may have been lacking in the gauche young colonial. Nevertheless, Brown-Séquard's resolve more than compensated for any social deficiencies.

From 1815, candidates had been required to obtain the *baccalauréat ès-lettres* (Bachelor of Arts degree) before the four-year course for the medical degree, and from 1823, students were required to hold both a Bachelor of Arts and a

---

[F] The École Normale Supérieure is a school of higher education apart from the public universities system. Established in 1794, it was originally intended to provide the Republic with a new body of teachers, trained in the values of the Revolution, but has since developed as an elite institution that grooms those destined for high office in the service of the nation.

Bachelor of Sciences degree to be eligible to sit the examinations for a doctorate in medicine. Brown-Séquard obtained the former toward the end of 1838 and, somewhat remarkably, the latter some months later. Thus it was that he entered the Faculty of Medicine, where the curriculum and content of the examinations were determined by the government. An excellent description of the life of a medical student at the time has been provided elsewhere.[8] The academic year was divided into winter and summer sessions. Clinical lessons were scheduled so that students could get from the Faculty to the various affiliated hospitals and were given mainly at the Charité and Hôtel Dieu, but also at other institutions. It was necessary to avoid conflicts between hospital duties, clinical courses, and courses at the Faculty—hospital rounds occurred between 7 and 10 A.M. in winter and 6 and 10 A.M. in summer, and included time for a clinical lesson delivered in a nearby lecture hall. Courses at the Faculty started at 10:30 A.M. or later, to allow time for students to gather from the various hospitals, the main ones being the Hôtel Dieu (next to the magnificent cathedral of Notre Dame), La Charité, and La Pitié, with a number of others throughout the city. Laboratory work or practical anatomy took place between noon and 3 P.M. to take advantage of the light. The dissecting rooms were in the École Pratique, immediately opposite the colonnaded Faculté de Médecine and just off the Boulevard Saint Germain, in the student quarter of Paris, with other rooms located near the Jardin des Plantes and at La Pitié. Lectures were between 10:30 A.M. and noon, or between 3 and 5 P.M.; evenings were reserved for further hospital rounds.

During Brown-Séquard's time, and for some time thereafter, graduation as a doctor in the Paris school required attendance at eighteen different courses over four years. No formal certification of attendance was required, however, but merely evidence of inscription (that is, of registration and payment of the appropriate fee) for the courses. In addition, many hours were spent in the dissection room to gain a firm understanding of human anatomy.[8] Time in the dissection room could be harrowing—limbs and other bodily parts seemed to be scattered about; animals roamed freely, attacking whatever remains were within reach; the smell of putrefaction was overwhelming; and a general sense of chaos was enhanced by the noise of other students. Nevertheless, students eventually developed an indifference to the horrors about them and an unfortunate disrespect for the dead that enabled them to move ahead with their studies. In addition, however, there was the risk to students of injury or infection with, in some cases, a fatal outcome. Indeed, an infection from a puncture wound in the dissecting room left Brown-Séquard ill with septicemia ("blood poisoning") for many weeks in 1842,[9,10] and was probably responsible for the permanent paralysis of two fingers of his right hand that occurred at about this time, although some have attributed this paralysis to one of his experiments upon himself.

Students were required to observe and assist hospital staff in medical care and dressing wounds for a year. During this time, they were supposed to develop clinical detachment, social graces, and communication skills, and they learned to quell any emotional unease as they walked the wards, mixing among the diseased and deformed. There were examinations in anatomy and physiology; pathology; chemistry, pharmacy and pharmacology; hygiene and forensic medicine; and clinical medicine.[8] Practical and oral examinations were given in anatomy, physiology, and clinical medicine and surgery. Graduation also required the preparation of a thesis that had to be defended in an oral examination before a jury of professors and assistant or associate professors. Although many theses were fairly mundane reviews of the published literature, exceptional students prepared theses that reported a major advance in medical science or thinking. So it was with Brown-Séquard's thesis, discussed later, which reported a substantial piece of original research concerned with the study of reflexes and with the sensory pathways in the spinal cord—and which marked the beginning of his scientific contributions.

It has been estimated that, in 1846, tuition fees amounted to 1260 francs for the four years of study at the Paris Faculty of Medicine. The total cost of a full medical education to obtain the MD degree—including living expenses for five years (the fifth year being taken up in passing the final examinations after completion of the four-year curriculum and in writing a thesis)—was approximately 10,000 francs, including fees for books and attendance at private courses of instruction.[8] During his early days as a medical student, Brown-Séquard—who had a quick mind and an excellent memory—organized tutorial-seminars for some of the other students to augment his meager financial resources, as well as to expand his own knowledge. He became a laboratory assistant to a professor of physics and chemistry, in whose absence he would have charge of the class. In his second year of medical studies, he joined the private laboratory of a physiologist, Dr. Martin-Magron, as a student.[9] This was a most fortunate move for Martin-Magron, a *professeur libre* (teacher without an official academic position) who seems to have been quite skilled in recognizing talent, tutored his students, encouraged discussion and debate, and maintained a well-equipped laboratory where students could gain personal experience in experimental physiology by experimenting on small animals. The more time he spent in the laboratory repeating the experiments of others, however, the more engrossed Brown-Séquard became in formulating new experiments to satisfy his own developing curiosity, for he was both imaginative and intuitive. Indeed, he began his experimental work on the nervous system in this private laboratory, often in collaboration with Dr. Martin-Magron, whose encouragement, guidance, and assistance he readily acknowledged. The work documented in his doctoral thesis (in 1846) was undertaken there, and in its introductory paragraphs he records his gratitude to his mentor "for the liberality with which the treasures of his heart and mind had been opened."[11]

It was as a student that Brown-Séquard developed the life-long habit of using himself as an experimental subject. One of his interests at the time was concerned with digestion, and he studied his own gastric juices by swallowing sponges to absorb them and then retrieving the sponges by pulling on the string to which they were attached. For years afterwards, an unfortunate tendency to belch and regurgitate food, probably as a result of these early experiments, detracted somewhat from his social graces. Many of the other experiments he performed on himself in later years also had unfortunate consequences, either personally (as when he nearly died after varnishing himself all over to investigate the function of the skin) or professionally (as when he injected himself with mashed-up testicles and obtained results that were attributed by others to self-deception).

In 1842, he became an extern to the Hospitals in Paris after succeeding in the competitive examinations for these much-prized positions—by his own report coming in fifth out of three hundred candidates.[12,G] However, ill with septicemia, he had to take time off while his 54-year-old mother nursed him back to health. Then, on July 10 of that same year, his mother died suddenly and unexpectedly, from an uncertain cause. His initial reaction was extreme and uncontained, as he sobbed and raged, unable to contemplate life without her.[10] Over the following days, he became increasingly withdrawn from a life that seemed to have no meaning to him. Despondent and lonely without her, he was unable to work for weeks and had nothing else to occupy his time except aimless travel within France. Finally abandoning his studies, he impulsively made his way back to Mauritius in December 1842,[12] taking passage with a friend (the Mauritian, Frederic Bonnefin, who also became a physician) on the *Bougainville* out of Le Havre and disembarking some three months later, on 24 March 1843, in Port Louis. This behavioral pattern—of depression, social withdrawal, and travel elsewhere in search of relief—was to become a common theme in Brown-Séquard's response to the stresses of his professional and personal life, and one that led him to further difficulties, for he failed to be

---

[G] Mailys Mouginot, archivist at the Assistance Publique—Hôpitaux de Paris, reports that Brown is listed eleventh on the list of sixty-six students who were selected as externs beginning on 1 January 1842.

identified in any lasting way with a particular country or major institution, but remained an outsider wherever he was. In any event, after about four months, he came to realize that his familiar surroundings in Mauritius were not a substitute for his mother's love or the intellectual challenges of his life in Paris. With the financial assistance of a friend, he therefore returned to France, arriving there in November 1843.[12] Life in Paris now became harder, and he lived in poverty with—at times—little to sustain him in the miserable lodgings at 5 rue Neuve-des-Beaux-Arts to which he had moved.[10]

Unlike many of the other medical students, he had no interest in drinking or womanizing, did not waste his time in the cafés, bars, or dance halls of the capital, and made no attempt to cultivate a social life. Many medical students had a *grisette*, a young working-class girlfriend, usually a shop assistant or seamstress, with whom they had an intimate but often short-lived relationship. Brown-Séquard avoided such entanglements, leading a solitary life with few friends among the middle-class French students or wealthy foreigners who were his classmates. At about this time, he developed what was to become a life-long habit of going to bed at 8 o'clock in the evening in order to arise at about 2 in the morning and work undisturbed while others slept. Whether this was the cause or consequence—or both—of his limited social life is uncertain. Regardless, it is clear that his first concern was with his professional advancement and that he was something of a social outcast.

Probably because of his difficult circumstances, it seems that he never sat the competitive examinations to become an intern in the Paris hospitals, an appointment that could be taken up either before or after graduation from medical school and was generally regarded as the passport to success in the clinical world of French medicine. He served his externship (with his friend Charles Robin, who became a respected microscopist) on the services of the great Trousseau and Rayer. The name of Armand Trousseau (1801–1867), an eminent physician at the Hôtel-Dieu Hospital of Paris, remains familiar to medical students the world over in connection with a clinical sign of tetany named after him. (Tetany is a condition in which a low level of calcium in the blood is associated with a characteristic combination of symptoms and signs including painful muscle spasms.) As for Pierre Rayer (1793–1867), this much-loved man—who eventually became physician to Emperor Napoleon III and, by imperial decree, Dean of the Faculty of Medicine in Paris—befriended, influenced, and helped many young physicians who were to attain great eminence in time, men such as Charcot, Claude Bernard, and Littré, as well as Brown-Séquard.

On 3 January 1846, Brown-Séquard qualified as a doctor of medicine, defending his thesis for the doctorate before a jury of professors presided over by Pierre-Eloy Fouquier (1776–1850), a senior, honored, and established clinical professor. The thesis provided an account of his studies in various animals of the reflex changes that follow section of the cord, and a description of his own studies to clarify the course within the spinal cord of the pathways subserving sensation. The work was dedicated simply to his mother.[11] It was published under the name of Brown, but thereafter he took to calling himself Brown-Séquard, adding his mother's family name to that of his father "to distinguish myself from all the other Browns" and to honor her memory, although the change in name was not formally legalized in France by a notary until 1859, some thirteen years after he had qualified as a doctor of medicine.[13] Somewhat unfortunately, the double-barrelled name went through several renditions in different publications, including Brown-Léquard, Brown-Séguard, and Brown-Séquart, before it finally appeared correctly. Over the next few years, the young man worked hard to establish himself as an experimental physiologist. Without his mother to consider, he was able to turn his back on the financial benefits that would normally reward the choice of a career in medicine and to look instead to the austere intellectual challenges of a scientific career.

Brown-Séquard's Thesis: The Spinal Cord and Sensory Pathways

To appreciate the importance of the work in Brown-Séquard's thesis, some background information is required concerning the nervous system and the evolution of concepts regarding its function. For nonmedical readers, a brief account is also provided here of the basic structure of the nervous system.

The nervous system, which regulates and coordinates the function of the body, is divided into the *central nervous system*, consisting of the brain and spinal cord (which extends down from the brain within the bony vertebral column or backbone), and the *peripheral nervous system*, which is made up of the nerves that run between the central nervous system and other parts of the body, such as the muscles, skin, bodily organs, and sensory organs. The nerves running to the trunk or limbs are connected to the spinal cord at every level by the nerve *roots*, which are designated as anterior or posterior roots depending on whether they are located more toward the front or back of the spinal cord. The peripheral nerves carry messages to and from the spinal cord in the form of electrical impulses. Nerves carrying impulses to the spinal cord are referred to as *afferent* or *sensory nerves*, whereas those bearing impulses from the spinal cord to the muscles or other effector structures are called *efferent nerves*. It is

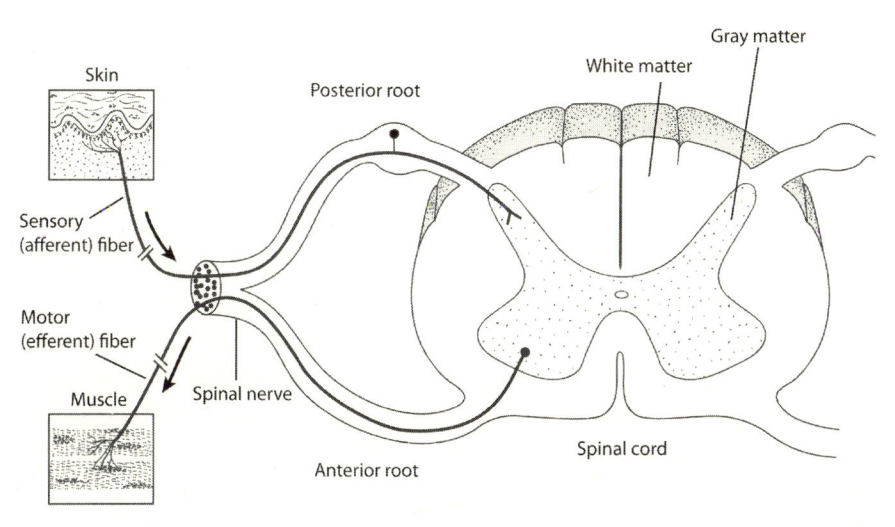

FIGURE 3.1 The spinal cord contains centrally situated gray matter that resembles a butterfly in shape and is composed of neurons, and an outer part that is white and composed of fiber tracts. An afferent (sensory) fiber from the skin passes via a spinal nerve and posterior root to the spinal cord. From the spinal cord, nerve cells send efferent (motor) fibers that traverse the anterior root and spinal nerve, passing to muscle.

now known that the posterior roots are essentially afferent, and the anterior roots are efferent (Figure 3.1).

Every nerve consists of a collection of nerve fibers, each of which arises from a nerve cell body or *neuron* and can also be classified as afferent or efferent in nature. Nerve fibers conduct impulses in only one direction. Most of the major peripheral nerve trunks contain intermingled afferent and efferent fibers, and the nerves are therefore called *mixed nerves*. The sensory (afferent) nerve fibers receive information from sensory receptors (specialized cellular structures) with which they connect or from the endings of the nerve fibers themselves. Such information may concern the external world and includes such factors as temperature (hot and cold), joint position, touch, and pain. (Certain other sensory functions, such as vision, hearing, position in space, taste, and smell are subserved by special nerves that are not considered here.) Sensory information may also relate to the body itself, to such matters as, for example, blood pressure, heart rate, the state of bladder fullness, and pain from internal organs. The sensory receptors or endings convert the information that they receive into electrical impulses that are then conveyed by the afferent fibers to the central nervous system. The efferent nerves run to muscles, blood vessels, sweat glands, and other structures such as glands, which they activate in response to the sensory input or input from the brain.

In addition to transmitting electrical impulses, each nerve fiber releases at its termination a chemical substance (or *neurotransmitter*) that influences the activity of the structure with which it connects. The nerve cells are thus like electrical generators (in producing electrical activity) and chemical factories (in manufacturing a chemical transmitter). The nerves themselves have been likened to telephone wires, containing bundles of insulated elements that conduct information at a constant rate over distance using an electrical (impulse frequency) coding system.

The brain and spinal cord are similarly composed of neurons and their fibers (as well as other supporting cell types), which are organized into neuronal aggregates (called *nuclei* and *gray matter*) and discreet fiber tracts. The brain looks gray on the outside (where its outer mantle is formed of nerve cell bodies) and white on the inside (where it is largely composed of nerve fibers running from one part of the brain to another, or to and from the spinal cord). A number of gray masses of nerve cells are also found within the brain and make up various *nuclei* or relay stations. If the skull of a human is removed, the most visible parts of the brain (Figure 3.2) are the paired cerebral hemispheres (which have been likened to the two halves of a walnut and are divided

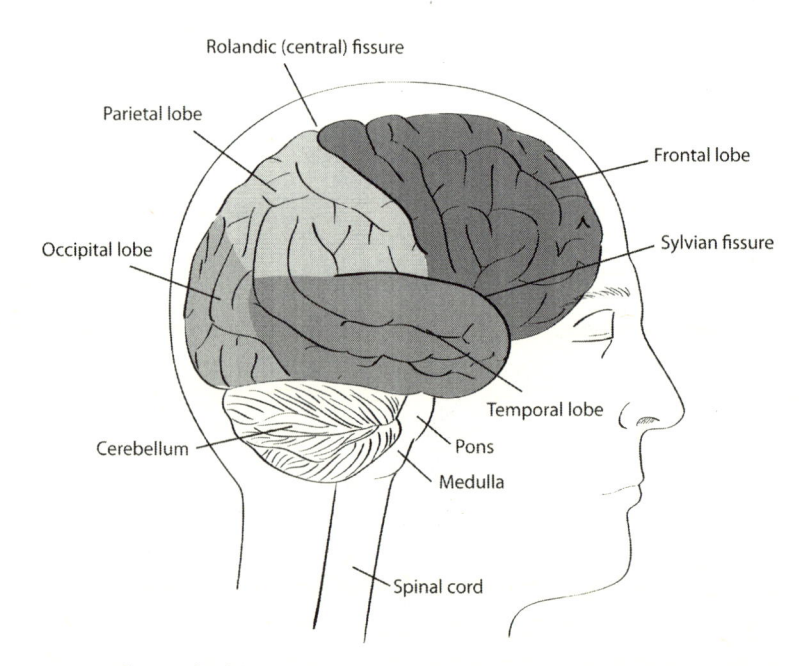

FIGURE 3.2 The cerebral hemispheres (comprised of the frontal, parietal, temporal, and occipital lobes) and the cerebellum overlie the brainstem (midbrain, pons, and medulla), which connects to the spinal cord.

into *frontal, parietal, temporal,* and *occipital lobes*). These are connected to the spinal cord by the *brainstem*, which is composed of the midbrain and hindbrain (*pons* and *medulla*, and by the *cerebellum* (or "little brain"), which covers the hindbrain. Nerve fibers within the spinal cord are said to *ascend* when they transmit impulses up toward the brain, or to *descend* when they conduct impulses from the brain toward the spinal cord.

For many years the spinal cord was neglected by medical scientists or regarded simply as the pathway permitting the brain to control the body. In the second century of the Christian era, Galen of Pergamon (in what is now Turkey), physician to the Emperor Marcus Aurelius in Rome and a medical writer and experimentalist of enormous repute, gained remarkable insight into the anatomy of the nervous system by his studies of different animals. Galen rejected the belief of Aristotle that the function of the brain is to cool the heart. He divided the nerves into those that felt soft and those that were hard, and related the function of the nerves to their consistency. The harder nerves, which came out of the brain more posteriorly, were held to have a motor function; he supposed that the softer consistency of the other nerves enabled them to receive sensory impressions. Although the effect of injury to the spinal cord was known to earlier writers, Galen initiated the experimental study of the function of the spinal cord by severing parts of it in nonhuman primates. Complete transection or division of the cord led to loss of power and sensation in all the bodily parts below the cut level; when only one-half of the cord was severed, paralysis was confined to the limbs or bodily parts on the sectioned (so-called *ipsilateral*) side.

Over the following centuries, anatomists noted that in cross-section (i.e., in a plane perpendicular to its length) the spinal cord was composed of centrally situated gray matter having a configuration resembling a butterfly, whereas the outer part of the cord was whiter in color and consisted of anterior (front), posterior (back), and lateral (side) columns of fibers oriented parallel to its length (i.e., running up or down the cord, with afferent fibers ascending toward—and efferent or motor fibers descending from—the brain). Apart from this, little knowledge was gained about the spinal cord until the eighteenth century. However, it came to be appreciated that the control by the brain of movement was incomplete, if only because headless animals were capable of some movements. Decapitated chickens, for example, were able to run about the farmyard until they died from loss of blood.

In the eighteenth century, Robert Whytt (1714–1766), physician to King George III in Scotland, described the contraction of a muscle that occurs in response to its sudden stretch. These reactions of muscle to stretch are among the simplest of reflexes, involving receptors and afferent fibers that convey information to the spinal cord (in this case, regarding the state of stretch of the muscle) and efferent fibers that pass from the neurons in the spinal cord to the muscle (and are therefore called *motor neurons*) to activate muscle contraction. In the spinal cord, there is a slight space between the end of the afferent fiber and the motor neuron to which it connects—the *synapse*. At the synapse, a chemical neurotransmitter is released from the afferent endings and excites the motor neuron to a fixed degree. When the motor neuron receives sufficient excitation (by input from many afferent fibers) after a sudden muscle stretch, it fires off to elicit a muscle contraction. Thus, this mechanism allows excitation from different sources to be added (and, conversely, inhibitory influences to exert their effect), so that the different influences on motor neuron function are integrated by the cell itself and determine its behavior. The stretch response described by Whytt was not due simply to some property inherent in the muscle, but depended upon the functional integrity of the spinal cord.[14] Whytt showed also that stimuli to the skin can elicit reflex responses even when only a limited length of the cord remains intact (*cutaneous reflexes*). In other words, simple reflex responses neither require the involvement of the brain or the cavities (the cerebral ventricles) within it, as supposed by Descartes, nor depend upon ill-defined connections between motor and sensory nerves in the periphery, as suggested in the seventeenth century by Thomas Willis (who, with Descartes, can claim credit for first conceiving of involuntary reflex actions, and for first using the term "reflex" to describe them; see footnote C, Chapter 5.)[15] However, immediately after complete transection of the cord, as when frogs are decapitated, Whytt found that reflex responses are initially lost, a phenomenon that subsequently came to be called *spinal shock*,[H] when it was rediscovered by Marshall Hall (1790–1857) in the nineteenth century.[16]

It was Marshall Hall,[I] in particular, who advanced the concept of spinal reflexes at the end of the eighteenth century and in the early years of the

---

[H] Spinal shock refers to the sudden loss of spinal cord activity (i.e., of neural function) below the level of an acute injury to the spinal cord. During spinal shock, the muscles are flaccid and paralyzed, and spinal reflexes are lost or markedly attenuated. The disorder is usually temporary, with recovery occurring over a period of up to about 6 weeks; patients are then left with permanent disability from the original injury to the spinal cord. The disorder is of clinical importance because it makes it difficult to determine the extent of any permanent loss of function immediately after an injury to the spinal cord. The precise mechanism underlying spinal shock is still unclear but it presumably relates to the loss of input to the spinal cord from multiple systems within the brain that affect the excitability of the spinal neurons.

[I] Hall studied medicine in Edinburgh, practiced for much of his life in London, traveled widely in Europe and the United States, learned Hebrew from a rabbi at the age of sixty-five, and

nineteenth century. Hall worked on sea snails, snakes, turtles, frog, toads, and a variety of other animals and showed, for example, that decapitated animals could move in response to touch or pain stimuli unless the spinal cord or the nerves to the muscles also were destroyed. His work was presented first to the Zoological Society, but a second paper submitted to the Philosophical Transactions of the Royal Society was not accepted for publication, apparently because its substance had already been reported elsewhere. Hall deserves credit for putting the concept of reflexes on a solid framework,[17,18] for extending the scope of reflex phenomena to include, for example, coughing, sneezing, and swallowing, and for bringing the autonomic nervous system into the same schema as the somatic nervous system.[19] He has not always received the recognition he deserved, however, and was accused by some of plagiarizing the work of others. The Royal Society, in particular, seemed to give his work scant attention, whereas his studies were well received in France and Germany.[19] His chilly reception and the apparent ill-will directed toward him in England may have related to his personality, for he did not make friends easily, was sometimes abrasive and irritable, had an overbearing confidence in the correctness of his own views, and did not take kindly to criticism.

Hall further showed experimentally that the "tone" (i.e., the state of tension) of resting muscles was governed by reflex activity—decapitation had only a relatively minor effect whereas destruction of the spinal cord led to loss of muscle tone (*flaccidity*), so that the muscles became floppy.[20] He also studied the spinal reflexes and related phenomena in patients with paralysis from disorders of the brain, spinal cord, nerve roots, or peripheral nerves, describing the clinical differences that reflect the site of the disturbance and urged that in cases of "cerebral or spinal disease, and disease of the nerves in their course, the condition of the reflex actions .... henceforth be carefully examined ....,"[16] as indeed they are to this day.

The anatomy of the motor and sensory nerves, and the pathways taken within the central nervous system of the various fiber tracts subserving sensation were poorly understood in the early nineteenth century. Two Edinburgh graduates had a major role in taking things further. The first, Alexander Walker

---

published papers on chemistry, thermometry, and other scientific topics, as well as on diverse aspects of medicine and physiology. His numerous medical books include works on disorders of the gastrointestinal tract, on diseases of women, and his celebrated *The Diagnosis of Disease*. His successful clinical practice did not stop him from taking a stand on what he perceived as social injustices or matters of public interest. Thomas Wakley, founding editor of *The Lancet*, is said to have described him as the most conscientious man he had ever met.

(1779–1852)—a brilliant eccentric and an anatomist[J] without any medical or surgical qualifications—adapted the Galenic concept to the spinal cord in 1809, suggesting that the anterior portion (front) of the cord was concerned with sensation and the posterior (back) half with movement. He therefore reasoned from their continuity with the cord that the anterior roots contained fibers transmitting sensory information fibers and the posterior roots were made up of motor fibers. Although he deserves credit for first suggesting a fundamental distinction between the anterior and posterior roots, the functions that he assigned them—without any experimental or clinical justification—were the exact opposite of those that subsequently received wide acceptance. He nevertheless clung stubbornly to his views on the function of the nerve roots until his death, becoming increasingly embittered that he did not receive more recognition for his contribution,

Charles Bell (1774–1842), another Edinburgh graduate, further advanced matters. Bell, an anatomist and surgeon who served at Waterloo, had settled in London, where he ran the Great Windmill Street School of Anatomy (founded by William Hunter) for several years. He was appointed Professor of Physiology and Surgery when the University of London was founded, delivering the Introductory Address in October 1828. In 1835, he urged the creation of the Middlesex Hospital Medical School,[K] which opened in London a few months later with 60 students.[L] Bell was a prolific medical author whose books were enhanced by his own artistic skill. In his now-celebrated pamphlet, *Idea*

[J] Walker is perhaps better known as a writer and novelist than as an anatomist. He contributed articles on science and the arts to several newspapers and periodicals, was an outstanding linguist, and founded a short-lived scientific journal and a literary magazine. He authored textbooks on the nervous system and on the medical sciences, and his nonmedical books included the trilogy *Beauty, Intermarriage,* and *Woman Physiologically Considered as to Mind, Morals, Matrimonial Slavery, Infidelity and Divorce*. He spent much of his professional life in London but returned to Scotland unwell and impoverished in 1842. *The Lancet* (7 July 1849, p. 26) subsequently launched a fund to help support him in his retirement; the editor himself contributed five pounds and a total of thirty pounds was eventually collected. The reader interested in Walker might do well to consult Courtney CP, Alexander Walker and Benjamin Constant: a note on the English translator of *Adolphe. French Studies* 29:137–150, 1975.

[K] The Middlesex Hospital Medical School merged with that of University College Hospital in 1987, and both are now part of an enlarged medical school based at University College London.

[L] Charles Bell has named after him a neurological disorder (weakness of the facial muscles resulting from a lesion of the nerve supplying them), a sign (a rolling up of the eye when a patient with severe facial weakness attempts to close the eye), and a nerve (the long thoracic nerve). He was knighted by King William IV. His *Essay on the Anatomy of Expression in Painting* (originally published in 1806) is said to have captivated Queen Victoria. He returned to Scotland at the end of his career, accepting a chair in surgery at the medical school of Edinburgh University, then one of the premier institutions in Europe.

of a New Anatomy of the Brain: Submitted for the Observation of His Friends,[21] which he published privately (with only one hundred printed copies) in 1811, he referred to certain experiments that he had performed on the nerve roots of animals. These experiments showed that the anterior roots had a motor function, because muscle contractions occurred when they were touched (and thereby stimulated) with the point of a knife. Similar motor responses did not occur when the posterior roots were stimulated. Thus, he showed experimentally that there are important differences between the anterior and posterior roots, although he did not determine the function of the posterior roots. Although his later writings indicate that Bell came to believe that the motor and sensory pathways are anatomically distinct, and that sensory fibers reach the spinal cord via the posterior nerve roots and then ascend in the posterior half of the spinal cord to the brain, he failed to provide adequate proof in support of his assertion.

François Magendie,[M] who was professor of medicine at the Collège de France, also felt that the different functions of the anterior and posterior spinal roots required clarification. Accordingly, when given a litter of puppies as a gift, he used them for experiments in which he cut through the bony vertebral column and then transected the nerve roots individually without disturbing the spinal cord. When he cut the posterior roots on one side in the lower region of the spinal cord (which supplies the legs), power was preserved but sensation lost in the limbs that these roots innervated. Transection of the anterior roots produced a paralyzed limb in which sensation was preserved. Confirmation of these findings by repeated experiments led him to conclude correctly, in 1822, in a paper that he published in his own *Journal de Physiologie Expérimentale et Pathologique,* that the posterior and anterior roots do indeed have different functions, the former conveying sensory fibers and the latter motor fibers.[22] Thus, Magendie claimed to have discovered the functions of, and differences between, the anterior and posterior nerve roots, a claim that was hotly contested by Bell,[23,24] who surreptitiously revised his earlier publications

---

[M] François Magendie (1783–1855), French experimental physiologist, vivisectionist, pharmacologist, and physician. He authored the first modern textbook of physiology, described an aperture (the foramen of Magendie) that permits the fluid bathing the brain (the cerebrospinal fluid) to circulate freely, and gave one of the earliest descriptions of the fluid itself. His work on the spinal roots is discussed above. He also studied the mechanics of vomiting, the effect of protein deficiency in the diet, the digestive properties of pancreatic juice, the role of the liver in detoxification processes, and the effects of various drugs, including strychnine. His work in demonstrating the presence of sugar in the blood led his assistant, Claude Bernard, to discover that the liver normally produces sugar or a substance (glycogen) readily converted to it.

in light of Magendie's work before republishing them in support of his own claim.[24] As Magendie later wrote

> Charles Bell had before me, but unknown to me, the idea of separately cutting the nerve roots; he also has the credit for discovering that the anterior root influences muscular contractility more than the posterior root. This is a question of priority in which I have, from the beginning, honored him. Now, as to having established that these roots have distinct properties and functions, such that the anterior ones control movement, and the posterior ones sensation, this discovery belongs to me ....[25]

Clearly, credit belongs to both men: to Bell for initiating the concept and approach and to Magendie for completing the work and confirming the deductions of Bell by experiments that to Bell seemed unthinkable in their brutality.[N] In any event, the important concept—that the anterior and posterior roots have different functions—is embodied to this day in the Law of Bell–Magendie, which recalls the contributions of both men.

As for Alexander Walker, he has quietly been forgotten. He believed to the end that he had been robbed of the credit for first suggesting the separation of function of the anterior and posterior nerve roots. His sentiments are quite apparent from part of the lengthy title of one of his own books, *The Nervous System, Anatomical and Physiological; in which the functions of the various parts of the brain are for the first time assigned; and to which is prefixed some account of the author's earliest discoveries, of which the more recent doctrine of Bell, Magendie, etc., is shewn to be at once a plagiarism, an inversion, and a blunder, associated with useless experiments, which they have neither understood nor explained.*

The motor and sensory fibers were generally believed to be anatomically distinct throughout their course in the central nervous system, where they are arranged into distinct fiber tracts. It was held—wrongly as it happens—that the posterior columns are the continuation in the spinal cord of the posterior roots, and thus constitute the single pathway taken by the sensory fibers as they ascend to the brain, whereas the anterior columns contain fibers that descend from the brain and permit the voluntary control of motor activity.

[N] Magendie's experimental methods were heavily criticized in England, including in Parliament, during the early nineteenth century for their cruelty and brutality, involving vivisection without anesthesia (which was then not available), often on a seemingly unnecessary scale. The approach was not helped by Magendie's public lecture-demonstrations in London, which provoked a public outcry and evoked strong antivivisectionist sentiment.

The young Brown-Séquard found himself in opposition to these beliefs in his doctoral thesis of 1846.[11] He returned to the issue in lectures that he delivered at the Royal College of Surgeons of England in 1858 and published in book form two years later.[26] He focused his attention on sensations arising in the skin and muscles, and on the control of muscles.[O] Beginning in the early 1840s, he repeated Galen's experimental work on the spinal cord, but extended it by describing the effect on sensation of sectioning one-half or more restricted segments of the cord. His initial work, performed in the laboratory of Dr. Martin-Magron and presented in his thesis, was divided into two parts.[11] The first part, performed in collaboration with his mentor, involved a study of reflex movements in frogs. These reflexes were found to be lost or diminished immediately after cord section, but subsequently recovered, and they ultimately became markedly enhanced. This unequivocal account of spinal shock was provided at about the same time that Marshall Hall gave the phenomena its designation, although some have suggested that it preceded Hall's account.[1]

The second part of the work embodied in Brown-Séquard's thesis was concerned with the functions of the various columns that comprise the spinal cord. It was introduced by a synopsis of the diversity of opinions regarding both the functions of different regions of the cord and the pathways taken by motor and sensory fibers within the cord. This was followed by an account of Brown-Séquard's own findings, with an experimental approach that involved making lesions selectively in different parts of the cord in several different animal species. The main conclusion from this work was that the posterior columns were not the main pathway taken by sensory fibers, because responses to sensory stimuli were not affected to any great extent by cutting the posterior columns if the rest of the spinal cord was left intact (Figure 3.3). His studies also suggested "the ease with which sensory impressions are transmitted from one side of the cord to the other," a remarkable and novel conclusion that he was able to justify by his experimental work over the following decade.

[O] The skin not only holds the body together but contains receptors that provide information—often that fails to reach consciousness—about the external environment. The information may relate to, for example, temperature, touch, pressure, skin movement, or pain, and includes details not just on the type but also on the intensity and location of the stimulus. The nature of the stimulus is revealed by the type of receptors and size of the nerve fibers activated; intensity by, for example, the rate at which impulses are conducted to the central nervous system; and location by the site of the stimulated receptors and by a phenomenon called *surround inhibition* (stimulation of one area leads to inhibition of adjacent areas, thereby focusing or sharpening the stimulus). Muscles contain receptors that are involved in the control of movement and posture, signaling muscle length and tension, and the rate of change in these parameters.

Posterior

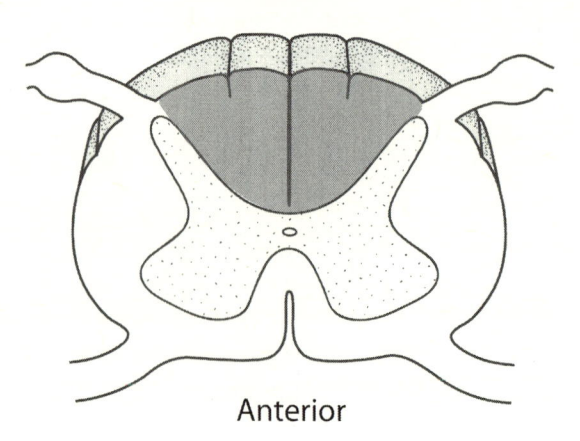

Anterior

FIGURE 3.3 Brown-Séquard found no sensory loss when he cut the posterior columns of the spinal cord in various animals. This suggested that—contrary to the prevailing belief—the posterior columns were not the main sensory pathway to the brain.

Thus, the Mauritian student of medicine, in his brief thesis, had not only described the phenomenon of spinal shock, perhaps before Marshall Hall, but had also shown that the prevailing concept of the sensory pathways was incorrect. Sensation was not dependent primarily on the posterior columns of the spinal cord, and sensory impressions passed from one side of the body to the other side of the central nervous system in the spinal cord rather than in the brain, as was then commonly believed. It was an original, courageous, and important thesis. It seems very likely that his examiners failed to realize quite what he claimed because, when he subsequently extended his work with further observations in animals and humans, he met with enormous opposition from a medical and scientific community that was not ready to accept new concepts that conflicted with the beliefs prevailing at the time. If the examiners had, in fact, understood his observations and their implications, the thesis would probably not have been accepted. The presiding professor, Fouquier, was a senior clinician and thus unlikely to have grasped the scientific significance of Brown-Séquard's observations. The virtually unknown young man had shown remarkable self-confidence in challenging the views of the established giants in the field, especially in the context of his doctoral thesis. He was to show such determination and integrity in much of his future work, regardless of the consequences to him, either personal or professional.

References and Source Notes

1. Coury C. The teaching of medicine in France from the beginning of the seventeenth century. In: O'Malley CD, ed. *The history of medical education. UCLA Forum in Medical Sciences: Number 12* (pp. 121–172). Berkeley: University of California Press, 1970.
2. Ackerknecht EH. Medical education in 19th century France. *J Med Educ*, 32:148–153, 1957.
3. Bonner TN. *Becoming a physician. Medical education in Britain, France, Germany, and the United States, 1750–1945* (pp. 106–114). New York: Oxford University Press, 1995.
4. Lesch JE. *Science and medicine in France: The emergence of experimental physiology, 1790–1855*. Cambridge: Harvard University Press, 1984.
5. Cited by Coury C. The teaching of medicine in France from the beginning of the seventeenth century. In: O'Malley CD, ed., *The history of medical education. UCLA Forum in Medical Sciences: Number 12* (pp. 121–172). Berkeley: University of California Press, 1970. See also Trousseau A. *Lectures on clinical medicine delivered at the Hôtel-Dieu, Paris*, 3rd edition. (Vol. 2; Introduction, pp. 3–45; translated by Cormick JR.) Philadelphia: Lindsay & Blakiston, 1869.
6. Anonymous. Hospital appointments in Paris: Concours. *Lond Med Rec*, 13:367–368, 1885.
7. Cawadias AP. The mid-nineteenth century clinical school of Paris. *Proc R Soc Med*, 45:306–310, 1952.
8. Palluault F. *Medical students in England and France, 1815–1858. A comparative study*. Thesis submitted for the degree of Doctor of Philosophy, University of Oxford, 2003.
9. Berthelot M. *Notice sur la vie et les travaux de M. Brown-Séquard*. Paris: Institut de France, 1898.
10. Role A. *La vie etrange d'un grand savant: Le Professeur Brown-Séquard*. Paris: Plon, 1977.
11. Brown CE. *Thèse pour le Doctorat en Médicine, présentée et soutenue le 3 Janvier 1846*. Paris, 1846.
12. Brown-Séquard CE. Autobiographic details provided in a letter dated 17 December 1852, and addressed to Lady Blanche [Ellen Fletcher], who was to become his first wife. MS 977/1. Archives, Royal College of Physicians, London.
13. Deed legalizing the change in name of Brown to Brown-Séquard, dated 12 December 1859. MS 987/4. Archives, Royal College of Physicians: London.
14. Whytt R. *The works of Robert Whytt M.D.* [Published by his son.] Edinburgh: Becket, Hondt & Balfour, 1768.
15. Sherrington CS. *Man on his nature*. Cambridge: Cambridge University Press, 1941.
16. Hall M. *On the disease and derangements of the nervous system*. London: Baillière, 1841.
17. Clarke E, O'Malley CD. *The human brain and spinal cord: A historical study illustrated by writings from antiquity to the twentieth century*. Berkeley: University of California Press, 1968.
18. Hoff HE, Kellaway P. The early history of the reflex. *J Hist Med*, 7:211–249, 1952.
19. Green JHS. Marshall Hall (1790–1857): a biographical study. *Med Hist*, 2:120–133, 1958.
20. Hall M. *Memoirs on the nervous system*. London: Sherwood, Gilbert & Piper, 1837.
21. Bell C. *Idea of a new anatomy of the brain; submitted for the observation of his friends*. London: Straham & Preston, 1811. Reprinted in *J Anat Physiol*, 3:147–182, 1869.
22. Magendie F. Expériences sur les fonctions des racines des nerfs rachidiens. *J Physiol Exp Pathol*, 2:276-279, 1822. Reprinted in Cranefield PF. *The way in and the way out: François Magendie, Charles Bell, and the roots of the spinal nerves*. Mount Kisco, NY: Futura, 1974.
23. Berkowitz C. Disputed discovery: vivisection and experiment in the 19th century. *Endeavour*, 30:98–102, 2006.

24. Cranefield PF. *The way in and the way out: François Magendie, Charles Bell, and the roots of the spinal nerves.* Mt. Kisco, NY: Futura, 1974.
25. Magendie F. Remarques de M. Magendie à l'occasion de la note de M. Flourens. *C R Acad Sci*, 24:319–320, 1847.
26. Brown-Séquard CE. *Course of lectures on the physiology and pathology of the central nervous system.* Philadelphia: Collins, 1860.

4

Great Expectations

Over the years following his graduation, Brown-Séquard—hyperactive and unfocussed in his work—did not follow a clinical career in Paris but used animals to study a variety of topics of biological interest. He authored numerous papers and notes on his researches in the scientific literature and, over the following ten years, came to typify the research-oriented physician who spends much of the time on laboratory-based research of clinical relevance. His work was to lead to a reinterpretation of various clinical phenomena despite the initial opposition of the medical profession. The methods that he used—animal vivisection—led him also into conflict with the antivivisection movement that was especially strong in Victorian England.

It can hardly be doubted that vivisection before the advent of anesthesia caused great pain to the animals being studied—leading to accusations of cruelty—and required remarkable technical skill on the part of the investigator. Anesthetics, once they did become available, were used very variably on animals during the mid-nineteenth century and often to lessen movement rather than prevent pain. Many were indignant about experimentation on living animals and scornful about the relevance of its findings to the conduct of clinical medicine. To them, the theological belief that the design of life was inspired by God implied not only that life was sacred in all its forms but that function should be inferred from structure (anatomy) and not by experiment.[1] In mid-century, then, medical science in Britain and the United States lagged somewhat behind the experimental approach being followed in France and Germany. This doubtless made Brown-Séquard an attractive candidate to consider for academic appointments in the English-speaking world, for he could give any medical institution to which he was appointed a scientific edge and bring to the clinic the latest advances from the laboratory. At the same time, attitudes began to change: animal vivisection performed with the sole intent of improving surgical skills or for educational purposes was hard for many to justify, although for research purposes it came to be more generally accepted, at least within the medical profession.[1] With the eventual introduction of anesthesia into the laboratory, the advance of physiological research was stimulated because studies on living animals were facilitated, and vivisection became less distasteful to investigators, many of whom eventually looked to experimentalists such as Brown-Séquard, Claude Bernard, and others as men whose example to follow.

The Early Days as a Physician-Scientist

Brown-Séquard continued to study the function of the spinal cord in many different animals including dogs, cats, sheep, guinea pigs, rabbits, and marmots. During the early 1850s, he showed more conclusively that the major pathways taken by sensory fibers traveling in the spinal cord to the brain were not at the back of the spinal cord in the posterior columns as previously believed (Figure 4.1) and that most sensory pathways cross from one side of the cord to the other as they ascend to the brain (Figure 4.2). His studies in animals and meticulous evaluation of patients with neurological disorders led him to conclude that a characteristic clinical disturbance results when one-half of the spinal cord is cut or otherwise affected by disease (Figures 4.3 and 4.4). The constellation of symptoms and signs that results is generally now named after him (Brown-Séquard syndrome) and consists of hyperesthesia (increased sensitivity to touch), impaired vibration and position sense, and weakness in the lower limb of the transected side, plus loss of pain (analgesia) and temperature appreciation on the other. A red-hot iron was sometimes used in animals to determine whether pain was appreciated. The hyperesthesia was demonstrated by the response to an electrical stimulus or to pressure or a slight pinch of the skin—before the spinal cord was cut, rabbits, for example, showed little response but after the transection they would shriek and become agitated. The degree of sensibility was judged not by the occurrence of limb movements (which might have been reflex in nature), but by the intensity of their shrieks and movements of the face, ears, and neck. The reason for this hyperesthesia was not readily apparent. In some instances, the animals were calmed by a little chloroform.[2]

Spinal Cord Lesion (shaded)　　　Clinical Result

A Posterior / Anterior

No sensory loss
Hyperesthesia

B

No sensory loss
Hyperesthesia

C

No "marked" sensory loss

D

Sensory loss

E

Sensory loss

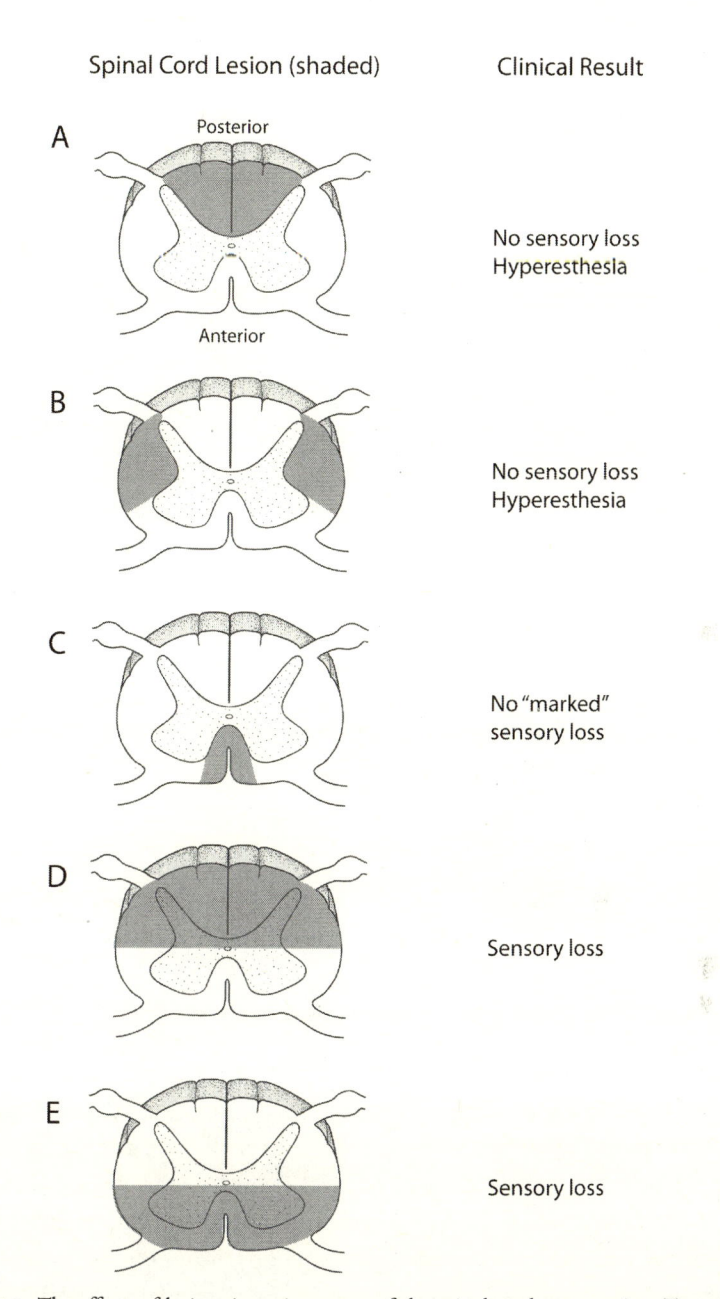

FIGURE 4.1 The effects of lesions in various parts of the spinal cord on sensation. Transection of the posterior (A) or lateral columns (B) caused no sensory loss but, instead, increased sensitivity (hyperesthesia) in the legs. Cutting the anterior columns (C) of the spinal cord produced no "marked" sensory loss (suggesting that perhaps there were mild or subtle sensory changes), whereas sectioning either the posterior (D) or anterior (E) one-half of the spinal cord led to loss of sensation in the legs. These findings suggested that sensory pathways involve the gray matter of the spinal cord, and perhaps also the anterior columns.

Spinal Cord Lesion (shaded)   **Clinical Result**

First lesion (right thoracic hemisection)

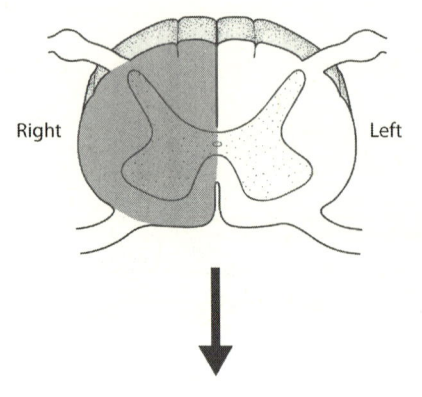

Contralateral (left) sensory loss

Ipsilateral (right) hyperesthesia and hindlimb paralysis

Second lesion (left cervical hemisection)

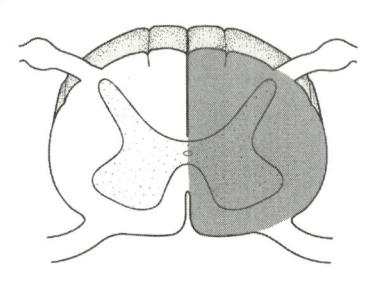

Sensory loss in right hindlimb

FIGURE 4.2 A lateral hemisection of the spinal cord in animals led to paralysis and increased sensitivity to touch (hyperesthesia) on the transected side and to sensory loss (loss of pain appreciation) on the opposite side of the body. These findings suggested to Brown-Séquard that sensory fibers cross from one side of the cord to the other. By making a second hemisection on the opposite side of the spinal cord a few segments above the original hemisection, Brown-Séquard was able to convert the hyperesthesia to sensory loss, suggesting that sensory fibers cross soon after entering the spinal cord.

Despite his meticulous work, his findings were initially disputed and even ridiculed. Ironically, in his later years—when his ideas finally were widely accepted—he actually changed his views about the organization of the sensory system, the manner in which sensory abnormalities occur in patients with neurological disorders, and the basis of the hyperesthesia; but, by then, the medical profession was not ready to accept his new concepts, and it remains slow to recognize their importance even today, as is discussed in Chapter 12.

Among his other experimental interests at the time was the phenomenon of rigor mortis and the consequences of irrigating animal corpses or severed

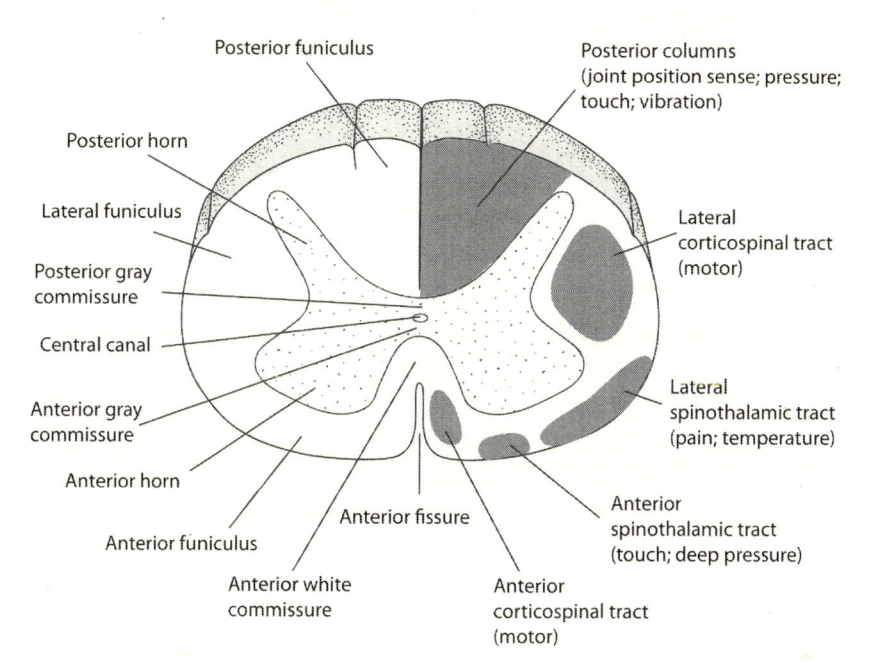

FIGURE 4.3 The spinal cord showing, on the left, its main anatomical subdivisions and, on the right, the main ascending sensory and descending motor pathways. A lateral hemisection of the spinal cord interrupts these (and other) pathways, leading to the clinical features of the Brown-Séquard syndrome.

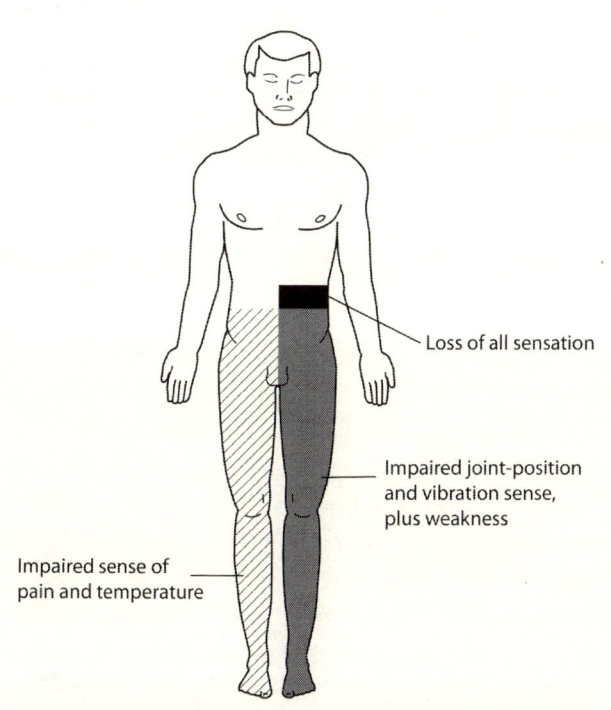

FIGURE 4.4 The clinical disorder that follows injury to one half of the spinal cord. On the injured side, all sensation may be lost at the level of the injury and, below it, paralysis is accompanied by impaired joint-position and vibration sense. Hyperesthesia also occurs but is usually not recognized. On the opposite side, pain and temperature appreciation are impaired.

limbs with fresh blood. Further, in 1850, he published the first of many papers dealing with different aspects of epilepsy, including work on experimentally induced epilepsy and on the inheritance of epilepsy in the offspring of animals with such seizures. Much of this work on heredity has now been discredited, however, because the conclusions to which it led were based on the erroneous interpretation of experimental observations, as discussed in Chapter 11.

During this time, few paid academic appointments were available, and most experimentalists therefore had to be independently wealthy or support themselves by private teaching, public lecturing, or clinical practice. Lacking private resources, the young Brown-Séquard attempted to maintain a private practice and economize on his daily expenses. He continued as an assistant to Martin-Magron, and was also helped in his endeavors by his old chief, Rayer, who gave him access to laboratory facilities and lent him equipment with which to perform experiments. Magendie similarly made facilities available to him and supported him in other ways; for example, when Brown-Séquard applied for the Montyon Prize of the Académie des Sciences but lost to Claude Bernard (who was Magendie's assistant), he received honorable mention and a financial award, probably at Magendie's insistence.[3] At about this time, he came into some money with which he bought a dog (almost certainly for one of his experiment) and also an extravagant dress-coat to wear to an appointment with an established medical man for whom he hoped to work as an assistant.[4,5] Somewhat unfortunately, however, both dog and coat were left unattended in the same room for several hours, and the dog—perhaps anticipating its fate—ripped the elegant clothing to shreds. The dog, of course, was always blamed for the young man's failure to obtain the sought-after post.

Nevertheless, Brown-Séquard continued in clinical practice, as well as pursuing his career in experimental physiology, and insisted—even as the years went by—that he was not simply a specialist in disorders of the nervous system, but rather that he had studied and continued to study every branch of medicine.[6] However, he never ceased in his struggle to be better than the average physician by recognizing the limitations of contemporary knowledge, and thus directed his efforts to learn more about the basis of human disease. His philosophy as a clinician is summarized by one of his more common comments, "I want to know something different, something better, than what the average doctors know," and his therapeutic approach was "if one way doesn't work, try another."[7] On one occasion, he looked after a friend of Sir James Paget (1814–1899), the distinguished British surgeon, after whom is named a disease of bone (osteitis deformans, which causes the bones to become weak, enlarged, and deformed), another of the nipple (a form of breast cancer), and a third of the penis or vulva (now called extramammary Paget's disease, an uncommon noninvasive tumor found in the genital and anorectal regions).[A] In a letter to Brown-Séquard, Paget wrote with his easy charm that "I have every confidence in yourself …. I have it all the more because … [you have some] uncertainty as to the exact nature of the case, for I have long learned to believe that in the real difficulties of medicine none but the ignorant feel quite sure."[8]

Brown-Séquard "never looked to make a fortune and it is not necessary to say that, having not looked, I did not find one."[9] Even the little that he earned was spent to further his work by the purchase of equipment or animals to be used in his experiments. Indeed, given his personal circumstances and the difficulties of his student days, it is hardly surprising that he became increasingly radical in his views, coming under the influence of the utopian socialist movement created by François Marie Charles Fourier (1772–1837), the social theorist and supporter of women's rights, who held that mutual cooperation (in special communities called "phalanxes") should be the basis of social success, with workers compensated for their labors based on their contribution. Fourier's ideas were carried forward by more pragmatic followers such as Victor Considérant (1808–1893), an engineer, writer, and editor of such periodicals as *La Phalange* and *La Démocratie Pacifique*, who wrote the *Manifesto of Peaceful Democracy*, which had some similarity to the *Communist Manifesto* published five years later by Marx and Engels. Brown-Séquard established ties with the Fourierists and was even given an editorial position on *La Phalange* that allowed him (in 1848) to communicate formally with the secretariat of the Institut de France concerning the works, letters, and papers presented at its Académie des Sciences, as documented in a letter to him by François Arago, Permanent Secretary of the Académie.[10]

It was at about this time that Brown-Séquard became increasingly close to César Daly (1811–1894), the illegitimate son of an Irish seaman and French noblewoman, who was also involved with the Fourierists and a contributor to *La Phalange,* and who became for a time the leading architectural writer

---

[A] Paget was a renowned pathologist as well as a surgeon and, while still a medical student at St. Bartholomew's Hospital in London, discovered the parasitic worm causing trichinosis, a disease acquired by eating infected pork. He later was appointed as surgeon to both Queen Victoria and the Prince of Wales, was one of the original three hundred fellows of the Royal College of Surgeons of England, became a fellow of the Royal Society and a friend of many eminent physicians and scientists of his day, and was created a baronet in 1871. His eloquence and following were such that Mr. Gladstone supposedly remarked that people could be divided into those who had and those who had not heard him speak.

in France.[B] Daly admired the young scientist and—in one of his notes to him—wrote of the "Dr. Brown-Séquard, who *should* be [a member] of the Institute [of France], which proves more than being of it."[11] Fortunately for the advance of science, Daly had a particular fascination for guinea pigs, which he kept in large number. Brown-Séquard would visit his friend, pick out a handsome animal, palpate its belly, and shaking his head, gloomily express his fears for its future unless he could take charge of the beast, which would never be seen again.[4,5] It is perhaps ironic, then, that he used the back of one of Daly's letters on which to scribble the draft of a manuscript concerning the results of experiments in which he removed the adrenal glands in various animals and showed that they were essential to life (see Chapter 6).[11]

Poverty was not the only problem with which he had to cope. He worked for 18 or 19 hours daily, slept very little, subsisted on the most meager of diets, and kept himself going with endless cups of coffee.[12] His health rapidly deteriorated on this harsh regime, he became increasingly weak and emaciated, and—because of the studies that he had undertaken on his own digestive juices—he suffered from postprandial gastric distension, flatulence, heartburn, and gastric regurgitation. At last, he had to give up work, take to his bed, and finally be removed by his friends to the country where, on a careful dietary regime, he gradually regained his vigor.[12]

In 1848—a year marked by revolution in many European countries including France, a year of poor harvests, increasing unemployment, and recession, and the year in which Marx and Engels published their *Communist Manifesto*—Brown-Séquard joined with several other anatomists and physiologists and two surgeons, Follin and Houel, to form the Société de Biologie, with Rayer as its first President.[13] Claude Bernard was appointed Vice-President, as also was Charles Robin, a histologist who had been an extern with Brown-Séquard on Trousseau's service just a few years earlier. Within a few months, Brown-Séquard was made one of the four Secretaries of the Society, and he later became President. He was always very active at its meetings, which he particularly enjoyed, speaking (as did his rival, Claude Bernard) at nearly all its sessions.[13,14] The Society attracted physicians and investigators such as anatomists and physiologists, chemists and anthropologists; its multidisciplinary nature was important for the advance of both clinical medicine and its scientific

---

[B] César Daly, French architect, author, and restorer of Albi cathedral, was the editor for nearly 50 years of the *Revue Générale de l'Architecture et des Travaux Publics*, a leading architectural journal during the nineteenth century. An influential architectural critic, his ideas were important in the eventual emergence of modern urban planning. He was also influential in discovering pre-Columbian ruins in Central America and encouraging pre-Columbian archaeology in Mexico.

underpinnings. Anyone could present an account of their work at the Society, and the text of the presentation was made available the day before the meeting to facilitate discussion, which was often lively and constructive—even heated— to Brown-Séquard's delight. The Society flourished, becoming a model for other learned bodies in England and Europe. It met every Saturday afternoon in the loft of the École Pratique,[C] and attendance of members was encouraged by imposing a fine of one franc on those absent without good cause.[13,15] It also appointed committees or commissions, on which Brown-Séquard served frequently, to examine contested scientific claims and report back to the Society. Such committees often met numerous times over many months, repeating experiments to verify their conclusions before submitting detailed reports of their findings.[16] Indeed, Brown-Séquard's findings on the sensory pathways in the spinal cord were so controversial that they—in turn—became subject to scrutiny by one such committee and received an unqualified endorsement. In the following year, he was elected to membership of the Société Philomatique, which had been founded in 1788 as a multidisciplinary scientific and philosophical society and was then one of the leading scientific societies in France (although its influence and prestige appear to have diminished in recent years). Shortly thereafter, he received a monetary award from the Académie des Sciences for his researches.[9]

In 1849, Brown-Séquard interrupted his experimental studies to work as an auxiliary physician under Baron Félix-Hippolyte Larrey (1808–1895), whose father had been chief surgeon to Napoleon and his armies,[D] at the military

---

[C] The so-called École Pratique, established in 1750, was designed for the practical education of surgeons. It contained the dissection rooms of the Faculty of Medicine and also various lecture halls; several hundred students were able to practice dissections there, but there were no teaching staff except for anatomy demonstrators who would put on special demonstrations and courses for a fee. Some students were selected to attend the school by competitive examination and were able to perform dissections without charge, whereas others paid for the privilege; the former had the first choice of bodies brought to the dissection rooms, taking precedence over regular students at the Faculty. Other dissecting rooms existed at La Pitié Hospital and on the grounds of a former cemetery close to the Jardin des Plantes.

[D] Dominique Jean Larrey (1766–1842), French military surgeon and chief surgeon of Napoleon's Grand Army, introduced field ambulances and hospitals to the battlefield (they had previously been about 3 miles behind the line) and originated the concept of first-aid by removal of the wounded from the battlefield immediately, rather than after the battle was over. He gave the first description of trench foot, advocated the use of maggots to prevent wound infection, and invented various surgical instruments and techniques. He was captured by the Prussians at the battle of Waterloo and sentenced to be shot, but a former student recognized him and pleaded for his life. It transpired that the son of Marshal Blücher, commander of the Prussian army, had been wounded and taken prisoner by the French in the Austrian campaign and that Larrey had saved his life. The Baron was released, breakfasted with the Marshall, and was given an escort back to France. On Napoleon's death, he was

hospital of Gros-Caillou during a cholera epidemic that began in the spring of that year and spread rapidly through France, Italy, and much of Europe to England, North Africa, and North America. Brown-Séquard remained in desultory contact with his chief for years thereafter. Indeed, in 1866, the Baron wrote that he had been made a corresponding Member of the Society of Surgery (Societé de Chirurgie)[17] and—as late as 1892—requested that they meet to go over Brown-Séquard's work, commencing with the salutation "Dear scientist, colleague, and friend" (*"Cher savant, confrère, et ami"*).[18] Larrey later became physician to Napoleon III and received many other honors; during the 1871 siege of Paris, he was surgeon-in-chief of the besieged armies. He wrote at length on military surgery and would often recall proudly that, in 1815, as a 6-year-old boy, he had met Napoleon I at a review: "the emperor came toward us. My sister, who was with me, made a gracious courtesy, while I inclined my head respectfully. Napoleon I, who was accompanied by my father, addressed him: 'Are those your children, Larrey,' and tapping me on the cheek with his right hand, he added, 'we will try and make something of him, won't we? As for the rest, he has only to resemble you.'"[19]

Cholera, characterized by acute and severe diarrhea, vomiting, and abdominal cramps, is caused by a bacterial infection. It is spread by food or water contaminated with infected human feces, is rarely transmitted directly from person to person, and flourishes in hot and humid conditions. If untreated, cholera can lead to severe dehydration, kidney failure, and death, often within a few hours. Epidemic cholera, perhaps originating in India, affected much of Europe and elsewhere during the nineteenth century, especially in the late 1840s and the 1850s, and led to many thousands of deaths. Indeed, in July 1850, Zachary Taylor, the twelfth president of the United States, died from cholera, to be succeeded by Millard Fillmore. Many contemporary physicians attributed the disease to direct exposure to dirty environmental conditions, a view seemingly supported by the more common occurrence of cholera in crowded, unsanitary slums and shantytowns than in prosperous areas. Medical treatment of the time included bleeding or the prescription of various medications to be taken by mouth, such as opium pills, Dover's powder (a mixture of ipecacuanha and opium), powdered chalk with opium, laudanum (an alcoholic tincture of opium), quinine, iron, calomel (mercury chloride), ipecacuanha, spirits (such as brandy) or other alcohols, camphor, ammonia,

---

bequeathed a large sum of money by the former Emperor with the comment "he is the worthiest man I ever met" and, years later, when Napoleon's body was brought home to France, Larrey, wearing the uniform of the Imperial Guard that he had worn at the battle of Wagram, followed the remains to its tomb. His name is inscribed on the Arc de Triomphe in Paris.

peppermint, and chloroform drops, or enemas (of opiates, broth, or such mixtures as gruel and salt). Various dietary and hygienic regimens, including cold shower-baths, also had their advocates.[20] Although a Dr. Thomas Latta recognized and successfully treated the dehydration occurring in cholera by copious infusion of saline and aqueous solutions into the veins during an epidemic in the early 1830s,[21] intravenous therapy was forgotten once that particular epidemic was over and appears not to have been used again for the treatment of cholera for almost 60 years.[22] Cramping was treated by ice, mustard, or turpentine placed on the abdomen or simply by briskly rubbing the skin. Brown-Séquard himself favored the use of laudanum, and his experience with cholera was to prove useful a few years later when he found himself in the midst of another epidemic on his return to Mauritius for a vacation.

The Move to America

The 1848 revolution in France led to the fall of the monarch Louis-Philippe and the establishment of the Second Republic, and later that year Louis-Napoleon Bonaparte (Napoleon's nephew) was elected its first president. As his term was drawing to an end, the National Assembly refused to accede to his request to revise the constitution to allow for his re-election so that, late in 1851, he seized dictatorial power in a coup d'état that began on the anniversary of Napoleon's victory over the Austrians and Russians at Austerlitz in 1805; within twelve months, the Second Republic was replaced by the Second Empire, with Louis-Napoleon assuming the title of Emperor Napoleon III. Brown-Séquard, with his ties to Fourierism, was an ardent republican and an opponent of the coup, which had led to popular gatherings and the barricades, followed by brutal repression and harsh punishment. With good reason, then, the high-principled physician—who was technically not French but British—fled to America in 1852. Given his impulsive nature, it is perhaps not altogether surprising that when he set sail he was unable even to speak English and indeed learned the language of the land to which he was traveling only while on the voyage.

The early days in America were difficult, and initially Brown-Séquard was compelled to give French lessons to make ends meet. It is said that his first medical activities were as an obstetrician, earning him five dollars per delivery, but there is little to support such an assertion. He is also reputed to have collaborated in the production of a textbook on obstetrics that subsequently did well and appeared in several editions,[23] but this too is unlikely. Instead, the results of his physiological work seem simply to have been referenced by the author of the textbook[24] to support clinical advice and provide a scientific basis for it. For example, based on Brown-Séquard's observations in animals, vaginal injection of carbon dioxide was advocated for provoking uterine contractions and in the treatment of uterine inertia during pregnancy.[25] Again, compression of the aorta was advocated as an efficient means of checking postpartum uterine hemorrhage, in part because this maneuver limits the amount of blood reaching the uterus, but also because uterine contraction was shown by Brown-Séquard to be stimulated by arrest of the arterial circulation. The experimentalist seems to have been appreciated widely by obstetricians and gynecologists. Some years later, with the founding of the Gynaecological Society of Boston in 1869, he was elected to honorary membership,[26] although this may have been because of his friendship with Horatio Storer (1830–1922), an antiabortionist and pioneer in the treatment of women's diseases, who had been his private pupil some years earlier and whose wife subsequently came under his care for a mental illness.[27] Indeed, Storer later dedicated one of his books to Brown-Séquard, so that it was associated "... with a name far more honored than his own [Storer's] can ever become."[28]

In any event, armed with letters of introduction from friends and colleagues to various prominent American personalities, Brown-Séquard rapidly returned to his interest in physiology and the nervous system, lecturing in Philadelphia, New York, and then Boston. The most revealing and interesting introduction was by Pierre Paul Broca (1824–1880), the French surgeon, anthropologist, and neurologist, who was intimately involved in the development of concepts concerning functional localization within specific convolutions of the brain and, in particular, with the notion that verbal expression depends on the integrity of the left third frontal convolution (Chapter 10). This cerebral convolution is still named after him, as is the disturbance of speech that follows its destruction (Broca's aphasia). His name also designates a cerebral region (area parolfactoria), a fiber tract (Broca's diagonal band), and several angles and points used in physical anthropology. He wrote to Dr. George B. Wood[E] of the University of Pennsylvania:

> Brown-Séquard is one of the most eminent physiologists of our time .... Still young, he has already enriched science with a number of new and important discoveries. I like to believe that the renown of his works has already crossed the seas and that ... he is not unknown to you .... Unfortunately, science today,

---

[E] George Wood (1797–1879) was one of the founders of the Philadelphia College of Pharmacy, where he held professorial appointments until he became Professor of Materia Medica and Pharmacy at the University of Pennsylvania, and then Professor of the Theory and Practice of Medicine until his retirement in 1860.

in the old world, is an unkind, harsh mother that does not support her children. France, embroiled in political upheavals ... has ceased to protect its artists and scholars .... Science is not possible for one who is not independently wealthy. Over the last eight years, Mr. Brown has used all his resources and endured unbelievable hardships to carry out expensive research work in experimental physiology. He now has only an honorable character, profound knowledge and has authored scientific papers that everyone can appreciate ...."[29]

Those whom he met him at this time encountered a lively and exuberant man of medium height, with dark hair, eloquent eyes, and the Latin habit of embracing the menfolk as well as the women,[30] although on occasions he seemed brooding and withdrawn. He loved argument, controversy, and debate. His early impressions of the United States can be gleaned from a letter written to a friend in New York, contrasting his experiences there and in Boston.[31] The inexperienced and shy bachelor from Europe found Bostonian women to be more attractive but less chic than New Yorkers, whereas the men (to whom he had paid less attention) had more of the style of gentlemen than their New York counterparts. Boston itself was a more peaceful city than New York, and had a charm reminiscent of a European town, with its less-planned, less-contrived layout reminding him particularly of Rouen, and its many gray and white buildings bringing back memories of Paris.

His letters to friends back in Paris emphasized his success and satisfaction with his new lot, to the extent that they became concerned lest he forget his French background and lose contact with them.[32] Indeed, Brown-Séquard was quick to grasp the opportunities for advancement offered him in America, and his lectures were an immediate success, not only with students but also with established practitioners and senior physicians. The *Boston Medical and Surgical Journal* described him as one of the most eminent of contemporary experimental physiologists and stressed that his lectures, and the experimental demonstrations accompanying them, were of immediate clinical relevance because they related the scientific discoveries of his experimental work to the phenomena of disease.[33] Similar notices of appreciation and gratitude were published in the *New York Tribune* for his novel and instructive course of lectures at the Medical Department of the University of New York,[33] and the two "brilliant and successful" courses by the "learned and able lecturer" at Pennsylvania College were received equally warmly, with a resolution of gratitude published in the *Medical News* and *Medical Examiner*.

It was during this first visit to America that Brown-Séquard first met Henry Feltus, a distant relative on his paternal side, with whom he developed a close and enduring relationship.[34] Feltus became a friend, confidant, and agent for the young scientist.[35]

Marriage

Ellen Fletcher was born in 1816 or thereabouts in Portland, Maine, an American of English descent and a niece of Grace Fletcher of New Hampshire, the first wife of the American statesman Daniel Webster.[F] She was one of four children; her mother, Mary, died while she was still a child, and her father, a merchant, died in 1842. Little is known about her early years or how she met Brown-Séquard, a man who seemed to have no interests other than in his work, but it was probably in Boston. He must have seemed stiff and shy to her. Anxious to please and impress her, Brown-Séquard asked her to attend his lectures on experimental physiology, and in his letters wrote of how his lectures had been received, the impressions he had made on others, and his theories on various clinical phenomena, including with them an occasional poem and even an account of his various expenses while lecturing. At times, however, his ardor was apparent: "... my love for you increases without pause. The more I think of you, and I cannot do anything but that, the more I admire the precious and rare qualities of your heart and mind .... I feel perfectly happy with the thought that my life will be associated with yours .... There is no devotion, no sacrifice of which I am incapable for you .... Oh, if it for me to find in you the tenderness that my mother had for me ...."[9]

He told her of his failure to make a literary career in France, his difficult life as a medical student, his success as a young scientist, and his poverty, but also made known his affection for her and eventually asked her to marry him. Nellie, as she was known to her friends, was the recipient of sound advice from friends to whom she wrote about their engagement. "Take things quietly and don't make [a] fuss, people have been married before and though for a day or so you may be somebody—you very soon relapse into your proper state and no-one cares whether you are a bride or not .... May you find your husband kind and affectionate but don't always be calling upon him for sympathy for a headache or a pain in your toe—don't have any unnecessary headaches—they are rather trying."[36]

As for Brown-Séquard, his letters generally remained focused on his work and professional concerns and achievements, and were curiously short on personal or domestic detail, even after they were married in March 1853. Four months later, in July, they returned to Paris, perhaps because he considered it his home but doubtless also so that he could claim credit for his important and original discovery, reported while he was in America, of the vasomotor nerves

---

[F] Daniel Webster (1782–1852), American lawyer, congressman, senator, presidential candidate, and Secretary of State to Presidents Harrison and Tyler.

(i.e., nerves supplying the blood vessels), credit that he feared others would claim, as discussed in Chapter 5. Ellen's early impressions of the French, both in France and later in Mauritius, reflected a simple upbringing. She wrote to her mother in Boston, "You cannot imagine how thankful I am when I see Frenchmen that Dr. S is so unlike them. To hear them speak lightly of religion, scoff at serious things, and discuss some points of morality would make me very wretched, but he is as particular and strict as any American ... he seems so grateful that I do not complain of being so far from my own country and that I am ready to like his friends ...."[37]

After he had shown his bride the Paris of his youth, caught up with professional matters, and renewed acquaintances and friendships, Brown-Séquard again immersed himself in his work as if he were still an unattached bachelor with little domestic responsibility.

The Cholera Epidemic of 1854

In 1854, the year that John Snow's experiments in London showed that contaminated water (rather than bad air) was important in the spread of the disease,[G] another epidemic of cholera occurred in Mauritius. This almost certainly was brought to the island by ships arriving from India with infected coolies (indentured laborers). The number of people who died in the epidemic that year is variously estimated at anywhere from seven to seventeen thousand, but the pattern of infection was seemingly haphazard in its spread. For example, nearly half of the female inmates of a local lunatic asylum died, whereas none of the inhabitants were affected in a nearby Indian camp of badly built and poorly ventilated huts.[38]

It was perhaps unfortunate that, early in 1854, Brown-Séquard—exhausted again—had decided to return to his native land in the Indian Ocean, probably to provide a break from the turmoil of his life in Paris. Together with Ellen and two other Mauritians (the physicians Frederic Bonnefin and Henri Lolliot) returning home after studying in France, he set sail in February from Nantes aboard the *Adolphe Lecourt*, a small cargo vessel loaded with livestock and carrying a few other passengers.[39,40] Many of his friends in France were concerned

---

[G] John Snow (1813–1858), British physician, the father of modern epidemiology, and a pioneer in the use of ether and chloroform for anesthesia. He administered chloroform to Queen Victoria during delivery of her last two children. By painstakingly mapping the distribution of infected cases and using statistical analysis, he showed that a cholera outbreak in London had spread in the water from a particular pump rather than by "bad air."

about his health, some feared that he would not survive the voyage, and Ellen was literally sick with worry on his account. The voyage was long and hot, although the tedium was punctuated by wondrous sunsets and the sight of distant lands; by unexpected encounters with passing ships, exotic birds, and marine animals; and by the occasional storms that left the travelers bruised and shaken. The imposed rest and sea air nevertheless revitalized the couple, and he seized the opportunity to study the temperature of humans and birds at different latitudes, while Ellen was kept busy in studying French and with dressmaking.

The excitement of their arrival in bustling Port Louis, with its backdrop of wooded hills and green mountains, was soon replaced by foreboding as they learned of the epidemic of cholera that had begun shortly before their arrival on May 12. The infection produced dread and panic as it spread: Those with means fled from the town to the country.[39,41] Shops rapidly emptied of fresh produce as farmers and market people kept away from the town, and those without anywhere else to go stayed indoors in the hope of avoiding the infection. Many local physicians, fearing for their own safety, refused to attend patients who contracted the disease.[41]

Local customs and superstitions were called on for protection.[39] Despite entreaties from the mayor, people made enormous fires at the edges of their properties or close to their homes to expel "bad air." Herbs and roots were added to the flames for good measure, dwellings were filled with the dense clouds, and loved ones approached the flames to inhale the purifying smoke. The burning of herbs was an Indian approach to warding off infection, and the many Indians who lived in Port Louis also hung garlands of sacred herbs around their houses and across the streets in those quarters where they lived. Indeed, the different groups forming the population organized many religious processions, ceremonies, and prayer-meetings in an attempt to stave off disaster. The more sophisticated citizens even arranged for all the guns on the island to be fired repeatedly to dissipate the bad air, but the constant crash and thunder simply added to the fears that beset the population. During the epidemic, the Indian mynah birds or starlings—"martins" as they were called locally— abandoned the main barrack square and other open spaces around the haunts of humans in Port Louis and were nowhere to be seen, perhaps frightened off by the noise and smoke of the preventive measures adopted by the citizenry. These birds, which had been imported from India and were protected as destroyers of certain insect pests in the sugarcane plantations, had apparently moved to the forest in the center of the little island and did not reappear until the epidemic had passed.[42]

With Brown-Séquard's reputation as physician and scientist, and given his previous experience in treating cholera at the Gros-Caillou Hospital in Paris, the eyes of his countrymen and of the colonial administration turned to him for help and guidance in treating the sick, controlling the spread of the disease, and determining the cause of the outbreak, which killed thousands of his countrymen.[43] He was, therefore, granted permission to practice medicine in the colony.[44] He and Ellen stayed at the country house of his godfather, together with about thirty family friends or relatives and some fifteen servants, and from there he made many visits to local hospitals and the sick. On one occasion, he returned to the house to find a carriage waiting to take him to the home of a very rich patient who had been deserted by all his servants other than his driver, so that the good doctor had himself to go into the town to find medicine for the unfortunate man, who died a short while later.[41] He gave his services without any thought of recompense or recognition, insisted that a hospital be opened for the poor, and took special charge of the Hospital of St. Mary, where he was able to save many unfortunate victims of the epidemic and ease the final hours of those too ill to survive.[40] Wherever he went, he was sought after for help, and he gave this freely as best he could and to the point of exhaustion. As Ellen wrote to her family, "his friends desire he should remain here [Mauritius] as he could make a fortune in two years."[41] She herself was "as happy as the day is long" once the danger of cholera was passed, and she spoke of the beauty of the land in letters to her family in the United States.[45]

In subsequently reporting to the local governing authorities the remarkably low death rate from the disease of the patients under his care, Brown-Séquard credited the devotion of the Sisters of Mercy and others, without mentioning his own effort.[40] Laudanum (tincture of opium) was the treatment he favored, in place of the traditional cold shower-baths, bloodletting, purging, or induced vomiting preferred by many physicians of that period, including Dr. MacPherson, an army doctor with whom he worked. For example, in a letter just a few years later to a friend, Gabriel Desiré Laverdant (1802–1884), a fellow Fourierist and the avant-garde author of a tract on art as an instrument of social radical change, he gave specific instructions about how cholera should be treated. He advised eight or ten drops of laudanum after each bowel movement for only a little diarrhea consisting of green or black stools, with variations in the regimen depending on the frequency of bowel-opening and the color of the stools; for cramping with coldness of the extremities, without diarrhea, ten drops of laudanum were to be taken every half-hour for two or three hours unless the cramps stopped sooner.[46] His mailed prescriptions are interesting for the detail he provided to cover every conceivable eventuality while the patient "awaited the arrival of a doctor." Even during the epidemic, however, Brown-Séquard found it difficult to resist the temptation to experiment. He is said to have swallowed the vomit of cholera patients and—feeling symptoms of the disease developing in himself—then taken laudanum, presumably to establish more clearly the utility of this approach to treatment. In fact, however, he took such large doses of the opiate that he became obtunded and had to be resuscitated with coffee.[40]

The epidemic reached its peak in June and was finally brought to an end in August. At the end of August, Brown-Séquard was appointed to a Commission of Enquiry to investigate the epidemic, from which he resigned in October as he prepared to leave his homeland once more, this time for the New World and Virginia. The popular press now called upon the citizens of the colony to present him with a medal commemorating his services. The response was immediate: He received a silver cup, and also a gold medal inscribed "The inhabitants of Mauritius to their compatriot Dr. Brown-Séquard, as a mark of esteem and in recognition of services rendered during the cholera of 1854."[47]

References and Source Notes

1. French RD. *Antivivisection and medical science in Victorian society*. Princeton: Princeton University Press, 1975.
2. Brown-Séquard E. *Experimental researches applied to physiology and pathology* (pp. 8–9). New York: Bailliere, 1853.
3. Role A. *La vie etrange d'un grand savant: Le Professeur Brown-Séquard* (pp. 60–64). Paris: Plon, 1977.
4. Anonymous. Brown-Séquard. Quelques notes intimes sur le célèbre physiologiste. *L'Eclair*, 4 April 1894.
5. Anonymous. The late Professor Brown-Séquard. Anecdotes of a great physiologist. *St. James's Gazette (London)*, 4 April 1894.
6. Francis SW. Biographical sketches of distinguished living New York physicians. V. C.E. Brown-Séquard, M.D., F.R.S., etc. *Med Surg Reporter (Philadelphia)*, 15:169–172, 1866.
7. Sayings of Brown-Sequard. MS 999/6 (p. 29). Archives, Royal College of Physicians, London.
8. Paget J. Letter to Brown-Séquard dated 30 April 1850 (?). MS 981/75. Archives, Royal College of Physicians, London.
9. Brown-Séquard CE. Letter dated 17 December 1852, addressed to Lady Blanche [Ellen Fletcher], who was to become his first wife. MS 977/1. Archives, Royal College of Physicians, London.
10. Arago F. Official letter dated 7 February 1848, authorizing Dr. Brown-Séquard to look at works, memoirs, and correspondence presented to the Académie des Sciences. MS 980/1. Archives, Royal College of Physicians, London.
11. Daly C. Letter to Brown-Séquard dated 31 October 1857. MS 980/10. Archives, Royal College of Physicians, London.
12. Brown-Séquard CE. On a new mode of treatment of functional dyspepsia, anaemia, and chlorosis. *Arch Sci Pract Med (NY)*, 1:30–33, 1873. [In this paper, Brown-Séquard described in detail the condition of "a patient" whom he allegedly encountered in 1851, but whom is undoubtedly himself.]
13. Gley E. Cinquantenaire de la Société de Biologie: Discours. *C R Soc Biol (Paris)*, 51: 1011–1080, 1899.

14. Berthelot M. *Notice sur la vie et les travaux de M. Brown-Séquard*. Paris: Institut de France, 1898.
15. Société de Biologie. Reglement primitif (1848). *C R Soc Biol (Paris)*, 20:XI–XIV, 1868.
16. Gley E. *Essais de Philosophe et d'Histoire de la Biologie* (pp. 168–312). Paris: Masson, 1900.
17. [Baron] Larrey F-H. Letter to Brown-Sequard dated 4 January 1866, informing him that he had been made a corresponding Member of the Society of Surgery. MS 984/15. Archives, Royal College of Physicians, London.
18. [Baron] Larrey F-H. Letter to Brown-Séquard dated 6 May 1892. MS 980/73. Archives, Royal College of Physicians, London.
19. Anonymous. Our Paris letter: Pasteur—Larrey. *Med Record*, 48:641–642, 1895.
20. Ayre J. *A memoir on the treatment of the epidemic cholera. Read before the members of the French Academy of Sciences; with their report thereon.* London: J Churchill, 1856.
21. Latta T. Letter to the Secretary of the Central Board of Health, London, affording a view of the rationale and results of his practice in the treatment of cholera by aqueous and saline injections. *Lancet*, 18:274–277, 1832.
22. Finberg L. The early history of the treatment of dehydration. *Arch Pediatr Adolesc Med*, 152:71–73, 1998.
23. Dupuy E. Biographies scientifiques. Brown-Séquard. *Rev Scientifique*, 2:737–743, 1894.
24. Bedford GS. *The principles and practice of obstetric* (pp. 395, 678). New York: Wood, 1863.
25. Brown-Séquard E. *Experimental researches applied to physiology and pathology* (p. 117). New York: Bailliere, 1853.
26. Gynaecological Society of Boston. Letter from Winslow Lewis and Horatio R. Storer to Brown-Séquard informing him that he had been elected an honorary member, dated 19 March 1869. MS 984/4. Archives, Royal College of Physicians, London.
27. Dyer FN. *Champion of women and the unborn: Horatio Robinson Storer, M.D.* (pp. 267, 352). Canton, MA: Science History Publications, 1999.
28. Storer HR. *Why not? A book for every woman* (p. iii). Boston: Lee & Shepherd, 1868. Cited by Dyer FN. Champion of women and the unborn: Horatio Robinson Storer, M.D. (p. 99). Canton, MA: Science History Publications, 1999.
29. Broca P. Letter introducing Brown-Séquard dated 15 February 1852. MS 986/5. Archives, Royal College of Physicians, London.
30. McCausland, Charlotte (née Brown-Séquard). Notebook relating to C.E. Brown-Séquard (her father), including letters to and about him (pp. 48–50). MS 999/7. Archives, Royal College of Physicians, London.
31. Brown-Séquard CE. Undated letter to a friend. MS 980/3. Archives, Royal College of Physicians, London.
32. Letter from a friend in Paris to Brown-Séquard, dated 21 July 1852. MS 980/4. Archives, Royal College of Physicians, London.
33. Notice concerning Dr. Brown-Séquard's lectures. *Boston Med Surg J*, 47:338–339, 1852.
34. Letter of introduction to Henry Feltus dated 14 May 1852, author uncertain. MS 981/128. Archives, Royal College of Physicians, London.
35. Feltus H. Miscellaneous correspondence to Brown-Séquard dated 1861–1869. MSS 981/129–164, Archives, Royal College of Physicians, London.
36. Bunker AJ. Letter to Miss Ellen Fletcher dated 16 January 1853. MS 999/6 (pp. 18–20). Archives, Royal College of Physicians, London.
37. Brown-Séquard, Ellen (née Fletcher). Letter to her mother dated 30 April 1854. MS 999/6 (pp. 20–23). Archives, Royal College of Physicians, London.
38. Babington BG. Presidential address. *Trans Epidemiol Soc Lond*, 1:135, 1863.
39. Anonymous (probably Ellen Brown-Séquard, née Fletcher). Notes on the Mauritius. A series of articles that appeared in *The New York Daily Tribune*, 1857.

40. Rouget FA. *Brown-Séquard et son oeuvre. Esquisse biographique* (pp. 15–20). Port-Louis, Ile Maurice: General Printing & Stationery Co., 1930.
41. Brown-Séquard, Ellen (née Fletcher). Letter to her mother dated 2 June 1854. MS 999/6 (pp. 23–25). Archives, Royal College of Physicians, London.
42. HMC. Birds and cholera. *Nature*, 28:366, 1883.
43. Barnwell PJ, Toussaint A. A short history of Mauritius (p. 167). London: Longmans, Green & Co. (for the Government of Mauritius), 1949.
44. Chief Medical Officer, Mauritius. Letter to Dr. Edward Brown-Séquard dated 30 May 1854. MS 980/6. Archives, Royal College of Physicians, London.
45. Brown-Séquard, Ellen (née Fletcher). Letter to her sister dated 6 July 1854. MS 999/6 (pp. 25–27). Archives, Royal College of Physicians, London.
46. Brown-Séquard CE. Letter to Gabriel Desiré Laverdant, dated 5 October 1865, regarding treatment of cholera. MS 981/71. Archives, Royal College of Physicians, London.
47. Newspaper articles from Mauritius (source not indicated), detailing correspondence between M. Fropier, Mayor of Port Louis and Brown-Séquard, 1854. MS 1000/161. Archives, Royal College of Physicians, London.

5

The Physics of the Circulation

Why We Don't Faint on Standing, and Why We Get Bedsores on Lying Still for Too Long

Brown-Séquard's hasty return to Paris in July 1853, just four months after his marriage, was almost certainly so that he could claim credit and receive proper recognition for his discovery of the function of the nerves supplying the blood vessels. He also wanted to be in Paris so that he could argue more persuasively about the function of these nerves, as his views differed from those of Claude Bernard (1813–1878), his powerful rival in France. The arteries are not simply inert pipes, but rather are muscular tubes that can be made to contract or dilate by the nervous system. The definition of the *vasomotor nerves*, that is, the nerves that control the caliber of the blood vessels, was achieved through the competing efforts of Claude Bernard and Brown-Séquard, two men whose careers had followed remarkably parallel courses, despite the differences in their experimental approach.

Claude Bernard, like Brown-Séquard, had had literary leanings that were dashed when first he came to Paris. A letter of introduction had gained him entry to the circle of Saint-Marc Girardin,[A] but his five-act play was not well

---

[A] Saint-Marc Girardin (1801–1873), French politician and literary critic. He was a long-time contributor to the *Journal des Debats*, became professor of history and then of poetry at the Sorbonne, and was elected to the Académie française in 1844. He was also active in politics for several years and became a leading opponent of the Republic and its President after the Franco-Prussian war of 1870.

received and the would-be man of letters went on to become an illustrious man of science, eventually succeeding the great François Magendie as Professor of Medicine at the Collège de France, where he came to personify the experimental approach to medicine. His studies were to show that the liver is able to manufacture sugar from a substance stored within it, which he called glycogen, and he initiated modern concepts of carbohydrate metabolism. His work also clarified the role of the pancreas in digestion and led him to formulate the concept of an internal environment that is kept constant by the interactions of different processes in the body.[1-3] Not surprisingly, then, he was led to the study of the nerves that supply the blood vessels and thus help to maintain the constancy of the internal environment, and his interests thus came to merge with those of Brown-Séquard. However, the two men differed markedly in the role that they conceived for the nerves supplying the blood vessels, and they were competitors rather than collaborators. Indeed, both competed for the chair of medicine at the Collège on Magendie's death; although Brown-Séquard was unsuccessful, he ultimately obtained the appointment on Bernard's death.

It is now known that the function of the heart and blood vessels is regulated by the nervous system. As mentioned in Chapter 3, the nervous system is divided into central (brain and spinal cord) and peripheral (nerve roots and nerves) components. In addition, however, a third component—the *autonomic nervous system*—that has both central and peripheral components is present in vertebrates and enables the body to adapt to its environment. If it were not for this system, for example, a person getting up from a bed or a chair would faint as the blood pooled by gravity in the legs, thus depriving the brain of an adequate blood supply. This third system regulates the activities of the various organs of the body, activities that occur automatically without conscious effort, such as those of the heart and gastrointestinal system. It controls the bladder, bowels, and sexual function; maintains the blood pressure; regulates breathing; and prepares the animal for "fight or flight," depending on external circumstances. The autonomic nervous system is itself divided into the *sympathetic* and *parasympathetic systems*, which are controlled by a portion of the brain called the *hypothalamus*, and the balance in activity of the two systems—which have opposing effects—governs certain behavior. This balance is altered depending on external events and emotions, and activity of either the sympathetic or parasympathetic system can be increased or diminished. (An additional component of the autonomic nervous system, the *enteric system*, has recently been recognized also, but is not germane to the present discussion.)

Although both systems operate continuously, the sympathetic system plays a major role in stressful situations, whereas the parasympathetic system is dominant at other times. The manner in which the system works is exemplified by the control of the heart. As is now understood, the heart beats normally at a low rate because its activity is controlled by the background activity of the parasympathetic system; with exercise, the heart rate increases because parasympathetic activity is reduced and, if the heart has to beat even faster, this is accomplished by an increase in sympathetic activity. Fear or anger activates the sympathetic system so that, for example, the heart beats faster and with greater strength; at the same time, blood flow to the skin is reduced (so that more blood can flow to the muscles, which may have to work strenuously to enable the animal to fight or run for its life), the blood pressure is increased, the hair may stand on end (to make the animal appear larger and more frightening to its enemies), the pupils dilate, the airways widen to allow for greater airflow in the lungs, the concentration of sugar in the blood is increased, and so on.

There are both afferent and efferent autonomic fibers in the various nerves of the body. The former carry sensory information from the blood vessels and major organs of the body to the spinal cord and various parts of the brain. The hypothalamus and other autonomic centers in the brain—which generate the reflex responses of the blood vessels, heart, and other organs to this sensory input—are connected directly or indirectly with autonomic nerve cells in the spinal cord. These, in turn, give rise to the efferent (motor) autonomic nerves, which stimulate their target organs (blood vessels, heart, etc.) by releasing chemical transmitter substances. Stimulation of the sympathetic nerves leads to release of the neurotransmitter *noradrenaline (norepinephrine)* at most nerve terminals, but of *acetylcholine* at some. Conversely, in the parasympathetic system only acetylcholine released. Noradrenaline and *adrenaline (epinephrine)* are also present in large quantities in the adrenal glands (small glands that lie close to the kidneys; Chapter 6), from which these neurotransmitters are released as needed. Receptors in the target cells respond to specific neurotransmitters, just like a lock that can be opened by one key but not another.

Discovery of the Vasomotor Nerves

In the first half of the nineteenth century, little was known about the autonomic nervous system or about the manner in which it controls the heart and blood vessels, and thus the circulation of blood. Many physiologists considered that the arteries had elastic properties rather than walls capable of active contraction. By the 1840s, however, the presence of nerves that appeared to pass to the blood vessels suggested to Jakob Henle (1809–1885; German anatomist and pathologist; see Chapter 11), Benedikt Stilling (1810–1879; German surgeon and anatomist[B]), and others that the circulation was regulated by the nervous system through nerves that Stilling first designated as vasomotor nerves (*nervus vasomotorius*).[4] The concept itself was not new, for Thomas Willis[C] in the seventeenth century believed that the nerve networks around blood vessels could contract, thereby constricting the vessels. What was new was the emerging belief that the blood vessels themselves could constrict or dilate under the control of the nervous system. Thus, the regulatory neural mechanism was postulated to act on muscle that comprised part of the wall of blood vessels, especially the wall of the small arteries; the muscle was so arranged that the contractile elements of the muscle formed a ring around the lumen of the vessel.

At the time, Claude Bernard was interested in the neural (nervous system) mechanisms regulating the temperature of localized regions of the body. He believed that heat was generated by local chemical reactions and that any neural influence was probably exerted on such chemical changes. He therefore decided to investigate the effect of interrupting the regional nerve supply.[5] He chose first to study the effect of sectioning the sympathetic nerves, because of their close anatomical relationship with the blood vessels, reasoning that these nerves might regulate the chemical reactions occurring in or about the vessels. Accordingly, he divided in rabbits and other animals the easily accessible sympathetic nerve on one side of the neck. He was surprised to find—contrary to his expectations, for he thought that the sympathetic system was responsible for animal warmth and that cutting the sympathetic nerves would lower the temperature of the face—a marked and rapid increase in skin temperature of the face and neck on that side, together with increased sensitivity and an apparent engorgement of the visible blood vessels in the thin ears of his rabbits. He presented this observation to the Société de Biologie in 1851, writing:

> I have seen that just after section of the cervical sympathetic nerve, the denervated structures become warmer .... When we put the thermometer either

---

[B] It was Stilling who invented the microtome, by which he cut frozen or alcohol-hardened spinal cords into a series of thin consecutive sections, as if slicing a salami; these serial sections were then inspected under the microscope.

[C] Thomas Willis (1621–1675), English physician, neuroanatomist, and a founding member of the Royal Society, is widely regarded as the father of neurology (a word that he coined). His published anatomical text on the central nervous system was illustrated by Sir Christopher Wren, architect of St. Paul's Cathedral in London. He described many anatomical features of the brain, and the arrangement of the major blood vessels at the base of the brain is named after him (the circle of Willis). He also provided seminal descriptions of several neurological diseases.

into the ears of the rabbit or into the nostrils of the animal, the temperature was higher (four to six degrees centigrade) on the side where the sympathetic nerve had been cut. Whereas the temperature increased, circulation became more active ....[6]

A few months later, he presented his findings to the Académie des Sciences,[7] emphasizing that the observed changes in temperature could not be the result of vascular engorgement as they had a different time course and were longer lasting than the changes in the blood vessels. However, he did not suggest any hypothesis regarding the role of the sympathetic nerves in heat production.

Bernard's work aroused a great deal of attention,[8] but Brown-Séquard had performed similar studies before leaving France for the United States in 1852, probably in Rayer's laboratory in Paris,[9] and these were published in August in the *Medical Examiner* of Philadelphia. His conclusions differed from those of Bernard. He noted:

If galvanism [electrical stimulation] is applied to the superior portion of the sympathetic after it has been cut in the neck, the vessels of the face and of the ear after a certain time begin to contract; ... the temperature and the sensibility diminish in the face and the ear, and they become in the palsied side the same as in the sound side .... When the galvanic current ceases to act, the vessels begin to dilate again and all the phenomena discovered, after sectioning the chain, by Dr. Bernard reappear .... I conclude that the only direct effect of the section of the cervical part of the sympathetic is the paralysis and consequently the dilatation of the blood vessels. Another evident conclusion is that the cervical sympathetic send motor nerve fibres to many of the blood vessels of the head.[10,D]

Brown-Séquard's conclusion was clear and unambiguous, and he established the relationship between the blood vessels and the sympathetic nervous system. The sympathetic nerves control the caliber of the blood vessels, which have contractile properties, so that they can narrow or widen. Regional temperature and sensibility change when the vessels dilate after interruption of the sympathetic nerve supplying them.

[D] The word *galvanism* was commonly used by physiologists at that time to mean electrical stimulation, without reference to the type of stimulation, although strictly it refers to galvanic (direct-current) as opposed to faradic (alternating-current) stimulation. In fact, Brown-Séquard used an induction coil, which delivers faradic stimulation; such coils, invented by the German electrophysiologist Emil du Bois-Reymond (1818–1896), were widely used in physiological studies after 1848, when the inventor published the first part of his *Researches on Animal Electricity*.

Claude Bernard subsequently—and independently—also stimulated the upper portion of the divided sympathetic nerve in the neck, thereby reversing the effect of nerve section, as also did Augustus Waller, an English physiologist. In 1853, Bernard gave a more detailed account of his findings and conclusions to the Société de Biologie,[11] but did not accept the vasomotor function of the sympathetic nerves, denying that the vasodilatation that follows sympathectomy was due to a "paralysis of the arteries." He continued to believe that these nerves influenced the regional temperature by a direct effect on the chemical reactions occurring in the tissues, and that the vascular changes were probably a consequence, rather than a cause, of the temperature change. He reiterated his view to the end of his career, although eventually conceding that the sympathetic nerves also had a vasoconstrictor effect.[5] In his 1853 paper, Bernard also referred to the fact that Brown-Séquard, on his return to Paris, had first told him of the work that he had reported earlier from Philadelphia and claimed credit for the contribution he had thus made.

> On his return to France, M. Brown-Séquard claimed as his theory stasis of the blood through paralysis of the arteries, and he announced that he had been the first to see in America that galvanization of the sympathetic leads to cooling of the parts and contraction of the arteries.[11]

And he added somewhat haughtily,

> I shall not enter into a discussion about priority concerning facts which all date from the same year .... I congratulate myself only on the urgency with which some experimenters ... have felt to follow me in this study on the phenomena of calorification ....[11]

Looking back on the exchange, it seems clear that credit rightly belongs to Brown-Séquard, not only for the originality of his observations but for correctly interpreting those observations. But Bernard was hard to convince, and persisted in attributing the increased temperature to a greater production of heat rather than to the change in blood flow. In the following year, he clarified his belief that the two phenomena were distinct, pointing out that they had a different time course. Moreover, he continued, at the time of sectioning the sympathetic nerve, an initial vasoconstriction (narrowing or contraction of blood vessels) is seen rather than a vasodilatation (distension of the vessels). Brown-Séquard's response was swift. He tartly reminded Bernard that when a nerve is being sectioned, as also during its electrical stimulation, that nerve is excited and the effects of its activity are therefore seen, whereas the long-lasting effects that follow nerve sectioning result from a loss of its function.[12]

Bernard did not answer or even refer to this critique of his views. Perhaps ironically, in that same year, it was announced that he was the recipient of the 1853 prize in experimental physiology from the Académie for his work.[13]

Brown-Séquard took the subject still further. Claude Bernard believed that abnormalities of the central nervous system or somatic nerves affected temperature of localized regions of the body in a manner opposite to that of lesions of the sympathetic nerves. "It is known," wrote Bernard "that injuries of the cerebro-spinal nervous system constantly produce a total or a partial diminution in the temperature of animals, either when a nerve has been divided or when the injury is made on the nervous centers."[14] Brown-Séquard, again, could not agree with Bernard, and found by experiment in birds and mammals that the temperature of a paralyzed extremity varied depending on the size of the regional blood vessels.[15] He cut the main nerve to the hind leg of guinea pigs, for example, and found an increase in temperature of the paralyzed limb that lasted for two or three days. The more dilated the arteries and other vessels, the higher the temperature.[15] In his own words,

> I have endeavored to prove that the local increase of temperature following the section of the sympathetic nerve is the result of paralysis of the blood vessels. I will now relate some other cases in which a local increase in temperature takes place after various other injuries of the nervous system, and apparently in consequence of the same cause ....[15]

There was no difference in this regard, then, between a lesion confined to the sympathetic nerves and a less restricted lesion (presumably because the latter also affected the sympathetic pathways as they traverse the spinal cord or the vasomotor nerve fibers that travel with the somatic nerves to the periphery).

The disagreement continued between the two physiologists with regard to the control of the circulation. Thus, Bernard, in 1858, reported that dilatation of the blood vessels could be induced in dogs by electrical stimulation of certain nerves.[16] In particular, stimulation of the sympathetic nerve in the neck caused vasoconstriction and thus a reduced venous outflow of blood, whereas stimulation of another nerve (the chorda tympani nerve) led to dilatation of the blood vessels (as well as increased production of saliva) in the salivary glands that he was studying (the submaxillary gland). He concluded that there are distinct vasoconstrictor and vasodilator nerve fibers.

It is more difficult to understand the action of a vasodilator than vasoconstrictor nerve, because vessels can dilate or become distended passively with a lessening of previous vasoconstrictor activity. Nevertheless, it seemed from

Bernard's experiment (and has since been confirmed) that vasodilatation can occur as an active phenomenon. Brown-Séquard, however, disagreed with Bernard, arguing instead that the neural control of the salivary glands involved vasoconstrictor fibers acting on the blood vessels and secretory fibers acting on the glandular tissue itself.[9,17] Vasodilatation, he suggested, resulted from a non-nervous mechanism that followed increased glandular activity, rather than from a direct effect by the nerves on the blood-vessel walls. This may seem somewhat similar to the argument that Bernard had used against the existence of the vasoconstrictor nerves described by Brown-Séquard, but it is now known that, in this latter instance, both men were correct. On the one hand, as Bernard suggested, in addition to the sympathetic vasoconstrictor nerves, vasodilator nerves do indeed exist. They may arise from either the sympathetic or parasympathetic component of the autonomic nervous system, depending of the target organ in which the vessels are situated; the sympathetic system may cause vasodilatation in the limb muscles, and the parasympathetic system in, for example, the salivary glands, genitalia, and gastrointestinal mucosa. On the other hand, as Brown-Séquard noted, vasodilatation also occurs in the salivary glands on stimulation of certain nerves (the chorda tympani in this instance) as a consequence of release into the gland of an enzyme that leads to the local production of a substance called *bradykinin*, a powerful vasodilator.[18] Each of the protagonists had thus correctly conceived of one physiological mechanism for the occurrence of vasodilatation and ignored another, Bernard on the basis of experimental evidence and Brown-Séquard based on intuition.

Vasomotor Reflexes

The state of the circulation, of the blood vessels, at any one time depends on both external circumstances and the internal milieu. Various reflexes come into play, so that internal or external stimuli lead to responses that maintain the circulation at an optimal setting. The vasomotor nerves have a crucial role in this context, and the importance of their discovery cannot be overemphasized. The ability to vary the distribution of blood in the body so that, depending on need, more blood is delivered to certain regions (with a corresponding reduction in the blood supplied to other parts) allows the best use of limited resources (i.e., the total amount of blood and output from the heart).

As to the reflexes that adjust the circulation, it was Brown-Séquard who first described such a vasomotor reflex.[9] With his friend Joseph Désiré Tholozan

(1820–1897), a fellow Mauritian and military physician who became the physician of the Shah of Persia, he reported that immersion of one hand in ice-cold water led to a substantial decline in temperature of the other hand but not that of the mouth.[19,20] Thus, he reasoned that the chilling of the nonimmersed hand

> exists in consequence, either of the arrival of a cooler blood, or in the diminution in the quantity of blood ... the blood that arrives in the hand is not cooler ... this we prove by the fact that the temperature is but very little changed in the mouth. The supposition then remains that the quantity of blood arriving in the hand is smaller than usual. This may happen by two modes, one of which is that the heart sends less blood, and the other that the blood-vessels of the hand are contracted and prevent, in part, the passage of blood. It is certain that the heart continues perceptibly to send the same quantity of blood. Therefore, we are induced to admit that the hand's blood-vessels are contracted ... the nervous centres are strongly excited, and they act ....[20]

In other words, the cold in one hand stimulated afferent fibers and thereby elicited a reflex vasoconstriction in the nonimmersed hand. Since this first description of the vasomotor responses to cooling of the skin, it has come to be widely recognized that the skin is an important organ for regulating body temperature. Blood flow to the skin can be reduced to diminish the amount of heat lost to the environment or—conversely—increased so that heat loss is enhanced (as when one is flushed in hot weather).

Brown-Séquard's discovery of this vasomotor reflex was followed by the recognition of many other vasomotor reflexes. The vasoconstrictor outflow to different organs and parts of the body is modulated or "tuned" by these reflexes, allowing for exquisitely fine adjustment in the circulation of blood depending on the state and activity of the organism. The regional blood supply—for example, to the skin, muscles, or intestines—can be selectively influenced by the brain through these reflexes. The central nervous system not only generates patterns of behavior but influences sympathetic nerve activity, so that the selected behavior can best take place. The startle response, for example, involves an increase in output from the heart and increased blood flow to the limb muscles, with a compensatory adjustment of the flow of blood to other parts of the body. Again, when we move to a standing position from a seated or recumbent posture, there is initially a slight decline in blood pressure, and this leads to a reflex increase in peripheral vasoconstriction and heart rate, so that the blood pressure is maintained and we do not faint because of an inadequate blood supply to the brain.

Pressure (Bed) Sores

Pressure or bed sores—or decubitus ulcers (from the Latin *decumbere*, to lie down), as they are called by physicians—plague the disabled and those confined to bed or a chair with chronic illness. They may cause pain, aggravate disability, and become infected, sometimes with a fatal outcome. They have been known since antiquity, and have been described in Egyptian mummies.[21] They are especially common in the elderly, in nursing home residents, and in those with spinal or other neurological injuries leading to paraplegia (weakness or paralysis of the legs) or quadriplegia (weakness or paralysis of all limbs). Avoidance requires skilled nursing and attention to a number of medical factors. Their cause has been disputed over the years: some have related them to nerve injury, others to pressure, and yet others to an impairment of the blood supply of the affected part.

It is now widely accepted that a variety of external and intrinsic factors are responsible. Pressure above a certain level limits the delivery of oxygen and nutrients to tissues and leads to the local accumulation of metabolic waste products. Pressure is generally greatest at sites where weight-bearing bony prominences come into contact with external surfaces, such as the mattress of a bed. Greater pressure for a period of time produces irreversible tissue damage. As the pressure rises, ulcer formation occurs with increased rapidity. Shearing forces may also play a role. When patients are placed on an incline, for example, muscle and fatty tissues are pulled downward by gravity, whereas the skin remains fixed in position by the pressure on it. Consequently, local blood vessels become stretched and angulated, adding to the risk of tissue damage. Friction occurs when patients are pulled across an external surface, such as the bed sheets, and may damage or cause a break in the superficial layer of the skin. Moisture on the skin leads to skin maceration and further predisposes to ulcer formation.

The intrinsic factors that predispose to bed sores can thus be surmised. Immobility is the most important, but skin maceration from urinary incontinence is also important. Bed sores are more likely to develop in the malnourished or those with inadequate dietary intake. Reduced blood flow to the skin may result from hypotension, dehydration, vasomotor failure, and excessive peripheral vasoconstriction (e.g., from shock or certain medications), and this makes the skin more vulnerable to injury, so that pressure for a relatively short time leads to its break-down. Certain disorders of the nervous system predispose to bed sores because they limit mobility (as in comatose patients or those with a stroke); when the neurological disorder has led to loss of sensation, patients do not feel any discomfort resulting from prolonged pressure and thus are less likely to move about.

Brown-Séquard recognized that pressure and moisture of the skin are major determinants for the development of bed sores, and was quick to relate his experimental work in animals to the clinical care of patients. When he cut the spinal cord of various mammals and birds, ulcerations occurred around the genital organs as a result of "continued pressure" and "the continual presence of altered urine and faeces."[10] Importantly, he also noted that pressure sores in normal and paraplegic animals healed equally well if the animals were kept dry and pressure on the affected part was avoided, and he could prevent the occurrence of these sores in animals in whom the spinal cord was cut when he "took care to prevent any part of their bodies from being in a continued state of compression, and of washing them many times a day to remove the urine and faeces."[22] Sir James Paget in England also applied these concepts to patient care, emphasizing to clinical audiences in the following years the importance of relieving external pressure on the skin and its blood supply and on the consequent need to ensure that the posture of patients is changed frequently.[23]

In lectures that he gave to the Royal College of Surgeons of England in 1858, Brown-Séquard also described ulcers that occurred in patients with compression of the spinal cord, not only at common sites of sustained pressure but at other sites where the effect of pressure was less obvious. He attributed these ulcers to abnormalities in the blood supply to the affected parts[24] and recommended alternating hot and cold applications to these parts.

> I apply sometimes eight or ten times a day, morsels of ice to the parts threatened or affected, and then after the application of the ice, which of course causes contraction of the blood vessels, I apply a kind of poultice which is very hot, and of course produces a reverse effect. By these alternations of extreme cold and heat, I produce a change in the circulation of the part .... [25]

Others used his approach with success. Silas Weir Mitchell[E] described a patient in whom

> The bed-sores were treated with alternate applications of iced-water for ten minutes, followed by a flaxseed-meal poultice as hot as could be borne. This local means, recommended by Brown-Séquard, succeeded marvelously, as it always does, the bed-sores healing easily within ten days.[26]

[E] Silas Weir Mitchell (1829–1914), American physician and literary writer, sometimes referred to as the father of American neurology. He became an authority on gunshot wounds during the American Civil War. He is discussed further in Chapter 8.

Clearly, Brown-Séquard had recognized the importance of maintaining the adequacy of the local circulation, although this aspect of his work was subsequently taken out of context by others and extended to apply more generally to the genesis of bed sores, particularly their occurrence soon after a severe spinal injury. Thus, as recently as the middle of the twentieth century, Munro attributed ulcers occurring in that particular context to an increased susceptibility to pressure necrosis caused by loss of circulatory reflexes.[27]

A somewhat different view was presented by Jean-Martin Charcot,[F] who discounted pressure or abnormalities of vasomotor function as a major causative factor in some instances and believed instead that damage to the brain or spinal cord could lead directly to the occurrence of acute ulceration. This "neurotrophic theory" was stated succinctly in his lectures:

> [W]e must relegate to a secondary position the influence of pressure; and also that of vasomotor paralysis, which may be completely absent .... To explain the production of trophic disorders which issue in sacral mortification, here again it is not to absence of nerve-action that we should appeal, but to irritation of the spinal cord. [28]

His hypothesis seems to have been prompted by the observation that "acute bed-sore may show itself independently of all neuroparalytic hyperemia, since we observe it forming upon that side of the body where the vasomotor nerves are not affected" in patients with damage to one side of the spinal cord (Brown-Séquard syndrome). This is not surprising, however, as the nonparalyzed side is where the perception of pain is impaired (see p. 46), so that mild recurrent injury or pressure may pass unrecognized by patients until skin damage is evident. Such a neurotrophic concept has now been discounted, but for a time may have discouraged an active approach by physicians to the prevention and treatment of pressure sores, as it implied that they were an inevitable consequence of damage to the central nervous system, rather than a marker of inadequate nursing care.[29]

[F] Jean-Martin Charcot (1825–1893), French clinical neurologist after whom is named a joint, an artery, a type of aneurysm (a balloon-like swelling of an artery that may rupture to cause a hemorrhage in the head), and at least three diseases (peroneal muscular atrophy, multiple sclerosis, and Lou Gehrig disease, as amyotrophic lateral sclerosis is known in the United States). He was a colleague and collaborator of Brown-Séquard, and is discussed further in Chapters 9 and 12.

The Vasomotor Theory of Migraine

Migraine has been known to afflict humankind since antiquity. It has affected people from all walks of life including military leaders (Julius Caesar, Napoleon), politicians (Thomas Jefferson), artists (Van Gogh and Monet), musicians (Debussy and Mahler), philosophers (Nietzsche), and writers (Cervantes and Lewis Carroll[G]). Migraine is characterized by headaches, often throbbing in character, that may be generalized or confined to one side of the head, are sometimes associated with nausea and vomiting, and may be worsened by light, sound, or even certain smells. They may last for several hours or more. They are sometimes preceded (*auras*) or accompanied by transient disturbances of brain function (causing, for example, limb weakness, language abnormalities, or pins-and-needles in an extremity) resulting from constriction of blood vessels to discrete parts of the brain. Visual disturbances are especially common and may consist of areas of temporary visual loss; of luminous visual hallucinations such as stars, sparks, unformed light flashes, or geometric patterns; or of some combination of these phenomena.

Accounts of migraine exist in Babylonian writings from 3000 BC. Hippocrates clearly described migraines and attributed them to vapors ascending to the head from the stomach; they were relieved, or so he thought, by vomiting. He described the visual symptoms sometimes occurring in migraine and the occasional association between headache and exercise or sexual intercourse. To Plato, by contrast, the head pain related to excessive absorption or preoccupation with the body. Galen's descriptive term "hemicrania" evolved slowly into "migraine," the current designation.[30] In medieval Europe, treatments for headache included drug-soaked poultices applied to the head and the local application of vinegar and opium solution, the vinegar being used to facilitate the absorption of the opium through the scalp. In the seventeenth century, Thomas Willis (see footnote C, p. 68) came to believe that migraine was caused by vasodilatation, and Erasmus Darwin (the grandfather of Charles Darwin) some years later proposed treatment by spinning the patient around in a centrifuge, so that blood passed from the head to the feet.

In the middle of the nineteenth century, Du Bois-Reymond (see footnote D, p. 69), a migraineur, noticed that his face became pale, the pupil small, and his eye bloodshot during an attack, whereas immediately after one his ear was reddened and hot on the affected side. He thus related migraine to sympathetic overactivity leading to a vasoconstriction of the blood vessels of the face

---

[G] It is likely that some of Alice's adventures in Wonderland were based on the visual distortions and misperceptions constituting the aura of Carroll's migrainous attacks.

and head. His paper, translated and published[31] in 1861 in the French-language journal (p. 97) that Brown-Séquard had founded and edited, led to a speedy response from the editor,[32] who felt it unlikely that contraction of blood-vessel walls could account for the pain of migraine. He pointed out that stimulation of sympathetic fibers does not cause pain in animals and that a reddened eye and small pupil suggest impairment rather than overactivity of sympathetic fibers. Indeed, in his experience, patients with migraine showed signs of reduced rather than increased sympathetic activity, with local vascular dilatation. In 1868, Edward Woakes (1837–1912), a British surgeon, introduced ergot, a chemical known to constrict the blood vessels (for example, of the uterus and thus used to control postpartum hemorrhage) for the treatment of migraine.[33] Subsequently, migraine came to be attributed to initial sympathetic overactivity, with narrowing of the intracranial blood vessels causing premonitory symptoms or auras such as visual complaints, followed by underactivity causing distension of the blood vessels and pounding headache.[34] Ergot, in the form of ergotamine and related compounds, continues to be used for migraine, although other effective agents have now been developed; it has complicated and mixed pharmacological actions but its most conspicuous effect is a vasoconstrictive one.

The basis of migraine remains uncertain. The vasomotor theory relating headache to the dilatation of blood vessels, and the preceding aura to vasoconstriction, is fine as far as it goes but presumably reflects instability in central neurovascular control mechanisms. It seems likely that certain structures within the brain are activated inappropriately, perhaps as a result of faulty sensory processing within the part of the brain—the brainstem—that innervates the face and neck through the so-called cranial nerves. Genetic and environmental factors also are clearly important in the genesis of the disorder.

The discovery of the vasomotor nerves and reflexes was important in suggesting how the functions of the organism are integrated into a cohesive unit. It led to suggestions about the pathogenesis of such disorders as bed sores and migraine that were of immediate clinical relevance. The young Brown-Séquard was much influenced in his conception of several other neurological disorders by the discovery of vasomotor nerves, as is exemplified by his approach to the pathophysiology of epilepsy (Chapter 11) and of paraplegia (p. 272). In addition, the observation that a disturbance of one part of the nervous system can affect the function of other parts of the nervous system and of distant parts of the body by influencing the local blood supply led to his later belief (Chapter 10) that one part of the brain can influence the function of other parts more directly by exciting or inhibiting them. This view—with its assumption that different parts of the nervous system integrate the various excitatory and inhibitory inputs that they receive and that this determines their behavior—is now widely accepted as a result of the elegant experimental work of Charles Sherrington, a later Nobel laureate.

References and Source Notes

1. Foster M. *Claude Bernard*. London: Fisher Unwin, 1899.
2. Olmsted JMD, Olmsted EH. *Claude Bernard and the experimental method in medicine*. New York: Schuman, 1952.
3. Tarshis J. *Claude Bernard: Father of experimental medicine*. New York: Dial Press, 1968.
4. Stilling B. *Physiologisch-pathologische und medicinisch-praktische Untersuchungen über die Spinal-Irritation*. Leipzig: Wigand, 1840.
5. Foster M. *Claude Bernard* (pp. 100–134). London: Fisher Unwin, 1899.
6. Bernard C. Influence du grand sympathique sur la sensibilité et sur la calorification. *C R Soc Biol (Paris)*, 3:163–164, 1851.
7. Bernard C. De l'influence du système nerveux grand sympathique sur la chaleur animale. *C R Acad Sci*, 34:472–475, 1852.
8. Hermann H. A propos d'un centenaire. Comment se fit la découverte des nerfs vasomoteurs. *Biol Med*, 41:201–230, 1952.
9. Laporte Y. Brown-Séquard and the discovery of the vasoconstrictor nerves. *J Hist Neurosci*, 5:21–25, 1996.
10. Brown-Séquard E. Researches on the influence of the nervous system upon the functions of organic life. *Med Exam (Philadelphia)*, 8:486–497, 1852. [*Experimental researches applied to physiology and pathology* (pp. 6–17). New York: Baillière, 1853.]
11. Bernard C. Recherches expérimentales sur le grand sympathique et spécialement sur l'influence que la section de ce nerfe exerce sur la chaleur animale. *Mem Soc Biol (Paris)*, 5:77–107, 1853.
12. Brown-Séquard CE. Note sur la découverte de quelques-uns des effets de la galvanisation du nerf grand sympathique au cou. *Gaz Med (3rd Series)*, 9:22–23 and 54–55, 1854.
13. Magendie F. Prix de physiologie expérimentale. *C R Acad Sci*, 38:193–195, 1854.
14. Bernard C. De l'influence du système nerveux grand sympathique sur la chaleur animale. *Gaz Med (3rd Series)*, 7:227–228, 1852.
15. Brown-Séquard E. On the increase of animal heat, after injuries of the nervous system. *Med Exam (Philadelphia)*, 9:137–141, 1853. [*Experimental researches applied to physiology and pathology* (pp. 73–77). New York: Baillière, 1853.]
16. Bernard C. De l'influence de deux ordres des nerfs qui déterminent les variations de couleur du sang veineux dans les organes glandulaires. *C R Acad Sci*, 47:245–253, 1858.
17. Brown-Séquard CE. *Course of lectures on the physiology and pathology of the central nervous system delivered at the Royal College of Physicians of England in May, 1858* (pp. 149, 172–173). Philadelphia: Collins, 1860.
18. Hilton SM, Lewis GP. The mechanism of the functional hyperaemia in the submandibular salivary gland. *J Physiol (Lond)*, 129:253–271, 1955.
19. Tholozan JD, Brown-Séquard CE. Recherches expérimentales sur quelques-uns des effets du froid sur l'homme. *J Physiol (Paris)*, 1:497–505, 1858.
20. Brown-Séquard E. On the influence exerted upon the general temperature of the body by a change in the temperature of one of the extremities. *Med Exam (Philadelphia)*, 8:556–559, 1852. [*Experimental researches applied to physiology and pathology* (pp. 32–35). New York: Baillière, 1853.]

21. Rowling JT. Pathological changes in mummies. *Proc R Soc Med*, 54:409–415, 1961.
22. Brown-Séquard E. Researches on the influence of the nervous system upon the functions of organic life (p. 16). In: *Experimental researches applied to physiology and pathology*. New York: Bailliere, 1853.
23. Paget J. Clinical lectures on bedsores. *Students J Hosp Gaz*, 10:144–146, 1873.
24. Brown-Séquard CE. *Course of lectures on the physiology and pathology of the central nervous system delivered at the Royal College of Physicians of England in May, 1858* (p. 176). Philadelphia: Collins, 1860.
25. Brown-Séquard CE. *Course of lectures on the physiology and pathology of the central nervous system delivered at the Royal College of Physicians of England in May, 1858* (p. 260). Philadelphia: Collins, 1860.
26. Mitchell SW. *Injuries of nerves and their consequences* (p. 263). Philadelphia: Lippincott, 1872.
27. Munro D. Care of the back following spinal-cord injuries: a consideration of bed sores. *N Engl J Med*, 223:391–398, 1940.
28. Charcot JM. *Lectures on the diseases of the nervous system delivered at La Salpêtrière* (pp. 87–89; translated by G. Sigerson). London: New Sydenham Society, 1877.
29. Levine JM. Historical perspective on pressure ulcers: the decubitus ominosus of Jean-Martin Charcot. *J Am Geriatr Soc*, 53:1248–1251, 2005.
30. Rapoport A, Edmeads J. Migraine: the evolution of our knowledge. *Arch Neurol*, 57:1221–1223, 2000.
31. Du Bois-Reymond E. De l'hémicranie ou migraine. *J Physiol (Paris)*, 4:130–137, 1861.
32. Brown-Séquard CE. Remarques sur le travail précédent. *J Physiol (Paris)*, 4:137–139, 1861.
33. Koehler PJ, Isler H. The early use of ergotamine in migraine. Edward Woakes' report of 1868, its theoretical and practical background and its international reception. *Cephalalgia*, 22:686–691, 2002.
34. Latham PW. *On nervous or sick head-ache—Its varieties and treatment*. Cambridge: Deighton, Bell, 1873.

6

Fame in the Making

BROWN-SÉQUARD LEFT Mauritius, where he had gone to relax after his battle concerning the vasomotor nerves, toward the end of 1854, this time for the New World and Virginia. As he observed of the country to which he was moving, "It is not permitted to be poor ... it is so easy with a little intelligence and energy not to be poor that I understand the blame that falls on those who do not make their fortune."[1] But it is unlikely that this explains his destination, for he was disinterested in—contemptuous of—the material benefits of his chosen profession. Why then did he choose to move to the apparent obscurity of Richmond, Virginia? The reason is hard to understand. He was a hero of the Mauritius cholera epidemic, an acclaimed scientist, and someone at home in the capital city of the French empire and in many of the leading centers of learning in the United States. Coming from a country where slavery had been abolished, with a mother who had befriended former slaves and worked as a seamstress, and as a believer in social justice and reform, he must have wondered about the style of life in the rural, declining state to which he traveled, with its paternalism and ready exploitation of those living at the margin of society. Perhaps he simply wished to return to his wife's homeland—but there were more attractive cities for a physician-scientist than Richmond, at least in the mid-nineteenth century. As a medical student in Paris, he would have assimilated the European belief that a marker of a successful career is appointment to an old and established hospital or medical school. But he was going not to an appointment at a prestigious academic center but to the newly created Medical College of Virginia in Richmond. He may have believed that he was more likely to get his way or whatever he wanted at a new institution but—if so—he was soon to be disappointed.

A medical school had been established in Richmond at Hampden-Sidney College some years earlier, and it fostered a close inter-relationship between teaching and patient care—hospital patients, laboratories, and lecture theaters, for example, were all accommodated in the same building. In 1853, however, a problem had developed with regard to the selection of a professor in the Institutes of Medicine [Physiology] and Medical Jurisprudence. Several physicians in Richmond approached a member of the Hampden-Sidney Board on behalf of one candidate, but the faculty insisted that it was their right to nominate their own colleagues and unsuccessfully proposed another. The ensuing dispute was finally referred to the state legislature and culminated in the granting of a charter to create a new medical college in February 1854.

Brown-Séquard had met several influential members of the Richmond medical establishment at the 1852 meeting of the American Medical Association. In May 1854, he was elected from among seven candidates to the new chair by eleven votes to two on the first ballot; the two dissenters immediately transferred their votes to make the final decision unanimous. The president of the board immediately wrote to him:

> At a meeting of the Board of Visitors of the "Medical College of Virginia," held at this city on the 26th instant, you were appointed to fill the chair of the vacant professorship of "Physiology and Medical Jurisprudence."
>
> The high estimate with which the Board have been impressed of your eminent attainments in medical science, and especially in those branches of it, which you are called on to teach in this institution, overcame all considerations of local pride and personal preference in tendering this Chair to you, although a stranger and a foreigner.
>
> As the organ of the Board, and in compliance with their resolution unanimously adopted, I announce to you your appointment and request that you will accept the office.[2]

It was a surprising choice because, at that time, most American professors were content simply with teaching generally accepted facts, rather than undertaking creative investigative work or teaching the importance of an experimental approach to their students. From the point of view of the college, it was perhaps a way of gaining immediate visibility in academic circles and of attracting new blood to the young institution. Commenting on the appointment, which Brown-Séquard was quick to accept, an editorial in the *Virginia Medical and Surgical Journal* indicated:

> In the great field of experimental physiology, M. Séquard and his celebrated co-labourer and rival, M. Claude Bernard, have gained equal reputation. M. Bernard, in reward for his investigations, has recently been appointed to the new chair of general physiology in the Faculty of Sciences at Paris. What more fitting compliment could we pay Dr. Séquard, American as he is on the maternal side (sic), and desirous of giving to this country the fruits of his future researches, than to select him for this position in our own College ....[3]

Some were angered by the appointment of an overseas candidate,[4] but the editor of the *Journal* responded tartly, "We are striving to build up a great College in Virginia, not to make fat offices to put our friends in. We look around for the best man to fill a professorship, and we take him, whoever he is."[5] Broca wrote from Paris to colleagues in America on learning of the appointment:

> Your young and great nation throws aside the prejudices which oppress old Europe. The narrow questions of nationality and boundary occupy you much less than the true merits of the man. How long will it be before we dare to follow your example? ... M. Séquard himself, is he not an instance of what I have said? ... he is not a Frenchman, and although educated in Paris, and speaking the language like one of us; although acknowledged to be possessed of eminent talent; yet he has been unable to attain any official position, only because he was a foreigner.[5]

Life in Richmond, Virginia

The new professor took up his position in the autumn of 1854, but his stay in Richmond was brief. The college authorities failed to provide him with laboratory animals for his demonstrations or for experimental purposes, apparently because of an administrative oversight, and his students therefore were sent to look for dogs, cats, and other suitable animals, which had to be kept in the college cellar, where their cries disrupted lectures during the day and sleep at night. The townspeople found it difficult to reconcile these goings-on with their belief in the college as a center of culture and learning, and began to regard it as a place possessed of the devil.[6]

The authorities became equally disenchanted with their new professor.[6] His renown failed to attract new students, faculty, or patients to their institution.

The students found it well-nigh impossible to follow some of his lectures because his English was accented and limited, with idiosyncratic turns of phrase, and the subject matter was pitched at a level well beyond their expectations. A former student, recalling his lectures, commented that "his agony in trying to make himself comprehended was, if anything, greater than ours in trying to comprehend him."[6] The lectures themselves were enlivened by experimental demonstrations on animals of points of especial importance that were often more entertaining than instructive, as when he implanted a dog's tail in the comb of a rooster and somehow managed to make it take root and grow[6]; the luckless rooster was unfortunately attacked by another, which promptly tore off the useless appendage. Such experiments have about them a certain exotic fascination—morbid or otherwise—but the reasons for undertaking them were never made clear. Perhaps they related to his work on the perfusion of fresh blood into severed animal tissues to maintain their viability, thereby allowing the reattachment of the tissues to their owner, as discussed in a later chapter. Brown-Séquard also had difficulty in fitting in with local society, for he lacked the charm and courtesy of the South, could be blunt to the point of rudeness, disliked inconveniencing himself for social reasons, and was interested only in his work. He disapproved of slavery and expressed himself so frankly on the subject that a malicious rumor eventually circulated that, with his dark complexion and foreign background, he himself was of black origin.

His experimental studies on himself led to gossip, excitement, or dismay. On one occasion, while attempting to determine the function of the skin, he covered himself from head to toe with varnish and was found unconscious on the floor in the animal room by a quick-witted student who saved his life by removing the varnish with alcohol or—some say—with sandpaper. He continued his early studies of digestion by swallowing sponges attached to a string, then withdrawing them at intervals for analysis. The belching and regurgitation that resulted made him a somewhat disagreeable dining companion. Nevertheless, Brown-Séquard did make influential friends in Virginia. Dr. McCaw, later dean of the college and editor of the *Confederate States Medical Journal* (the only medical journal published under the Confederacy) wrote, "... simple-minded and guileless, he was truth itself as far as he saw it. His most affectionate nature made dear friends wherever he was."[7] Still, his unhappiness was readily apparent to Ellen, who wrote to a friend: "... [I] keep up his spirits which sometimes are low enough here. There is no sympathy and little politeness shown him. I wish we had remained in the Mauritius ...."[8]

Bored, disillusioned, and missing the intellectual excitement of his life in Paris, Brown-Séquard submitted his resignation at the end of his first term, and this was formally accepted on 30 March 1855. His reaction was typical, and was repeated at many other institutions in later years—rather than working through the issues, he simply packed up and left. In spite of his shortcomings as a lecturer, his students were disappointed to see him go, for to them he was caring, well-meaning, brilliant, and a strong-minded eccentric who had fired their imagination. In any event, after attending the May meeting of the American Medical Association and spending a short time in New York, Brown-Séquard set sail for France once more.

Setting the Record Straight About the Sensory Pathways

Back in France, his work on the route taken by sensory pathways within the spinal cord (discussed in Chapters 3 and 4) continued to meet with opposition, conflicting as it did with the prevailing view of the time. The Société de Biologie therefore established an independent committee, at Brown-Séquard's request, to examine the issue. Paul Broca was appointed chairman of the committee, which included Claude Bernard and Edmé-Félix Alfred Vulpian[A], as well as several other medical scientists (Bouley, Giraldès, and Goubaux).[B] The selection of Broca was fortunate because he was not only an admirer of Brown-Séquard but at one time had been tutored by the same Martin-Magron who had introduced Brown-Séquard to the laboratory and collaborated with him in his early studies on reflexes. The committee not only reviewed the original account of the work, but repeated certain experiments. Its report, in July 1855, supported unequivocally the conclusions reached by Brown-Séquard:

> The doctrine [that sensory fibers travel in the posterior half of the cord, and the motor fibers in the anterior half], so seductive and widely accepted, is only one more deception ... whose debris is scattered on the grounds of history.

[A] Edmé-Félix Alfred Vulpian (1826–1887), French neurologist and scientist, became a professor and then dean of the Faculty of Medicine at the University of Paris. In addition to his work on the adrenal glands, discussed later in this chapter, Vulpian demonstrated that curare caused paralysis by affecting a point between nerve and muscle (the so-called neuromuscular junction). He was a friend of Brown-Séquard and later co-founded a journal with him, as indicated in Chapter 9.

[B] Henri Bouley (1814–1885), a founder-member of the Société de Biologie and later president of the Académie des Sciences, was interested in the scientific aspects of veterinary medicine, as also was Armand-Charles Goubaux (1819–1890). Joaquim Albino Cardoso Casado Giraldès (1808–1875), born in Portugal, was a learned Parisian surgeon and anatomist, some of whose work was published in Brown-Séquard's first journal, and after whom is named a vestigial structure found in the testis.

> The beautiful experiments of M. Brown-Séquard have just brought down forever this well-cemented edifice, the foundation of which was laid by Charles Bell and the last stone by M. Longet. It is indeed true that appearances are often misleading .... For a long time, as you know, our colleague has studied without a break the functions of the cord, and six years ago he communicated to you his first work on the subject .... But minds were so biased in favor of the doctrine of Charles Bell that the first work of M. Brown-Séquard was received with a certain disbelief and received only passing attention ....[9]

Thus, the committee confirmed Brown-Séquard's conclusions that the posterior columns of the cord are not the main or sole pathway taken by sensory fibers ascending to the brain. Curiously, although it studied the effects of sectioning the various columns of the spinal cord, sometimes at different levels, the committee did not investigate the effect of a lateral hemisection of the cord. The omission is surprising, because Brown-Séquard had not only challenged doctrines that were widely believed at the time, but had also shown that, by making hemisections at different levels of the spinal cord, certain sensory fibers crossed from one side of the cord to the other. The report of the committee did refer, however, to the extraordinary surgical skill of Brown-Séquard, for autopsy confirmed the unexpected precision with which his lesions were made, so that he had cut "... not one fiber too few, not one molecule too many ...." In any event, Broca subsequently wrote of the committee's report that

> [It] had produced quite a commotion in the scientific world .... This revolution ought to have taken place five years ago, but Brown was then ... unknown, awkward in his speaking and writing, and with the only merit of simply being the foremost physiologist of our time .... A conspiracy of silence was organized around him, and the unfortunate fellow, without bread or support, was forced to leave France and find a living in America. Two months ago he returned with some savings. I found this nonsense had gone too far and that it was time to stop it. When Brown came back to the Société de Biologie to speak about his experiments, I started a vigorous campaign for him, which has occupied the Society during several meetings. The president ... had to make up his mind and pursue the matter by appointing a committee. And so I made my report—not for the physiologists who would have liked to shelve it—but for the general medical public, who is indifferent to scientific information only when such is not available. Public opinion has spoken in favor of Brown. All of a sudden he is as important as he deserves to be; it is even being said that the Institut will have to give him the grand prix for physiology.[10]

The description that Brown-Séquard had provided on the effects of cord hemisection and on the sensory pathways within the spinal cord thus gained wide acceptance after 1855, and the clinical consequences of such lesions came to be designated the *Brown-Séquard syndrome*. The syndrome—of weakness or paralysis of the limb below and on the side of the hemisection and of impaired pain and temperature appreciation on the opposite side—is known to all medical students and anatomists, if only because it seems to be explained so beautifully by the now-known pathways within the spinal cord of the descending motor and ascending sensory fibers. Nevertheless, certain medical authorities, such as Charcot (see Chapter 12), seemed almost disinterested in the basis of the clinical findings, dismissing them as imponderable and not even mentioning Brown-Séquard's name when discussing the experimental studies, including cord hemisections, that clarified the course of the sensory fibers in the spinal cord.[11] It seems likely that the formidable clinician came eventually to view as a rival the experimental neuroscientist with whom he also clashed on various other academic issues and that he seemed bent on denying him any credit for his scientific achievements (as discussed in Chapter 12).

Despite their general acceptance, certain of Brown-Séquard's findings remained difficult to explain, such as the heightened sensitivity (hyperesthesia) that occurred on the same side of the body below a lateral hemisection of the spinal cord. Most physiologists and clinicians, therefore, continue to ignore its occurrence while accepting the general principles to which his work had led. Similarly, the contralateral sensory loss that he found was more complete than is generally accepted, and the discrepancy was quietly neglected. In fact, however, his findings have been confirmed by others,[12] and cannot simply be cast aside. They are discussed further in Chapter 12.

Work, a Prize, and a Baby

Toward the end of 1855, James Paget—the British surgeon with whom he had corresponded previously over a patient—wrote to encourage Brown-Séquard to apply to the Royal Society for a grant to support his scientific work, and he took the opportunity to invite him to lecture in England, both in London and at Cambridge.[13] A friendship had developed between the two men, and several more letters passed between them before Brown-Séquard visited London. A close friendship had by now also developed between Brown-Séquard and Charles Robin. The two had been externs together on Trousseau's hospital service and were active in the Société de Biologie, and they organized a small private laboratory of their own in the rue Saint-Jacques in Paris, where they could accept students and pursue their own research interests. Among their students were some who subsequently became quite distinguished, including Carl Friedrich Otto Westphal (1833–1890), the German neuropsychiatrist who coined the term "agoraphobia" to describe the anxiety of some of his patients in open spaces, and who gave his name to a collection of nerve cells at the base of the brain (the Edinger-Westphal nucleus) that influences the function of one of the cranial nerves (the third cranial nerve, which is concerned with eye movements and the pupillary reflexes). Another was Johann Czermak (1828–1873), the Austrian physiologist who introduced the laryngoscope into clinical medicine.

In October 1855, François Magendie died. He had been the Professor of Medicine at the Collège de France for almost a quarter-century, for much of which Claude Bernard had been his assistant, collaborator, and deputy. Not surprisingly, Brown-Séquard applied for the vacant chair,[14,15] but the appointment went appropriately to Claude Bernard. Thus, the year that began with disappointment in Richmond ended with disappointment in Paris.

1856 was a happier year for Brown-Séquard, both professionally and domestically. In January, he was awarded the 1855 Montyon Prize in Experimental Physiology[C] by the Académie des Sciences for his work on the sensory pathways in the spinal cord.[16] The annual award was made on the recommendations of a committee that, ironically, was now chaired by Claude Bernard as successor to Magendie. Brown-Séquard had competed for the prize previously and, although unsuccessful, had received an honorable mention on one

---

[C] Antoine Jean Baptiste Robert Auget, Baron de Montyon (1733–1820), the French philanthropist, provided funds anonymously to various institutions and hospitals, including the Académie des Sciences, for various prizes, one of the earliest (1818) being for experimental physiology; his identity was revealed after his death. He also left the Académie a substantial legacy. The Académie gave these prizes in various subjects, with a subsidiary *récompense* for the runner-up, and an honorable mention for an especially commendable work that received no actual award. In the 1830s, the Montyon legacy was also used to support the cost to the Académie of publishing works such as its weekly proceedings (the *Comptes Rendus*). In the 1840s, the size of the main and subsidiary prizes was limited, and in some years the main prize was not awarded at all if the entries did not meet the expected standard. Over the following years, the Montyon legacy came also to be used to enhance the value of lesser prizes awarded by the Académie and to provide small grants supporting scientific research. Among the grantees was Brown-Séquard who, on March 22, 1858, received 1,500 francs for expenses. The legacy was subsequently used for a number of other general purposes, as described by Maurice Crosland (*Minerva*, 17:355–380, 1979). Montyon also gave funds for prizes to reward courageous acts of virtue by the poor, as determined by the Académie française. Despite his philanthropy, however, some accounts of Montyon are not flattering. A report in the *New York Times* of December 9, 1883, shows him to have been a calculating, mean man who would, for example, write to the superintendent of his farm, telling him how much hay he ought to take away from his horses when they were not at work.

occasion for his work on the function of the nervous system and on another for his studies on the sensory pathways, with the prize going then to Bernard himself.[17,18] On February 19 of this same year, Brown-Séquard's only son, Arthur Désiré Jules Charles Edouard (the several names conforming to French custom), was born in Paris.[19] To give Ellen an opportunity to show off the baby to her family, the latter half of 1856 saw Brown-Séquard back in America, giving a series of lectures on epilepsy in Boston that were published in the *Boston Medical and Surgical Journal*[20] and subsequently in book form.[D] He lectured also at the New York Academy of Medicine and, early in the New Year, in Baltimore and in Charleston to enthusiastic and appreciative audiences of physicians and students. Professionally, however, 1856 was particularly important as it was the year that Brown-Séquard published the results of his experimental work showing the adrenal glands to be essential to life, work that met with disbelief but was eventually substantiated by others and initiated the science of experimental endocrinology.

The Adrenal (Suprarenal) Glands

As Rolleston has described elsewhere,[21] the anatomy of the adrenal (suprarenal) glands was first described in the sixteenth century by Bartholomaeus Eustachius (ca. 1520–1574)[E] in Rome under the title of *glandulae renibus incumbentes* (glands on the kidneys). Casserius (1561–1616), who taught William Harvey in Padua, designated them *renes succenturiati* (secondary kidneys), and his successor Spigelius (1578–1625) referred to them as *capsuli renales*. The familiar term *suprarenal capsules* was introduced in 1629, by the French anatomist Jean Riolan (ca. 1580–1657), who regarded these structures as functionally active originally in fetal life, perhaps because of their relatively larger size in the fetus. Caspar Bartholinus "the elder" (1585–1629), the Danish physician and theologian, called them the *capsulae atrabilariae* and believed that contained within a central cavity was a "humor" (black bile or atrabilia) that passed by communicating channels to the kidneys and was then excreted in the urine. These organs are now generally known as the adrenal glands; they lie in close relation to the kidneys and consist of two parts: an inner section (or medulla) and an outer portion (cortex) that have different functions. The medulla

---

[D] The *Boston Medical and Surgical Journal* later became the *New England Journal of Medicine*, one of the most influential medical journals in the world.

[E] Bartholomaeus Eustachius (ca. 1500–1574), Italian anatomist who clarified the anatomy of the ear, teeth, cranial nerves, and other bodily structures.

secretes norepinephrine (noradrenaline) and epinephrine (adrenaline) at times of stress (see p. 67), whereas the cortex secretes various corticosteroids including aldosterone, which is involved in regulation of salt and water balance (and is thus termed a *mineralocorticoid*); glucocorticoids such as cortisol, which regulate fat, carbohydrate, and protein metabolism, modulate various cardiovascular and behavioral functions, and affect the immune system's inflammatory response; and certain so-called sex steroids, which influence the reproductive system and gender-related activities. The adrenal glands are *endocrine* glands; that is, they secrete their products directly into the blood rather than through a duct. It was only in 1905 that Ernest Starling introduced the term *hormone* for the secretions of the endocrine glands.[22] The name was apparently suggested to him by a classicist, W.T. Vesey (an authority on Pindar, the Greek poet), over dinner with the biologist William Hardy (who is sometimes mistakenly credited for the suggestion) at Gonville and Caius College, Cambridge, and is derived from the Greek word "to excite."[23]

The function of the adrenal glands remained unknown for more than three hundred years after these structures were described by Eustachius. A common view in the eighteenth century was that, during fetal life, the adrenal glands served to accumulate urine or to divert blood from the kidneys. In 1841, Magendie included them as structures without a known function. Then, in 1849, Thomas Addison (1793–1860) described several patients with adrenal destruction in a presentation before the South London Medical Society and, in 1855, he published his famous monograph, *The Constitutional and Local Effects of Disease of the Supra-renal Capsules*.[24] In this work, he described the occurrence of anemia, ease of fatigue, malaise, weakness, a bronze discoloration of the skin, and "remarkable feebleness of the heart's action," associated with apparent disease (usually tuberculosis) of the adrenal glands in eleven cases that came to autopsy. Other symptoms include weight loss, diminished appetite, nausea, low blood pressure, low blood sugar, muscle aches, irritability, and depression.[F] The monograph made reference to three of his colleagues, each of whom had contributed to the subject matter of his monograph and were so illustrious that they also have diseases named after them: Richard Bright,[G]

[F] President John Kennedy is said to have had Addison's disease.
[G] Richard Bright (1789–1858), British physician who worked at Guy's Hospital in London, focusing his studies on kidney disease and noting its association with swelling of the ankles and the presence of protein in the urine. Bright's disease was until recently a common term for disease of the kidneys. He also wrote a well-known medical textbook with Addison (although most of the work was done by Addison) and was appointed Physician Extraordinary to Queen Victoria.

Thomas Hodgkin,[H] and Sir William Gull.[I] Of these great physicians, Addison himself was perhaps the most celebrated. Born in the north of England, the son of a grocer, he was a shy, remote, and unhappy man, but a remarkable clinician whose name is also associated with a type of anemia that he described (now called pernicious anemia), as well as with disease of the adrenal glands. Sadly, he suffered bouts of severe depression and, in 1860, took his own life.

Addison's clinical account of the disease that now bears his name (i.e., of insufficiency or failure of the adrenal glands) led Brown-Séquard to investigate the functions of the adrenal glands. In August 1856, he reported to the Académie des Sciences in Paris that excision of both glands in cats, dogs, guinea pigs, and rabbits led invariably and rapidly (within a day or so) to weakness and a fatal outcome, indicating that these glands were essential to life.[25] Although death sometimes followed removal of just one of the adrenal glands after a longer interval, Brown-Séquard believed—and subsequently showed—that survival was possible in such circumstances.[26] However, animals then died rapidly after the later removal of the second adrenal gland. Brown-Séquard emphasized that death was not due to hemorrhage, peritonitis, or damage to organs adjacent to the adrenal glands.[25] The animals developed profound lassitude, loss of appetite, and increasing weakness until, shortly before death, they lost the use of first the hind limbs, then the forelimbs, and lapsed into coma. The heart and respiratory rates increased but then became more feeble, and the body temperature declined. Convulsions sometimes occurred.[25] He did not observe any pigmentation but assumed this was because of the short interval between removal of the glands and death. Transfusion of blood from a normal animal allowed animals to survive for a period after the adrenals had been removed.[25]

[H] Thomas Hodgkin (1798–1866), one of the "great" British physicians at Guy's Hospital, remembered for the cancerous disease of the lymph glands—Hodgkin's disease, a malignancy—named after him. A radical, Hodgkin encouraged the education of working-class men, was a founding member of the Senate of the University of London, and was concerned about the degradation of indigenous peoples by colonists. His arrival at Guy's in a carriage "with a half naked native American" is said to have caused much consternation among the hospital authorities and may have prevented him from receiving a permanent clinical appointment there. He accompanied Moses Montefiore, a wealthy philanthropist, patient, and friend, on a visit to Palestine, where he died of dysentery.

[I] Sir William Gull (1816–1890), outstanding clinician on the staff at Guy's Hospital, remembered for his seminal descriptions of hypothyroidism (the consequences of an underactive thyroid gland) and anorexia nervosa. He is said by some to have been a suspect in the notorious and unsolved Jack-the-Ripper murders in the east end of London (other suspects have included a member of the British royal family).

The belief that the adrenal glands were essential to life was challenged immediately by many other investigators, such as Philippeaux, Gratiolet, George Harley, and Moritz Schiff (see p. 244), who published seemingly conflicting findings in which certain animals survived for months (but ignored the fact that others did not) despite the removal of both adrenal glands.[27] Even Brown-Séquard's old tutor, Martin-Magron, opposed his views.[27] Thus, Philippeaux showed that white rats survived the operation,[28,29] to which Brown-Séquard countered by suggesting that the functions of the adrenal glands must have been taken over by other glands.[26] Philippeaux then proceeded to remove other organs from his unfortunate rats, but they still failed to succumb:[30] (In fact, their survival was later explained by the presence of accessory or additional adrenal glands.) The speed with which Brown-Séquard's animals died suggested to some that infection or other secondary effects of the surgery (such as damage to adjacent nerves and blood vessels) may have been responsible, despite his assertions to the contrary. Brown-Séquard, in turn, pointed out that the duration of survival after removal of the two adrenal glands depended on the age and species of the animals being studied, and on whether the two glands were removed simultaneously or at different times.[31] In addition, in a systematic study, he operated on rabbits as if to remove their adrenal glands but without actually doing so, examining instead the effects of deliberately induced peritonitis, and of damage to the kidneys, liver, renal veins, and inferior vena cava.[32] The time course of subsequent survival was quite different (being considerably longer) than in animals undergoing removal of both adrenal glands, even when all these other structures were damaged during the same operative procedure, thus supporting his original contention. Later work using strictly aseptic techniques confirmed the view that the glands were indeed essential to life. It was subsequently shown by others (such as Tizzoni, Abelous and Langlois, de Domenicis, and Cybulski)[27,33] that the original opinion of Brown-Séquard was correct; various animals died after complete removal of both adrenals. The interval before death varied, as Brown-Séquard had noted, from a few hours to several weeks.

The functions performed by the adrenal glands were unclear. Brown-Séquard initially believed that these glands removed a toxic chemical from the blood, but later, in an 1869 course of lectures at the Paris Faculty of Medicine, he suggested instead that the "glands have internal secretions and furnish to the blood useful if not essential principles" that act at sites distant to that of their manufacture.[34]

In 1856, Vulpian (see footnote A, p. 85) concluded that the medulla synthesized a substance that was related to its function.[35] He applied a solution of ferric chloride to slices of the adrenal glands and noted that the medulla—but not the cortex—stained green; the same reaction occurred with samples of blood leaving the adrenal, but not with blood entering it. Some years later, in 1893, George Oliver (1841–1915), a British physician practicing in Harrowgate, observed that adrenal extracts from sheep and calves, prepared from material supplied by his local butcher, caused a marked narrowing of the arteries (he did not have a device to measure the blood pressure but measured the caliber of the radial artery at the wrist with a special device) when his son took some of the extracts by mouth. He went with his adrenal extract to Edward Schäfer (1850–1935), professor of physiology at University College London, and is said to have found him measuring the blood pressure of an anesthetized dog. Schäfer was incredulous about Oliver's claim, but nevertheless injected some of the extract into the dog's veins. To Schafer's astonishment, the blood pressure increased dramatically. Subsequent studies by Oliver and Schäfer[36] led eventually to the first isolation of a hormone (epinephrine or adrenaline) from the adrenal medulla and confirmed that the function of the adrenals was not to detoxify the blood but to secrete chemical agents into it. However, it was only in the twentieth century that Addison's disease was found to result from deficiency of hormones secreted by the adrenal cortex, and treatment came to consist of taking hormones to replace those normally made by the adrenal glands.

As for Brown-Séquard, after 1858, he turned his attention to other topics but his studies on the adrenal glands remain an important milestone, marking the initiation of modern experimental endocrinology. They also exemplify the importance to the advance of medicine of clinician-scientists who can grasp the significance of clinical phenomena (such as the unusual disease and pathological findings described by Addison) and turn to the laboratory to gain fresh insight into their basis.

References and Source Notes

1. Brown-Séquard CE. Autobiographic details provided in a letter dated 17 December 1852 and addressed to Lady Blanche [Ellen Fletcher], who was to become his first wife. MS 977/1. Archives, Royal College of Physicians, London.
2. Newspaper article from Mauritius (source not indicated), announcing Brown-Séquard's appointment to the Medical College of Virginia and reproducing the letter addressed to him by J.M. Patton, 1854. MS 1000/161. Archives, Royal College of Physicians, London.
3. Editorial and Miscellaneous. *Virg Med Surg J,* 3:173–175, 1854.
4. Haag HB. Charles Edouard Brown-Séquard: his Richmond sojourn. *Virg Med Monthly,* 86:311–313, 1959.
5. Editorial and Miscellaneous. *Virg Med Surg J,* 3:276–278, 1854.
6. Taylor WH. Old days at the old college. *Old Dominion J Med Surg,* 17:57–100, 1913.
7. Ott I. Dr. Brown-Séquard. *Med Bull,* 18:361–366, 1896.
8. Brown-Séquard, Ellen (née Fletcher). Letter to a friend dated 17 March 1855. MS 999/6 (27–28). Archives, Royal College of Physicians, London.

9. Broca P. Rapport sur les expériences de M. Brown-Séquard relatives aux propriétés et aux fonctions de la moelle épinère. *C R Soc Biol (Paris)*, 7:23–50, 1855.
10. Schiller F. *Paul Broca*. Berkeley: University of California Press, 1979.
11. Charcot JM. *Lectures on the pathological anatomy of the nervous system: diseases of the spinal cord*. (pp. 88–89; translated by Comegys CG). Cincinnati: Thomson, 1881.
12. Denny-Brown D. The enigma of crossed sensory loss with cord hemisection. In: Bonica JJ, Liebeskind JC, Albe-Fessard DG, eds., *Advances in pain research and therapy*. (Vol. 3, pp. 889–895). New York: Raven Press, 1979.
13. Paget J. Letter to Brown-Séquard dated 14 December 1855. MS 981/74. Archives, Royal College of Physicians, London.
14. Brown-Séquard E. Letter to the Director, Collège de France, dated 17 November 1855. MS G-IV-C, 32B. Archives, Collège de France, Paris.
15. Brown-Séquard E. Indication des principaux travaux originaux du Dr. E. Brown-Séquard. [Document submitted by Brown-Séquard in support of his candidacy for the vacant Chair of Medicine at the Collège de France, 1855.] MS G-IV-C, 32C. Archives, Collège de France, Paris.
16. Bernard C. Rapport sur le concours pour le Prix de Physiologie Expérimentale de l'année 1855. *C R Acad Sci*, 42:137–141, 1856.
17. Magendie F. Rapport de la commission chargée de décerner les Prix de Physiologie Expérimentale pour les années 1847 et 1848. *C R Acad Sci*, 30:209–210, 1850.
18. Magendie F. Prix de Physiologie Expérimentale. Rapport sur les prix de l'année 1851. *C R Acad Sci*, 34:418–419, 1852.
19. Birth certificate issued by the Mairie du XIe Arrondissement and dated 21 February 1856. MS 987/2. Archives, Royal College of Physicians, London.
20. Brown-Séquard E. Experimental and clinical researches applied to physiology and pathology. *Boston Med Surg J* 55:337–342, 377–380, 421–427, 457–461, 1856; and 56:54–58, 112–115, 155–158, 174–176, 216–220, 271–278, 338–340, 433–437, 473–478, 1857.
21. Rolleston HD. *The endocrine organs in health and disease with an historical overview* (pp. 301–358). London: Oxford University Press, 1936.
22. Starling EH. The Croonian lectures on the chemical correlation of the functions of the body. *Lancet*, 166:339–341, 1905.
23. Henderson J. Ernest Starling and 'hormones': an historical commentary. *J Endocrinol*, 184:5–10, 2005.
24. Addison T. *On the constitutional and local effects of disease of the supra-renal capsules*. London: Highley, 1855.
25. Brown-Séquard E. Recherches expérimentales sur la physiologie et la pathologie des capsules surrénales. *C R Acad Sci*, 43:422–425, 1856.
26. Brown-Séquard E. Nouvelles recherches sur les capsules surrénales. *C R Acad Sci*, 44:246–248, 1857.
27. Vincent S. *Internal secretion and the ductless glands* (pp. 134–142). London, Arnold, 1912.
28. Philipeaux JM. Note sur l'extirpation des capsules surrénales chez les rats albinos (*Mus ratus*). *C R Acad Sci*, 43:904–906, 1856.
29. Philipeaux JM. Sur l'extirpation des capsules surrénales chez les rats albinos. *C R Acad Sci*, 43:1155–1156, 1856.
30. Philipeaux JM. Ablation successive des capsules surrénales, de la rate et des corps thyroides sur des animaux qui survivent à l'opération. *C R Acad Sci*, 44:396–398, 1857.
31. Brown-Séquard E. Nouvelles recherches sur l'importance des fonctions des capsules surrénales. *C R Acad Sci*, 45:1036–1039, 1857.
32. Brown-Séquard E. Recherches expérimentales sur la physiologie des capsules surrénales. *C R Acad Sci*, 43:542–546, 1856.

33. Anonymous. Progress of medical science: Experiments on the supra-renal capsule. *Med Record*, 26:545, 1884.
34. Major RH. Charles Edouard Brown-Séquard. In: *Essays in biology in honor of Herbert M. Evans* (pp. 371–377). Berkeley, University of California Press, 1943.
35. Vulpian A. Note sur quelques réactions propres à la substance des capsules surrénales. *C R Acad Sci,* 43:663–665, 1856.
36. Oliver G, Schäfer EA. The physiological effects of extracts of the suprarenal capsules. *J Physiol,* 18:230–276, 1895.

7

Fame and Fortune in Britain

A Piece of Cake

IN 1856, THE Académie des Sciences awarded Brown-Séquard one thousand francs for his experimental work on epilepsy,[1] described in Chapter 11, and shortly thereafter the Montyon Prize in Experimental Physiology for work on the irrigation of tissues with arterial blood (Chapter 14).[2] The Montyon Prize in experimental physiology had been created in 1818 and provided formal recognition of the field by the Académie; in the nineteenth century, it was one of the most prestigious prizes open to medical scientists. Toward the end of 1857, Brown-Séquard returned to New York to lecture, but he did not take up an academic position there despite claims to the contrary.[3]

In 1858, he started his own French-language periodical—the *Journal de la Physiologie de l'Homme et des Animaux*—which he dedicated to Biot, Rayer, Flourens, and James Paget. He had recognized the importance to his career and reputation of keeping his name in print, and he ensured this by the succession of books, articles, and notes that he authored, as well as by taking on the responsibility of editing a journal. He also used his journal to support the work of colleagues and others in whose work he believed. When his friend Broca developed certain controversial theories concerning the definition and significances of animal species, theories that were a potential source of embarrassment and a possible cause for a clash with the authorities, Brown-Séquard published the work in several articles in his journal.[4] Unfortunately, however, the work involved in editing a journal and supervising its production proved too demanding and, even though he enlisted the assistance of several colleagues (including Martin-Magron, Broca, and Robin) and of his wife, the sixth and final volume of the *Journal* appeared in 1865, two years later than its cover date.

Success in the United Kingdom

In May 1858, Brown-Séquard delivered a now-famous course of six lectures at the Royal College of Surgeons of England for a fee of fifty pounds. These were a remarkable blend of experimental and clinical observations, demonstrating the facility with which he could pass between the laboratory and the clinic, using knowledge gained from one to advance work in the other. For example, based upon both his studies in animals and the clinical cases seen by him or published by others, he was able to point out that the various sensory modalities (such as light touch, pain, hot, and cold) are mediated by separate nerve fibers. In his own words, "the various sensitive impressions—of touch, of pain, of temperature, of muscular contractions, etc. are transmitted by conductors which are quite distinct from one another, and so much so that the conductors of painful impressions for instance, are not more able to convey other kinds of impressions than to transmit the orders of the will to muscles."[5] He spoke on the physiology and pathology of the nervous system before the most eminent medical and scientific personalities of the day, and they received his commentary with excited approval. His audience[6] included Thomas Huxley (p. 138); William Gull (p. 91); R. Bentley Todd,[A] the greatest British neurologist of the period, whose name is still associated with the transient, localized weakness that may follow certain epileptic seizures; Lionel Smith Beale, Todd's pupil and disciple, a microscopist who was appointed to the chair of physiology at King's College London in preference to Huxley and subsequently to the chair of medicine at King's College Hospital, and who is sometimes described as the father of scientific medicine in England[7]; John Burdon Sanderson, the physician and physiologist who held chairs at University College London and then at Oxford and also did much to promote a scientific approach to medicine; and William Bowman, a friend and collaborator of

---

[A] R. Bentley Todd (1809–1860), clinician and medical educator who had a particular interest in the nervous system and began to distinguish different disorders affecting the spinal cord. He championed the view that effective treatment requires accurate diagnosis, a view that was not generally accepted at the time. Unfortunately, he was rather too fond of alcohol, which he took liberally himself and prescribed freely to his patients, and in consequence he is often caricatured as a drunk. He died young, of cirrhosis of the liver.

Todd's,[7] often regarded as the "father of general anatomy" in Britain, whose work on the structure of the eye, the kidney (recalled by the term Bowman's capsule), and the muscles has ensured his reputation. Notable for his absence, however, was James Paget, the friend of Brown-Séquard who had done so much to organize the lectures.[8] He had developed pneumonia a few days before they were to be delivered[9] and at one point it was feared that he would die; he finally rallied and, after convalescing by the sea, was able to take up his life again.

Brown-Séquard sold his lectures to a journal, *The Lancet*, for fifty pounds and the printer's blocks (valued at another thirty pounds),[10,11] and they were subsequently published in book form in the United States.[12] *The Lancet*, first published in October 1823 by Thomas Wakley, a physician, radical reformer, and member of parliament, reached out to medical and surgical practitioners and students. As was stated in the preface that appeared in the first issue of the journal,

> We are well aware that we shall be assailed by much *interested* [sic] opposition. But, notwithstanding this, we will fearlessly discharge our duty. We hope the age of "Mental Delusion" has passed and that mystery and concealment will no longer be encouraged.[13]

In reproducing Brown-Séquard's lectures,[14] *The Lancet* (in July) announced

> When we consider that what are denominated nervous diseases are still the opprobria of the profession, and afford opportunities to a class of quacks for plundering the public, we earnestly hope that these lectures will not be read for mere motives of curiosity, but that they will be studied with that degree of attention which their immense importance merits.[15]

While in London, Brown-Séquard lectured also at the Royal Society and at the ancient St. Bartholomew's Hospital (the oldest surviving hospital in London, being founded in 1123). He wrote to Ellen, who had remained in France, of his success in England, saying that he had spoken before the largest audience ever assembled at the College of Surgeons, and one that included "all the men of distinction in London." He added that the daily papers mentioned him, that Queen Victoria enquired about him, and that he had never before enjoyed such acclaim.[11] "It is said everywhere that there is no example of such a success as mine. From all quarters the most flattering compliments. I hear that the question has been agitated yesterday to create a chair for me with large emoluments. I do not know where: they have not been willing to tell me ...."[11]

Nevertheless, despite his success, he remained worried about money and repeatedly calculated his likely earnings to determine whether they would cover their expenses.[16] He shared his monetary concerns with Ellen, not in a constructive way but as if by causing her disquiet he somehow lessened his own ruminations and foreboding. His letters also reveal troubling swings between despondency and anxiety on the one hand and elation on the other. He was preoccupied with his own health,[16] referring constantly to his chronic fatigue, frequent headaches, and troublesome heartburn, but he rarely asked after hers. He sent an unending stream of instructions concerning his journal and publications, as well as petulant complaints about her perceived minor failings and petty irritations. He was jealous about her closeness to their son Edouard and instructed Ellen to "show him my likeness and speak of me to him, as frequently as you can."[17] Several months later, he felt the need to add "I do not like Monsieur Edouard not to mind more than he seems to do the absence of his father .... He will [get] no cakes if he does not care about me."[18]

During his stay in London in that spring of 1858, the possibility was raised of his securing a Chair of Physiology at Oxford, with a starting annual salary of about five hundred pounds (then twenty-five hundred American dollars),[19,20] to Ellen's seeming dismay. He responded to her: "Your objections about Oxford are not insurmountable .... Now as to the future I will certainly have any chair I choose in the United States and we shall go and live at home after three, four, or five years passed at Oxford—Oxford is a relay—and an agreeable one which gives the certitude of arriving safe at home. Our child will be an American: there is no fear about that."[21] In any event, the chair in England never materialized.

While in London, in 1858, he met the leaders of the Scottish medical establishment and made plans to lecture there. He also met with Mr. Wakley, the founding editor of *The Lancet*, who offered him the annual sum of five hundred pounds if he would become a subeditor of the journal, with plenty of time set aside for his own clinical and scientific works.[22] According to Paget, the object was to have Brown-Séquard's name on the cover of the journal to give it scientific respectability.[23] The expectations of him were opaque, and they were not clarified over the following months. If the promised salary were for scientific papers and reviews of books, Brown-Séquard wrote in April 1859, he would probably accept it, but if he were expected to write editorials he determined to decline.[24] The details of any subsequent discussions are unknown, but there is no record that he ever accepted Wakley's offer.

In any event, flushed with success and armed with further invitations to the British Isles, he returned to Paris in June. It was not until April 1859 that he began a series of twelve lectures in Edinburgh and Glasgow before large and enthusiastic audiences.[25] They went well, and he enjoyed his visit despite grumbling that he would have "to submit to many dinner and supper parties, which are not agreeable things to me."[26] The Scots were "kind, polite, and gay as possible" and as such "differ[ed] from New Englanders in many respects."[26] Whether his American wife ever came to share this view is unclear. After completing his lectures, Brown-Séquard returned to London, and then to France, but not for long. In mid-May he arrived in Dublin for a ten-day visit to lecture on a variety of neurological topics including paraplegia (weakness of both legs),[25] epilepsy, galvanism (electrical stimulation), the spinal cord, vasomotor nerves, and the effects of stimulating the auditory nerve, and the course was warmly received by an audience that increased in number and importance with each lecture.

The lectures that he gave in Edinburgh, Glasgow, and Dublin focused in part on disorders of the spinal cord, and he summarized his views on weakness of the lower limbs in a monograph that he published in 1861.[25] In these lectures, Brown-Séquard described the clinical changes in various disorders of the spinal cord, including myelitis (inflammatory disorders), tumors, hematomas (collections of blood either within or adjacent to the cord), and meningitis. He discussed various clinical features such as flexor spasms, paraspinal rigidity (i.e., stiffness or spasm of the muscles adjacent to the backbone or vertebral column), sensory disturbances, trophic changes, reflex erections of the penis, and disturbances in the control of the bladder and bowels, and he examined their value in differential diagnosis. (Trophic changes are changes that occur in the skin, blood vessels, bones, muscles, or other tissues because of loss of their nerve supply; for example, the skin may become thinned, shiny, or discolored, the muscles wasted or atrophied, and the tissues swollen.) He did not mention the tendon reflexes, that is, the reflex contraction of a muscle when it or its tendon is stretched. These are the reflexes that are tested when a physician taps various places on the arms and legs with a small rubber-tipped hammer, thereby stretching the tendons of selected muscles; evaluation of these did not become a routine part of the neurological examination until some twenty years later. He did, however, refer to the reflex movements elicited, for example, by touching the soles of the feet, and by any "irritation" of the rectum by fecal matter, the bladder by urine, or the urethra by a catheter.

In his 1859 lectures, Brown-Séquard documented the clinical evidence in support of the entity of "reflex paraplegia," a speculative but widely held diagnosis in the early nineteenth century, but one that has since fallen into disrepute.[27] In brief, it was a designation for weakness or paralysis of the legs occurring in relation to disease of various organs (such as the uterus, urethra, bladder, prostate, kidneys, bowels, or lungs) or to a variety of other circumstances, in none of which there was any evidence of direct involvement of the spinal cord. Brown-Séquard believed that a reflex constriction affected the blood vessels to the spinal cord, and perhaps also those to the nerves or muscles. In discussing this disorder,[27] he recalled many of his illustrious predecessors and peers who had published cases exemplifying it and in which the cord was normal at autopsy. Unlike cases with direct involvement of the spinal cord by disease, there was usually little or no pain, sensory disturbance, sphincter dysfunction, or muscle atrophy. In many instances, the cause of the neurological deficit was probably psychogenic: there were no objective neurological signs other than weakness, and recovery occurred rapidly after cure of the primary condition, regardless of its nature.[27] Why did Brown-Séquard uphold the existence of an entity lacking any convincing scientific foundation, even though it was widely accepted at the time? Perhaps it appealed to him because it brought together his views on the importance of reflex actions and on the control of the blood vessels by the nervous system (see Chapters 5 and 14).

His success in London, Scotland, and Ireland encouraged Brown-Séquard to look at the possibility of a more permanent appointment in Britain, although he remained active in the academic environment of Paris. He was one of the first of a few physicians and scientists to rally around Broca in his attempts over some two years to establish a new learned society that would integrate a variety of disciplines concerned with the human subject.[28-30] Such an organization was viewed with suspicion as possibly subversive by the authorities,[29] but in May 1859, the Société d'Anthropologie was finally established with Brown-Séquard as a founder-member, Martin-Magron (his old mentor) as its first president, and Broca as secretary.[30]

Queen Square and the National Hospital for the Paralysed and Epileptic

London in the middle of the nineteenth century was a city in transition, the center of a culture of commerce and empire, and—like Paris—a place that nurtured new ideas and scientific advances. More and more people were crowding in to find work, living in the dingy rooms and tenements that made up the dreary slums or suburbs of the metropolis, away from the majestic center of empire. The grandeur of Regent Street, Piccadilly Circus, Trafalgar Square, and Oxford Circus, and the more muted elegance of Belgravia and Mayfair were havens for the affluent or well-born and signs of the prosperity of the period. Nevertheless, much of the city smelled of soot, sewage, dirt, and decay, and crime was common despite the "bobbies" patrolling the streets. The port of London was thriving, but the Thames—its commercial aorta—was clogged with sewage as well as ships. Queen Victoria had taken up residence in Buckingham Palace, the first British monarch to do so; the Great Exhibition of 1851, in the Crystal Palace, had been a sensation; and—by 1859—Big Ben had made its appearance over parliament, the nation's debating house, and India had come under the direct rule of London. The capital was connected to other parts of the country by railroads, but the metropolitan underground railway system that was to connect different parts of the city had yet to be built; the first leg, from Paddington to Farringdon Road, was completed in 1863.

The city had many beautiful squares. Set in the Bloomsbury region of London, Queen Square had first been set out in 1716 and was named after Queen Anne, whose son—the delicate Duke of Gloucester—lived there.[31] The church of St. George the Martyr, at the south end of the square, dates from 1706. Other buildings facing the square housed the high-born and the wealthy. Elihu Yale—who made his fortune, some say corruptly, while with the East India Company in Madras (Chennai) and gave goods and part of his library to the institution that was to become Yale University—reportedly lived close by, at least for a period. The building that is No. 1 Queen Square dates from 1710 and was once a beer shop. King George III is supposed to have stayed nearby to see his doctor, and his wife Charlotte rented a cellar beneath the beer shop to store food for him; the pub now located there is still known as The Queen's Larder. Originally, the north end of the square was undeveloped, with unobstructed views of the Highgate and Hampstead hills but, by the middle of the nineteenth century, new building put an end to this panorama, and various hospitals came to be located in the square, as did the St. John's Nursing Services established by Florence Nightingale.[B] Robert Louis Stevenson famously described it as

> a little enclosure of tall trees and comely old brick houses, easy enough to see into over a railing at one end but not very easy to enter for all that, unless the visitor has profound knowledge or the instincts of an arctic explorer. It seems to have been set apart for the humanities of life and the alleviation of all hard destinies. As you go around it, you read upon every second door-plate, some offer of help to the afflicted. There are hospitals for sick children where you may see a little white-faced convalescent on the balcony talking to his brothers

---

[B] Florence Nightingale (1820–1910), pioneer in nursing, accomplished writer, and applied statistician, earned the designation "the Lady with the Lamp" from the wounded during the Crimean War for her remarkable achievements when she worked among them as a nurse. She reformed hospital care and initiated sanitation reforms that led to markedly reduced death rates.

and sisters and the baby, who are below there, on a visit to him and obstruct your passage not unpleasantly ....[31,32]

The center of the square had been placed in the care of the residents by an Act of Parliament, and a handsome statue of Queen Charlotte—wife of King George III—dominated the northern portion of its gardens. It was in this square that a new hospital was established in 1860, for the care of the paralyzed and epileptic.

In addition to poor-law hospitals and charity-supported general hospitals, some with affiliated medical schools, more than sixty specialist hospitals existed in London in the late 1850s. This in itself is surprising as, during much of the Victorian era, specialized hospitals were regarded with suspicion by many authorities, including the editors of *The Lancet*, because many had been established with the sole object of furthering the welfare of their founder-physicians. The specialist hospitals already in existence in the capital at mid-century included those for "consumption" (tuberculosis) and diseases of the chest; for fistulas and other diseases of the rectum; for stones and disorders of the urinary organs; for diseases of the bones and joints; for disease of the heart, skin, eyes, ears, and teeth; for venereal diseases, smallpox, and cancer; and for "lying-in" (childbirth). There were hospitals for the nationals of foreign countries such as the French and Germans, and later the Italians; hospitals for women, sick children, abandoned children (foundlings), lunatics, merchant seamen, and soldiers who were chronically ill or retired; and even hospitals for those practicing special forms of medicine, such as homeopathy. But there were few facilities in the metropolis for the care of the neurologically disabled, who had to manage as best they could or languish in long-stay poor-law hospitals and asylums for the insane. Then a middle-aged spinster—Miss Johanna Chandler—was inspired to take matters into her own hands[31-33] after her beloved aging grandmother was paralyzed by a stroke. Once she realized the paucity of support for those with special needs because of infirmity, she resolved to devote her life to help them. Together with her sister Louisa, she began to collect money from the sale of trinkets and small ornaments to provide facilities for the disabled. Progress was slow until they were able to interest the Lord Mayor of London, Alderman David Wire, who had himself recently developed weakness down one side of the body[33] and, indeed, was to die shortly thereafter. At a meeting held in the Mansion House in November 1859, it was decided to establish a new hospital specializing in the care of neurological illness. A Committee of Management was formed with the Lord Mayor as chairman and Edward Chandler, Johanna's brother, as secretary, and public subscriptions amounting to some 800 pounds were received.[32]

Although the Chandler sisters wanted to establish an institution to care for the chronically disabled, Wire wished instead to avoid creating simply another board-and-care facility. Instead, he preferred the new hospital to be a center for active treatment, and among the original resolutions set down by the founders it was noted that

> Indoor patients will be, exclusively, those persons whose cases do not appear to be incurable. For these a probationary period of residence in the hospital will be granted; but if at the expiration thereof, or earlier if such persons shall be considered incurable, they will be removed in order to make room for others whose cases may be more hopeful. The persons so removed will still be eligible to become outdoor patients.[32]

A Board of Management, consisting mainly of business men, was established, with Wire as its first chairman, to serve as the governing body of what became known as the National Hospital for the Relief and Cure of the Paralyzed and Epileptic (now the National Hospital for Neurology and Neurosurgery).

Suitable premises had to be found in London for the new institution. Early in 1860, an empty house was rented at 24 Queen Square for 110 pounds annually, its size permitting accommodation for eight inpatients. The front and back parlors of the house were converted into a consulting (examining) room and waiting room for outpatients, and the butler's pantry became the dispensary. Later in the spring, the new hospital opened, and patients were admitted at once. Perhaps surprisingly, a second institution, the London Galvanic Hospital, was founded in 1861 by Harry Lobb (about whom little is known). Located in Cavendish Square, it was dedicated to "the treatment, with the aid of Electricity, of all forms of Nervous and Muscular Diseases, for which this force is particularly adapted."[34] *The Lancet* articulated its unequivocal disapproval with some asperity:

> One gentleman, as though the whole range of diseases had been exhausted, founds an hospital which he conducts for carrying on a special form of treatment; not a new method, certainly not a universal method, but one which is well understood by the profession; which has been the subject of innumerable essays, papers, and books; and which is practised within its proper limits at all our hospitals. This institution is denominated the Galvanic Hospital and is conducted by Mr. Harry Lobb. Next may come a Quinine Hospital, an Hospital for Treatment by Cod-liver Oil, by the Hypophosphites, or by the Excrement of Boa-Constrictors.[35]

It seems that the hospital did not flourish, and little was subsequently heard of it despite the attraction it held for certain of the aristocracy. Yet another hospital, The London Infirmary for Epilepsy and Paralysis,[36] was opened in the 1860s close to Harley Street, in the medical heartland of London. It did well, moving to larger premises next to Regent's Park after a few years and subsequently changing its name to the Hospital for Diseases of the Nervous System to distinguish it from the National Hospital.[C] The impetus to develop this new—third—hospital for neurological diseases came from an émigré from Germany, Julius Althaus, a physician of the brain and an electrotherapist (i.e., a believer in the use of electricity for the management of certain disorders of the nervous system and muscles).[D]

Despite the competition and the antispecialist fervor of much of the establishment, the new neurological institution at Queen Square soon aroused the interest of the medical profession, and certain physicians sought a position on its staff. Indeed, one well-respected medical man was apparently prepared to pay 1,000 pounds for an appointment.[37] Fortunately, the Board of Management insisted that appointments be made solely on the basis of medical ability and scientific expertise, realizing that the hospital would be concerned with the treatment of patients with obscure and poorly understood disorders.

Among the first appointments made to the National Hospital were John Zachariah Laurence, a philanthropist, linguist, and surgeon whose name is memorialized in the mysterious Laurence-Moon-Biedl syndrome, a hereditary disorder that is characterized by obesity, pigmentary changes in the retina, mental retardation, polydactyly (the presence of extra fingers or toes), and hypogonadism. Jabez Spence Ramskill—a friend of the Chandlers with an interest in epilepsy—was appointed a physician, but he is little known today. The other founder-physician to be appointed was Brown-Séquard. James Paget wrote personally to Alderman Wire on his behalf almost as soon as he heard of the proposed hospital, in early December 1859: "You are probably already aware that it is the intention of Dr. Brown-Séquard to offer himself as a candidate for the office of physician .... I beg you to let me assure you that I know nothing by which, so much as by the election of Brown-Séquard, you could promote the best object of the proposed hospital, surely the advancement of the knowledge of the diseases for the relief of which it is designed. If the

---

[C] The hospital eventually moved again, this time to Maida Vale. The Maida Vale Hospital amalgamated with the National in 1948 and closed in 1983, its patients being transferred to the Queen Square site.

[D] Julius Althaus (1833–1900), was born and educated in Germany and spent time in Paris, Berlin, and other European centers before emigrating to England. In addition to his instrumental role in the founding in London of what was to become the Maida Vale Hospital, he wrote on a variety of medical topics including a popular *Treatise on Medical Electricity* and the well-known *On Failure of Brain Power*.

medical profession *everywhere* [emphasis in original] could be polled to return the man most suited for this object I have, no doubt whatsoever, that Brown-Séquard would be elected by a great majority."[38] Wire replied that he fully intended to vote for him but that it would make things easier and also unanimous if Brown-Séquard would make formal application for the post.[38]

Brown-Séquard, now in his forty-third year, then wrote from Paris to apply for the position on the staff.[39] He listed his qualifications and the various organizations to which he belonged including, among others, the Faculty of Physicians and Surgeons of Glasgow; the Société Philomathique, Société d'Anthropologie, and Société de Biologie of Paris; the American Philosophical Society and the Academy of Natural Sciences of Philadelphia; and the Royal Society of Arts and Sciences of Mauritius. He also made mention of five prizes or awards he had received from the Académie des Sciences in Paris, two small awards (part of the grant of the Queen for the advancement of science) in 1856 and 1857 from the Royal Society of London, and the gold medal he had received in Mauritius for his work during the 1854 cholera epidemic. He went on to summarize his various publications, and recalled the course of six lectures delivered at the Royal College of Surgeons of England in 1858 and the many other lectures he had given in England, Scotland, Ireland, Paris, and North America.

Supporting letters were sent by many men of distinction who had heard his lectures and met him in various contexts. The Physician-in-Ordinary to the Queen in Ireland and the Regius Professor of Medicine at Dublin University wrote jointly to indicate that "Dr. Brown-Sequard is not only a scientific investigator of the first class, but is, to our knowledge, a most judicious and sound physician …." and that "the appointment of this distinguished physician to an hospital for the treatment of diseases of the nervous system would have an important effect in improving the knowledge and the treatment of those affections."[40] From Glasgow, several professors, lecturers, and physicians, including the president of the Faculty of Physicians and Surgeons of Glasgow, expressed their conviction that "the permanent settlement of Dr. Brown-Séquard in this country would be a valuable and important acquisition to British medical and physiological science,"[41] and stressed that his recent lectures had embraced not only physiological topics but also their pathological and clinical applications. Their counterparts in Edinburgh made a similar point and wrote also of the remarkable originality of his views and their high esteem for him "both as a man of science and as a gentleman."[42] They went on, "… the acquisition of Dr. Brown-Séquard for this country … will greatly tend to advance the study of physiology, and to make more accurate the knowledge of nervous disease and pathology in general, as well as to improve the treatment of a large and important class of diseases." A number of eminent medical men signed this testimonial, including Joseph Lister (who introduced antiseptic techniques into operative practice) and John Struthers (after whom is named a ligament in the elbow). Dr. Laurence, the ophthalmologist who himself was to be appointed as surgeon to the staff, similarly emphasized to Alderman Wire the outstanding qualities of Brown-Séquard, adding that as a British subject he was not eligible to receive an appointment in the Paris hospitals.[43] Many other letters were received on behalf of Brown-Séquard's candidacy, including one from Henry Bence Jones,[44] the noted physician, chemist, and biographer (of Michael Faraday, whose lectures he had attended at the Royal Institution), whose name remains familiar to succeeding generations of medical practitioners because of the "Bence Jones protein" that he discovered in the urine of a patient with myelomatosis (a cancer of certain cells in the bone marrow) in 1848.

Struthers wrote also to Brown-Séquard himself that, "As the brilliancy of your fame in physiology might throw into comparative shade your claims as a practical physician, I wish to say particularly how assured I am of your unsurpassed claims on that ground also. I knew how much your writings had tended to elucidate disease, but I had no idea until I heard those excellent lectures which you delivered here last summer, that you could throw so much light on the subjects of epilepsy and paralysis—diseases which hitherto have either been treated at random or confessed as hopeless .... I may add that I have met you at the bedside, and have noticed the very careful manner in which you examine and treat disease .... I trust we will be able to secure your permanent settlement among us. I only wish it was Edinburgh rather than London for our own sake here, and we will quite envy London the possession of one so famous."[45] James Paget similarly wrote to him that an appointment to the new hospital would be an "excellent occasion for your starting to practice in London."[46]

The hospital records indicate that on 29 December 1859, Brown-Séquard was elected to the hospital staff,[37,47] and a telegram was immediately sent to him in Paris informing him of his appointment.[48] It was not until the new year, however, that Brown-Séquard acknowledged the news of his appointment in a letter from Paris to Mr. George Reid, now secretary to the hospital, and wrote to Alderman Wire to express his thanks.[37,47] He had been distracted, he indicated, by "distressing circumstances over the last ten days" that related almost certainly to the birth of a daughter, named Charlotte after his mother. She died when only 7 weeks old at the end of February, and is buried in Paris, in the cemetery where he too was later buried.[49]

The appointment to the hospital was unpaid, as was then customary. The staff engaged in private practice, and only visited the hospital on certain days and for emergencies. Brown-Séquard himself built up a large private practice during his stay in London over the next four years and continued his teaching role both at the hospital, where he gave clinical lectures every Monday afternoon, and elsewhere.

It is at this time that he was reputed to have been one of the first to use bromides as a treatment for epilepsy and advised his students to prescribe treatment for at least twelve to fifteen months after the last attack and to continue it through any concurrent illnesses,[50] an approach that is still followed today.[E] An enterprising pharmacist in New York is said to have made a fortune when he made up in hogsheads a copy of a prescription given by Brown-Séquard to an epileptic outpatient at the hospital, and advertised it as Brown-Séquard's specific for epilepsy, presumably because his name was so widely recognized among the medical fraternity and general public. In fact, although he may have been among the first to use it for this purpose, bromides were actually introduced as a treatment for seizures in the 1850s, by Sir Charles Locock, Queen Victoria's physician-accoucheur. Locock originally used it to treat women with what he termed "hysterical epilepsy," but which in most instances was probably epilepsy occurring in relation to the menstrual period. He believed it calmed their "sexual excitement," which was held to be a contributory factor in their epilepsy. As masturbation (and its associated excitement) was widely regarded as one of the causes of seizures at the time, the drug came into more general use to control seizures, continuing to be used for this purpose until the advent of phenobarbital in 1912 and phenytoin in 1937. Radcliffe, who was to succeed Brown-Séquard at the National Hospital, and Sir Samuel Wilks, an eminent physician at Guy's Hospital, also deserve much of the credit for ensuring that bromides had a place in the treatment of epilepsy.[51–53] Perhaps it was because of episodes such as this—in which his name was attached to therapies or cures for which he himself claimed no priority—that among the records at the National Hospital is a minute from June 1860 of a note read by Dr. Ramskill on behalf of Brown-Séquard to the effect that "the names of the Physicians shall not be published nor allusion made to their cures in future advertisements."[47]

Although renown for his scientific expertise, Brown-Séquard was, among his generation, one of the most outstanding and rigorous of clinicians specializing in disorders of the nervous system. He was meticulous in obtaining a

---

[E] Patients typically continue on antiseizure medication until they have been free of attacks for at least one or two years, depending on the circumstances. It is important that they continue with their medication during any intercurrent illness over this time, as such illnesses may precipitate further seizures.

complete history of his patients' complaints, enquiring after seemingly irrelevant or petty details in the belief that they could provide fresh insight into the disease process or a guide to the individual diagnosis and prognosis. He remained in close contact with his patients, even when he was away on his travels, sometimes writing to them several times over a few days to clarify the course of events or offer advice and guidance, and even sending lists of questions in order to amplify the information available to him from the initial consultation.[54]

Brown-Séquard's success as a medical practitioner in London was such that he was soon overwhelmed by the demands on his time of a busy clinical practice, and he eventually decided that he had to limit his activities if he were going to pursue his interest in physiology. Nevertheless, wherever he went, his opinions were sought after by the rich and powerful, and were given freely to all without regard to position or status. He stressed the importance of rehabilitation for neurological patients and pressed for the establishment at the hospital in Queen Square of a gymnasium for physical therapy and for apparatus to administer electrotherapy to patients. Such a department was eventually set up and came to be regarded as the finest in England.

As a clinician and clinical teacher, he was one of the earliest to stress the importance of studying the reflexes in evaluating patients with neurological disorders, although his immediate interest was in reflex disturbances of secretory, vascular, cardiac, and trophic functions, rather than the muscle stretch reflexes (or so-called tendon reflexes) that are now a standard part of the clinical examination, as explained earlier. His skill as a clinician is illustrated also by certain of his teachings that are now well established. Throughout his professional career, for example, he stressed the importance of quantifying the clinical findings, recognizing that this provides a more objective measure of functional status than simple descriptive terms and facilitates comparisons of the findings of different observers or those obtained at different times. As early as 1852, he wrote on a means of quantifying certain sensory deficits.[55] E.H. Weber[F] had found that if the two blunted points of a compass are applied simultaneously to the skin, either one or two points will be perceived depending upon the distance between the points and the region to which they are applied. Brown-Séquard suggested that this technique of determining the

---

[F] Ernst Heinrich Weber (1795–1878), German physiologist, studied the sensory responses to stimuli and published a classic monograph on the subject (*The Sense of Touch and the Common Sensibility*) that is considered by some to be the foundation of experimental psychology. Weber himself is regarded as the father of psychophysics; that is, the branch of psychology concerned with studying the relationship between physical stimuli and their psychological effects, especially the sensations that they elicit.

threshold for two-point discrimination could be used as a means of measuring the degree of touch sensitivity in disease states, stressing its value in determining the presence and extent of anesthesia or hyperesthesia, and in following the changes occurring over time.[55] He had clearly appreciated the need for quantitative clinical assessment of sensory function in patients with neurological disease, a need that remains to be satisfied several generations later (although computerized techniques are now available and in use at specialized centers). Similarly, he frequently made use of a dynamometer to record the power of muscles in the limbs. Such early attempts at precision in the emerging specialty of clinical neurology were important. The need is widely recognized today, and rating scales have been developed for many neurological phenomena (such as muscle power, the state of the stretch reflexes, and muscle tone, i.e., their stiffness or resistance to passive movement), as well as for level of disability and disease severity.

His approach to patients with neurological disorders embodied concepts that are now widely held but were not always received favorably. In the first place, he believed that symptoms do not necessarily result only from a loss in function of a part of the nervous system, but may relate instead to an overactivity or "irritation" of the affected region that produces abnormal motor activity or sensory phenomena. Second, he emphasized that the affected region of the brain may act upon some other, distant part, thereby producing a variety of additional symptoms and signs. Indeed, as early as 1861, he discussed the remote effects of focal cerebral lesions, initially attributing these to reflex actions. He wrote, "... when it is impossible to explain, by a loss of function of the part altered in the brain, the symptoms which are generated ... we are bound to acknowledge, at least, that there is some peculiar influence upon other parts of the encephalon starting from the inflamed part."[56] In time, however, Brown-Séquard came to believe that localized disease of the brain produced an "irritation" that spread to other parts of the brain, where it affected activity through excitatory or inhibitory processes. The direct sequelae of a focal lesion were thus consistent and predictable, whereas the indirect sequelae (remote effects) were more variable in their occurrence and severity. As he came to place increasing emphasis on the remote effects of cerebral lesions mediated through the processes of excitation and inhibition, he was led to believe that a relationship did not necessarily exist between them and the site and nature of the primary cerebral lesion. Such a view led him to a conclusion by the 1870s that seemed to remove any orderly framework from his approach to patients with neurological diseases, namely that a lesion located anywhere in the brain may produce any of the symptoms of cerebral disease.[57] The basis for and validity of this belief is considered further in Chapter 10.

Brown-Séquard also correctly stressed to his students and colleagues the utility of distinguishing between symptoms reflecting focal cerebral dysfunction and those resulting from more diffuse disturbances, recognizing at the same time that discretely localized pathology, such as a brain tumor, may have more widespread effects if, for example, it increases the pressure within the head. Among the symptoms of such diffuse disturbances he included "... vertigo, general cephalalgia [headache], delirium, loss of consciousness, diminution of intelligence going as far as idiocy, coma, trembling or irregular spasms of muscles [myoclonus, in modern terminology], general debility, vomiting, and slowness of pulse and of respiration. Local affections of the brain are generally characterized by the absence of most of the above symptoms and also by the fact that one side of the body is alone affected ...."[58] Such distinctions are still made today, and are known by all students of medicine.

In 1860, Brown-Séquard became a Fellow of the Royal College of Physicians of London which, incorporated by Royal Charter in 1518, is the oldest of English medical foundations. He was also elected a Fellow of the Royal Society of London. Among the names of his supporters on the nomination form for Fellowship of the Royal Society are those of Paget (to whom he had dedicated the *Journal de la Physiologie de l'Homme et des Animaux*, which he founded in 1858), James Arnott (President of the Royal College of Surgeons), Francis Sibson (physician, surgeon, author, and medical artist), and William Benjamin Carpenter (a physiologist and zoologist who was one of the first to emphasize that alcoholism is a disease and proposed a part of the brain known as the thalamus as the seat of consciousness).[47] Brown-Séquard's name appears in the Charter Book of Fellows' signatures in the same column as Joseph Lister[G] and Francis Galton.[H,47]

In 1861, he delivered the Croonian Lecture at the Royal Society, discussing the relationship between rigor mortis, putrefaction, and muscle activity prior to death. He reported his findings that in rested, cold, or paralyzed muscle,

---

[G] Joseph Lister (1827–1912), English surgeon, knighted by Queen Victoria, introduced antiseptic techniques into surgical practice and insisted that surgeons wear clean gloves and gowns and use instruments cleaned with antiseptics—this at a time that preceded wide acceptance of the germ theory of disease.

[H] Sir Francis Galton (1822–1911), English meteorologist, explorer, psychometrician, statistician, and promoter of eugenics, and a cousin of Charles Darwin. He devised modern techniques of weather mapping and was the first to describe anticyclones; he explored parts of Africa, provided a scientific system for classifying fingerprints that came to be used widely by police forces, and introduced or expanded many statistical concepts (such as of correlation and regression) and applied them to the analysis of biological phenomena. He was a pioneer in the use of identical twins to study the role of heredity and the environment ("nature and nurture") in development.

rigor mortis was delayed in onset but persisted for longer before the beginning of putrefaction compared to muscles that had been violently exercised prior to death.[59] This work so impressed John Stuart Mill, the philosopher of science, that in later editions of his *System of Logic* he used it to exemplify his four methods of experimental inquiry, and singled out Brown-Séquard's researches on the nervous system for further commentary and praise.[60] In 1861, Brown-Séquard also gave the prestigious Gulstonian Lectures at the Royal College of Physicians of London. The lectures were published in *The Lancet*, combined with clinical lectures he had delivered at The National Hospital, and summarized his views on the manner by which symptoms originate with cerebral disorders.[61] In particular, he emphasized that symptoms may result from loss of function of a region of the brain or from increased or abnormal cerebral activity, a concept that is now generally accepted but which, in 1861, provided a novel framework for understanding neurological disorders.

As Brown-Séquard's influence increased, his circle of acquaintances began to expand to include some of the leading intellectuals of the capital. Charles Darwin (1809–1882), for example, whom he first met in 1858 as a guest speaker at the Philosophical Club of the Royal Society,[1] wrote to him in the hope of a favorable review in France of his *Origin of Species*: "... I shall be truly glad to read any criticisms from one who stands so very high in one of the very highest branches of Science as you stand ...."[62] Darwin wrote again, "... I look with profound interest for the judgement of such men as yourself ...," perhaps because the views of Brown-Séquard were so close to his own.[63,J] A longer-lasting relationship developed between Brown-Séquard and T.H. Huxley (1825–1895), the apostle of Darwinism. Indeed, Huxley wrote to Darwin in 1862 that "I am very glad to hear about Brown Séquard; he is a thoroughly good man ...."[64]

Nevertheless, Brown-Séquard's social life was largely restricted to professional interaction with the leaders of the medical and scientific community, and he preferred not to waste time on the frivolities of city life or the formalities of

---

[1] The Philosophical Club of the Royal Society, a dining club, was founded in 1847, by certain fellows who believed that the society was not occupying its proper role in the country. The new club was intended to maintain the standards of the society, stimulate the intellectual activity of its members, and promote the influence of science in Britain. The rules limited the number of members and permitted no strangers, except "scientific foreigners temporarily visiting this country," to attend any of the club meetings. It merged with the larger Royal Society Club in 1901. For further information, see Bonney TG. *Annals of the Philosophical Club of the Royal Society written from its minute books*. London: Macmillan, 1919.

[J] Brown-Séquard intended to publish a review of Darwin's *Origin of Species* in his journal, but no such review appeared.

the drawing room, had no interest in entertaining, and had no wish to be associated with high society. He was awkward and charmless in most social gatherings, did not seem at ease with people, was uncomfortable at the dining table, and found distasteful such widespread habits as the use of tobacco. "I never smoke," he once said, "and have seen the most evident proofs of the injurious effects of tobacco on the nervous system."[65]

In May 1862, the hospital records first refer to a protégé of Brown-Séquard who was destined to become the father of modern British neurology, John Hughlings Jackson (1835–1911).[37] Brown-Séquard proposed that Jackson be elected an assistant physician, and this was indeed resolved "on the understanding that he should visit the Hospital twice a day and see the out-patients at their homes for which extra service he will be allowed the remuneration of fifty pounds per annum." Within a few years, the melancholy Jackson was made full physician, and he made major contributions over many years to the academic reputation of the hospital, with reports that have become some of the most treasured classics of neurology, providing descriptions and insight to the physiological underpinnings of various neurological phenomena. He was born in the country, found unsatisfying his early years in medicine, and thought of leaving the profession. Once in London, however, he met Brown-Séquard, although in unclear circumstances, and was persuaded not to waste his time on unfocussed observations of disease in general, but instead to keep to the nervous system.[66] Jackson remained in close contact with Brown-Séquard for perhaps three or four years, but he was deeply influenced by the older man.[67] He referred frequently to Brown-Séquard's work in his own writings over the years, and he followed Brown-Séquard in attempting to interpret clinical phenomenology in light of current scientific concepts.[67]

The hospital itself thrived. In 1863, the second floor of the building was converted into accommodation for ten more inpatients, and the outpatient area was also enlarged. In the following year, an adjoining house was purchased, thereby permitting the hospital to accommodate thirty-five beds.[32] Other innovations in its first decade included the establishment of day rooms that were attached to each ward and the employment of male nurses before other institutions in England.[33] Not all the neighbors were thrilled at these developments. When patients took to sitting in the Square just beyond the railings of his house, Lord Chief Justice Pollock threatened legal action against the hospital.[31]

Because the men appointed to the staff were generally outstanding, the hospital avoided much of the hostility directed at that time by the medical establishment toward new institutions serving special interests. Nevertheless, there were some delicate moments. Gordon Holmes, in an historical account of the hospital, recalls that when Samuel Wilberforce, Bishop of Oxford, came to dedicate its first extension, he had apparently been briefed inadequately and used the occasion to denounce all special hospitals, cursing the enterprise that he had been called in to bless.[32] This was the self-same Wilberforce who, in 1860, had crossed swords with Thomas Huxley at a famous Oxford debate on evolution.[K]

Brown-Séquard first lived at 82 Wimpole Street, then moved to a fine house in fashionable Cavendish Square, with a good-sized consulting room on the ground floor that looked out onto the plane trees in the square.[L] As success came to him, he found that his private practice was making increasing demands on his time. He thereupon refused to see patients without an appointment, and when this failed to lighten his load, he doubled his fees. This probably enhanced his eminence in the eyes of the lay-public, and he found his house besieged by anxious patients; a friend who visited him in Cavendish Square on one occasion found the large reception rooms filled with patients and their friends, and after a brief chat on the stairs, was asked to "come and have a talk over old times, but come at night for fear of the patients." Despite the privations of his early life, however, he refused to profit unduly from clinical practice. Thus, when offered the princely sum of one hundred guineas to consult on a patient in Liverpool, he responded that he would be there shortly on his way to New York and would then see the patient for his customary fee of five guineas.[68,69]

It is said that Brown-Séquard finally decided to leave London after looking from his consulting-room window to see a line of carriages belonging to his

---

[K] Samuel Wilberforce (1805–1873), son of William Wilberforce (politician and antislavery activist), English bishop, public speaker, and opponent of Darwinism, clashed heatedly with Thomas Huxley in that debate. Legend has it that Wilberforce asked of Huxley whether it was through his grandfather or grandmother that he claimed his descent from a monkey, to which Huxley responded that if he had to choose between being descended from an ape or from a man who would use his great powers of rhetoric to crush an argument, he would prefer the former rather than the shame of the latter.

[L] The house, 25 Cavendish Square, was taken over by Brown-Séquard's successor at the National Hospital, Dr. Charles Radliffe, and then, in 1892, by Sir Victor Horsley (1857–1916), the eminent neurosurgeon and physiologist who studied the function of the brain in animals and humans by electrical stimulation, was the first to remove a spinal tumor, was interested in thyroid function, and was responsible for many other surgical innovations, including an apparatus for stereotactic neurosurgery. He died of heatstroke in Mesopotamia during World War I. The house and those adjacent to it are no longer in existence, having been replaced by a large department store, and the character of the square has been changed by modern London's traffic.

fashionable patients filling the street outside. He had turned to medical practice only for reasons of financial expediency and felt that he was wasting his time on it rather than pursuing more scientific studies.[70] Furthermore, Ellen, in poor health for some time, was anxious to return to her native country, where Abraham Lincoln was overseeing the bitter campaigns of the Civil War to overthrow the seceding states of the Confederacy. The year 1863 was a momentous one in North America, ushered in by Lincoln's Emancipation Proclamation, declaring that all slaves in rebellious states or parts of states were free. It was the year that "Stonewall" Jackson, the brilliant but eccentric Confederate general, was mistakenly shot by his own men. His left arm had to be amputated, and General Robert E. Lee, his commander, is reputed to have sent a message saying "he has lost his left arm but I my right." Jackson died a few days later of a chest infection. The story spread rapidly in the South that a legion of angels had left Heaven to fetch him, but returned empty-handed; Jackson had outflanked them and was already there. The costly but important Union successes at Vicksburg and Gettysburg occurred also in 1863 and were turning points in the war, but they were followed soon after by riots in New York City against new laws passed by the Congress to draft men into military service.

It was at this time, then, that, Brown-Séquard's relationship with the National Hospital and with the development of neurology in England drew to a close. In a minute dated 15 July 1863—at the height of the violence in New York City, which resulted in several hundred deaths and enormous property damage—it was noted by the Committee of Management that he intended to give up practice in England and resign as a physician to the hospital and accordingly wished that a successor be named as soon as was convenient.[37]

Hughlings Jackson applied unsuccessfully for the vacant position, but the appointment went instead to Dr. Charles Bland Radcliffe (1822–1889), a provincial man noted more for abstract thought than any investigative work, although he did contribute to the literature on epilepsy, helped to establish the popularity of bromides as effective antiepileptic agents, and undertook experiments on the electrical properties of nerve and muscle. In addition to succeeding him on the hospital's staff, Radcliffe took over Brown-Séquard's house in Cavendish Square. He died of a "ruptured varicose vein." As for Brown-Séquard, he was elected an Honorary Physician to the hospital and stayed in contact with Hughlings Jackson[71] and other members of its staff over matters of common interest, as well as with the leaders of the British medical profession. According to *The Lancet,* there was much regret at his decision to leave London, where his success as a practitioner had been spectacular and where he had quickly acquired a large circle of admirers.

References and Source Notes

1. Cloquet J. Rapport sur le concours pour les Prix de Médecine et de Chirurgie pour l'année 1856. *C R Acad Sci*, 44:174, 1857.
2. Coste J. Rapport sur le concours pour le Prix de Physiologie Expérimentale pour l'année 1857. *C R Acad Sci*, 46:281, 1858.
3. Anonymous. Honors to science. *Boston Med Surg J*, 56:526, 1857.
4. Schiller F. *Paul Broca* (pp. 128–131). Berkeley: University of California Press, 1979.
5. Brown-Séquard CE. *Course of lectures on the physiology and pathology of the central nervous system* (p. 39). Philadelphia: Collins, 1860.
6. Brown-Séquard CE. Undated letter to a friend, providing biographical details. MS 994/2. Archives, Royal College of Physicians, London.
7. Cartwright FF. Robert Bentley Todd's contributions to medicine. *Proc R Soc Med*, 67:893–897, 1974.
8. Paget J. Letters to Brown-Séquard dated 29 March and 30 April 1858. MSS 981/76 and 981/77. Archives, Royal College of Physicians, London.
9. Brown-Séquard CE. Letters to his wife Ellen dated 8 May and 11 May 1858. MSS 977/11 and 977/12. Archives, Royal College of Physicians, London.
10. Contract between the Messrs. Wakeley and Dr. Brown-Séquard dated 3 June 1858. MS 984/3. Archives, Royal College of Physicians, London.
11. Brown-Séquard CE. Undated letter to his wife Ellen, probably written in May or June 1858. MS 977/24. Archives, Royal College of Physicians, London.
12. Brown-Séquard CE. *Course of lectures on the physiology and pathology of the central nervous system*. Philadelphia: Collins, 1860.
13. Anonymous. Preface. *Lancet*, 1:1–2, 1823.
14. Brown-Séquard E. Course of lectures on the physiology and pathology of the central nervous system: Delivered at the Royal College of Surgeons of England in May 1858. *Lancet*, 2:1–4, 27–31, 53–56, 109–112, 137–140, 165–168, 219–220, 245–247, 271–274, 295–297, 345–347, 367–369, 391–393, 415–416, 441–443, 467–468, 493–494, 519–520, 545–547, 571–573, 599–601, 625–626, 651–653, 1858.
15. Anonymous. Dr. Brown-Séquard's lectures. *Lancet*, 2:25, 1858.
16. Brown-Séquard CE. Correspondence with his wife Ellen, 1852–1864. MS 977/2–43. Archives, Royal College of Physicians, London.
17. Brown-Séquard CE. Letter to his wife Ellen dated 29 May 1858. MS 977/25. Archives, Royal College of Physicians, London.
18. Brown-Séquard CE. Letter to his wife Ellen dated 5 April 1859. MS 977/30. Archives, Royal College of Physicians, London.
19. Brown-Séquard CE. Letter to his wife Ellen dated 14 May 1858. MS 977/13. Archives, Royal College of Physicians, London.
20. Brown-Séquard CE. Letter to his wife Ellen, undated but probably May 1858. MS 977/15. Archives, Royal College of Physicians, London.
21. Brown-Séquard CE. Letter to his wife Ellen dated 17 May 1858. MS 977/17. Archives, Royal College of Physicians, London.
22. Brown-Séquard CE. Undated letter to his wife Ellen. MS 977/28. Archives, Royal College of Physicians, London.
23. Brown-Séquard CE. Undated letter to his wife Ellen. MS 977/27. Archives, Royal College of Physicians, London.
24. Brown-Séquard CE. Letter to his wife Ellen dated 10 April 1859. MS 977/34. Archives, Royal College of Physicians, London.
25. Brown-Séquard E. *Lectures on the diagnosis and treatment of the principal forms of paralysis of the lower extremities*. Philadelphia: Collins, 1861. [The substance of this book, in a

condensed form, was part of the course of lectures delivered by Brown-Séquard in April and May 1859, in Edinburgh, Glasgow, and Dublin.]

26. Brown-Séquard CE. Letter to his wife Ellen dated 3 April 1859. MS 977/29. Archives, Royal College of Physicians, London.
27. Brown-Séquard E. *Lectures on the diagnosis and treatment of the principal forms of paralysis of the lower extremities* (pp. 5–56). Philadelphia: Collins, 1861.
28. d'Échérac. Jubilé du cinquantenaire de la Société d'Anthropologie de Paris: 7 Juillet 1859–7 Juillet 1909. Discours. *Bull Soc d'Anthropol (5th Series)*, 10:299–301, 1909.
29. Schiller F. *Paul Broca* (pp. 131–135). Berkeley: University of California Press, 1979.
30. Broca P. Séance d'ouverture: 19 Mai 1859. *Bull Soc d'Anthropol*, 1:1–2, 1860.
31. The Chartered Society of Queen Square. *Queen Square and the National Hospital 1860–1960*. London: Edward Arnold, 1960.
32. Holmes G. *The National Hospital, Queen Square, 1860–1948*. Edinburgh: Livingstone, 1954.
33. Critchley M. The beginnings of the National Hospital, Queen Square (1859–1860). *Br Med J*, 1:1829–1837, 1960.
34. Advertisement for the London Galvanic Hospital. *Electrician*, 5: between pp. 120 and 121, 1863. Cited by Morus IR. The measure of man: technologizing the Victorian body. *Hist Sci*, 37:249–282, 1999.
35. Editorial. The march of specialism. *Lancet*, 81:183, 1863.
36. Bladin PF. Julius Althaus (1833–1900). Neurologist and cultural polymath; founder of Maida Vale Hospital. *J Clin Neurosci*, 15:495–501, 2008.
37. Gooddy W. Some aspects of the life of Dr. C.E. Brown-Séquard. *Proc R Soc Med*, 57: 189–192, 1964.
38. Paget J. Letter to Mr. Alderman Wire dated 10 December 1859. MS 988/8. Archives, Royal College of Physicians, London.
39. Brown-Séquard CE. Letter to the Governors of the Hospital for Paralysis and Epilepsy dated 1859, applying for the office of Physician. MS 988/1. Archives, Royal College of Physicians, London.
40. Letter of support (undated) for Brown-Séquard's application, signed by the Physician-in-Ordinary to the Queen in Ireland and the Regius Professor of Medicine in the University of Dublin. MS 988/2. Archives, Royal College of Physicians, London.
41. Letter of support for Brown-Séquard's application, dated 14 December 1859 and signed by senior members of the medical profession in Glasgow. MS 988/3. Archives, Royal College of Physicians, London.
42. Letter of support for Brown-Séquard's application, dated December 1859 and signed by a number of practitioners and teachers of medicine in Edinburgh. MS 988/4. Archives, Royal College of Physicians, London.
43. Laurence JZ. Letter to Mr. Alderman Wire dated 12 December 1859. MS 988/9. Archives, Royal College of Physicians, London.
44. Bence Jones H. Letter of support for Brown-Séquard's application, dated December 1859. MS 988/11. Archives, Royal College of Physicians, London.
45. Struthers J. Letter to Brown-Séquard dated 20 December 1859. MS 988/5. Archives, Royal College of Physicians, London.
46. Paget J. Letter to Brown-Séquard dated 11 December 1859. MS 981/78. Archives, Royal College of Physicians, London.
47. Gooddy W. Charles Edward Brown-Séquard. In: Clifford Rose F, Bynum WF, eds., *Historical aspects of the neurosciences* (pp. 371–378). New York: Raven Press, 1982.
48. Depêche Télégraphique, 29 December 1859. To Dr. Brown-Séquard. MS 988/13. Archives, Royal College of Physicians, London.

49. Tombstone of Charlotte Ellen Brown-Séquard, died 29 February 1860, aged 7 weeks and buried in the cemetery of Montparnasse, Paris.
50. Bowditch HP. Lecture notes taken at Harvard Medical School 1866–1867: Dr. Brown-Séquard. Harvard Medical Archives, CB 1869.9. Countway Library of Medicine, Boston.
51. Pearce JMS. Bromide, the first effective antiepileptic agent. *J Neurol Neurosurg Psychiatry*, 72:412, 2002.
52. Friedlander WJ. The rise and fall of bromide therapy in epilepsy. *Arch Neurol*, 57:1782–1785, 2000.
53. Pearce JMS. Sir Samuel Wilks (1824–1911): on epilepsy. *Eur Neurol*, 61:124–127, 2009.
54. Brown-Séquard CE. Letter of 27 November 1862 to an unnamed patient, with a list of questions concerning his symptoms and signs. MS 980/16. Archives, Royal College of Physicians, London. [Contained in the Archives are a number of other letters that passed between Brown-Séquard and his patients.]
55. Brown-Séquard E. On a means of measuring degrees of anaesthesia and hyperaesthesia. *Med Exam (Philadelphia)*, 8:503–504, 1852. [See also *Experimental researches applied to physiology and pathology* (pp. 23–24). New York: Bailliere, 1853. This book consists of a collection of papers that were published in the *Medical Examiner* of Philadelphia between August 1852 and August 1853.]
56. Brown-Séquard CE. Lectures on the diagnosis and treatment of the various forms of paralytic, convulsive, and mental affections, considered as effects of morbid alterations of the blood, or of the brain or other organs. Lecture 1 – Part 1. On the mode of origin of symptoms of disease of the brain. *Lancet*, 2:1–2, 1861.
57. Brown-Séquard CE. Introductory lecture to a course on the physiological pathology of the brain. *Lancet*, 2:75–78, 1876.
58. Brown-Séquard CE. Lectures on the diagnosis and treatment of the various forms of paralytic, convulsive, and mental affections, considered as effects of morbid alterations of the blood, or of the brain or other organs. Lecture 1 – Part 2. On the mode of origin of symptoms of disease of the brain. *Lancet*, 2:29–30, 1861.
59. Brown-Séquard CE. On the relations between muscular irritability, cadaveric rigidity, and putrefaction. [The Croonian Lecture]. *Proc R Soc Lond*, 11:204–214, 1861.
60. Mill JS. *A system of logic, ratiocinative and inductive*, 8th edition (pp. 270–279, 313–314). London: Longmans, Green & Co., reprinted 1947.
61. Brown-Séquard CE. Lectures on the diagnosis and treatment of the various forms of paralytic, convulsive and mental affections, considered as effects of morbid alterations of the blood, or of the brain or other organs. *Lancet*, 2:1–2, 29–30, 55–56, 79–80, 153–154, 199–200, 391–392, 415–416, 515–516, 611–613, 1861.
62. Darwin CR [Charles]. Letter to Brown-Séquard dated 2 January (? year). MS 981/96. Archives, Royal College of Physicians, London.
63. Darwin CR [Charles]. Letter to Brown-Séquard dated 16 April (? year). MS 981/97. Archives, Royal College of Physicians, London.
64. Darwin Correspondence Project Database. Accessed on 8 January 2010 at http://www.darwinproject.ac.uk/entry-3396/ (letter no. 3396, Huxley TH to Darwin CR, 20 January 1862).
65. Francis SW. Biographical sketches of distinguished living New York physicians. V. C.E. Brown-Séquard, M.D., F.R.S., etc. *Med Surg Reporter (Philadelphia)*, 15:169–172, 1866.
66. Hutchinson J. The late Dr. Hughlings Jackson: recollections of a lifelong friendship. *Br Med J*, 2:1551–1554, 1911.
67. Greenblatt SH. The major influences on the early life and work of John Hughlings Jackson. *Bull Hist Med*, 39:346–376, 1965.

68. Anonymous. Désintéressement d'un savant. *La Republique Française*, April 13, 1894.
69. Anonymous. Obituary: Professor Brown-Séquard. *Lancet*, 1:975–77, 1894.
70. Brown-Séquard CE. Undated letter to a friend, providing biographical details. MS 994/2. Royal College of Physicians, London.
71. Hughlings Jackson J. Letter to Brown-Séquard dated 27 January 1866. MS 980/22. Archives, Royal College of Physicians, London. [Discusses various cases and refers to Brown-Séquard's promise concerning the Epileptic Hospital.]

8

Broken Dreams and Promises

BROWN-SÉQUARD DID not finally leave the measured calm of England until May 1864,[1] in part because of Ellen's poor health. No job or appointment awaited him in the New World. When eventually the family arrived in America, the Civil War was tramping to its eventual close and the country was in disarray. Not surprisingly, Brown-Séquard's sympathies were with the North, and he expressed the hope from its very start that "soon the rebellion will be crushed."[2]

Brown-Séquard, Medicine, and the Civil War

The medical services available to Civil War combatants were wanting, although the war had led to many changes in medical care and provided an opportunity for the American military to learn how to handle casualties.[3] Many of these casualties had resulted from gunshot and other high-velocity projectiles from ever-more-sophisticated armaments placed in prepared defensive positions, fired often over great distances at troops advancing without cover or adequate protection. At the onset of war, only a small number of surgeons were available to care for troops at a regimental level, usually in garrison hospitals. After a battle, a hospital would be established near the battlefield to care for the injured until they were able to return to duty or could be moved away from the front to general hospitals. In these hospitals, infection was widespread, conditions were poor, and surgeons lost control over the care of their patients.

The surgeons themselves were largely inexperienced and learned their business by trial and error; the concept of asepsis had yet to be born, medication to alleviate pain or induce anesthesia was in short supply, and hospitals reeked of fear and suffering. In time, the railroads came to be used to evacuate the wounded to rear-area hospitals, but often in pitiful conditions and after much delay. In an effort to improve matters, William A. Hammond[A] was appointed surgeon-general of the army by President Lincoln in 1862, and the treatment of the wounded was streamlined: regimental aid stations evacuated the wounded to a field hospital close to the front, from which they would be sent within three or four days to a large depot hospital. Once it was clear that that they could endure the trip, soldiers unlikely to return to their units were then moved by special ambulance trains to single-storey pavilion general hospitals further to the rear or to large metropolitan hospitals, where accurate medical records were kept, care was optimized, and the outcome of specific treatments noted.[3]

Brown-Séquard's contributions were minor, but he did what little he could, speaking to army surgeons and others about the care of the wounded. In June, within a few weeks of his arrival in the America—while Sherman was on his ruinous march through the South—he lectured at the Smithsonian Institute to army surgeons and others.[4] Tetanus ("lockjaw") was a major infective complication of war wounds, resulting in death among most of those who developed the disease. The cause of the disease was then unknown, but was usually attributed to physical factors such as the cold.[B] Brown-Séquard stressed the importance of cleansing wounds, ensuring sleep, and controlling spasms with potassium bromide, and sometimes the need to cut nerves passing between the injured part and the brain or spinal cord or even to amputate the injured limb.

[A] Hammond returned to New York City after the Civil War and, in 1866, was appointed Professor of Diseases of the Mind and Nervous System at Bellevue Hospital Medical College, a position that he held until his resignation in 1873, following a series of disagreements with other faculty and the administration. He remained in contact with Brown-Séquard and supported his later efforts to introduce organ extracts into clinical practice.

[B] Tetanus is an infectious disease of the nervous system caused by the toxin of the tetanus bacillus (*Clostridium tetani*), which enters the body through injuries that puncture the skin. It is now preventable by immunization ("tetanus shot"). It is characterized by painful muscle stiffness and spasms (especially of muscles that close the jaw, leading to "lockjaw"), irritability, sweating, and an increase in heart rate and blood pressure. There is difficulty in swallowing and breathing. Modern treatment involves cleansing the wound, antibiotics, tetanus immune globulin or antitoxin (to neutralize toxin as much as possible), and a booster dose of tetanus vaccine (or a full course in those not previously vaccinated). Muscle spasms are controlled by medication but may lead to the arrest of breathing; care is otherwise supportive. More than a million cases of tetanus occur annually, mainly in developing countries where immunization is not available routinely, and many have a fatal outcome.

He discussed also the emergency management of hemorrhage, a common complication of any wound. Hemorrhage leads to a reduction in the volume of circulating blood; in consequence, the tissues receive inadequate perfusion and thus insufficient oxygen, organs fail, and death eventually results from collapse of the circulation (so-called "shock").[C] At regimental aid stations, active bleeding was controlled usually by bandaging and application of pressure at appropriate points but sometimes by more radical means, such as by tying off an artery. Styptics such as silver nitrate, gallic and tannic acids, "persulphate of iron," alum, and turpentine were also used to arrest bleeding. The wounded were then sent on to a field hospital, where their wounds, often infected or gangrenous, could be treated more fully, sometimes by amputation, to prevent further bleeding. Brown-Séquard pointed out that pressure on the main arteries to the four limbs for three or four minutes may be a life-saving measure in desperate situations, as it sometimes increased significantly the effective volume of blood remaining in the system, allowing time for the source of hemorrhage to be identified and bleeding controlled. It is of interest that previously, in 1857, he had transfused blood from one animal species to another: "Into dog I have transfused, by the jugular vein [a vein in the neck], the blood of the rabbit, guinea pig, cat, cock, hen, pigeon, duck, turtle (three species), frog and eel. When I have used fresh arterial blood or defibrinated venous blood charged with oxygen, I have not observed trouble other than the momentary alteration of the respiration and circulation that follows transfusion into the jugular vein."[5,6] He now advocated the slow transfusion of a small amount of human blood (no more than about an ounce at a time, with the total in the order of five ounces), claiming that this often led to clinical improvement in cases of hemorrhage and in certain other contexts. Quite how this was supposed to do so is not entirely clear. In any event, blood transfusion was generally not used to treat the wounded, with few exceptions, because of the catastrophic reactions that sometimes followed.[D] Two cases

---

[C] Shock leads to an increase in heart and breathing (respiratory) rates, and then to low blood pressure and mental changes (confusion, irritability, indifference, limited responsiveness, and eventually coma). The patient appears pale, cold, and lifeless. Modern treatment involves maintaining breathing and the circulation, rapid transport to hospital, provision of oxygen, preventing further blood loss, and giving blood or other fluids intravenously to maintain and restore the circulating blood volume.

[D] Blood or blood products can be transfused from one person to another and, in the first half of the nineteenth century, several reports of successful transfusion were published. In other instances, however, "transfusion reactions" occurred, with a fatal outcome. Various substitutes for blood were also transfused at that time, such as milk, egg albumen, and salt solutions, with mixed results. In 1901, Karl Landsteiner, an Austrian, discovered the existence of human blood groups, work for which he received the Nobel Prize for Physiology or Medicine in 1930. Red

that involved blood transfusions are in the military records. A private, wounded in June 1864 and requiring leg amputation to control hemorrhage and gangrene, reportedly underwent transfusion of about two ounces of blood from a "strong healthy German" in order "to test the method ... as recommended by Brown-Séquard," with immediate improvement such that he recovered.[E] The other case was of another private who underwent a leg amputation for uncontrollable bleeding and received sixteen ounces of blood from a healthy man; he seemed to do well for about eight or nine days, but then succumbed from recurrent hemorrhage and dysentery.[7]

Dysentery and diarrhea were frequent and often fatal. A favored remedy for such "fluxes" among generalists, and also for the relief of pain, was that advanced by Brown-Séquard, namely a combination of morphine and atropine given by injection underneath the skin. The combination allowed greater doses of morphine to be given and tolerated safely, and seemed to enhance the benefit of treatment.[8,9] A preparation with a similar composition (containing extracts of opium, belladonna, cannabis, stramonium, and aconite) but taken by mouth for the relief of pain, known as Brown-Séquard's Antineuralgic Pills, also became popular, and became widely available in the shops, where within a few years it cost two dollars for a hundred pills.[F]

Among other topics that he covered, Brown-Séquard spoke about spinal injuries, a subject about which he had lectured and written previously, including in the now-famous book of his 1858 lectures,[10] stressing that they were often caused by the pressure of displaced bone on the spinal cord rather than

---

blood cells carry certain inherited major protein markers (known as "antigens") that affect how they react with other tissues. These antigens allow the blood to be characterized into "blood types." The major markers are designated A, B, AB, and O (when none is present). Additional markers for the so-called Rhesus factor allow blood to be classified also as Rhesus (Rh) positive or negative. If blood of an incompatible type is transfused, chemicals (antibodies) in the recipient's blood will attach to the transfused cells, causing them to clump together, disintegrate, or obstruct the circulation. Blood is now cross-matched before transfusion to ensure that such adverse reactions do not occur. Other complications of transfusion, such as infection, may still occur. The first transfusions were direct from donor to recipient before the blood could clot; in other instances, blood was "defibrinated" (i.e., fibrin—a protein involved in the clotting of blood—was removed from the blood) to reduce the risk of clotting. In the early twentieth century, anticoagulant substances ("blood thinners") were added to the blood, so that it could be stored for later use, and this led to the development of blood banks.

[E] The surgeon, Edwin Bentley (1824–1917), later delivered Douglas MacArthur, the World War II hero, on an army post (1880) and was one of the founders of what is now the College of Medicine at the University of Arkansas. He is buried at Arlington National Cemetery.

[F] The content of each pill was as follows: 0.67 grain of extract of hyoscyamus, 0.67 grain of extract of conium, 0.5 grain of extract of ignatia, 0.5 grain of extract of opium, 0.33 grain of extract of aconite leaves, 0.25 grain of extract of cannabis, 0.2 grain of extract of stramonium, and 0.16 grain of extract of belladonna leaves.

by direct injury. Similarly, many cases of post-traumatic epilepsy (i.e., seizures following head injury) were the result of pressure on the brain from displaced bone fragments, the removal of which could lead to the cessation of seizures. He accepted that the literature on the utility of surgical decompression was incomplete, but emphasized that some patients, at least, not only survived but did well. To his chagrin, however, his colleagues seemed reluctant to accept that the removal of such bony fragments could save life or minimize neurological damage—even though Brown-Séquard had previously shown by his work in animals that opening the spinal canal to expose the spinal cord and its covering meninges (membranes) is not dangerous—and the noninterventionist approach of the conservatives was favored by many.

As the war continued, the treatment of spinal cord injuries evolved. First, it became increasingly clear that patients with spinal cord injury needed to be immobilized before they were moved, to prevent extension of their injury, and that care of the bladder, bowels, and skin was important to prevent fatal complications, such as bedsores. Many with spinal cord injuries were transferred to Turner's Lane General Hospital in Philadelphia,[G] which specialized in neurological and nervous complications, and were treated there by S. Weir Mitchell, William W. Keen, and George R. Morehouse. Second, experience with spinal cord injuries increased and management improved; operative intervention became more common, although it still depended on the idiosyncrasies and clinical experience of the surgeon, despite the influence of Brown-Séquard and other like-minded physicians. Several years after the end of the war, an official *Medical and Surgical History of the War of the Rebellion* was published.[11] It included reports on 642 gunshot wounds of the spine, associated with a mortality of 55 percent. The death rate associated with surgery was 43 percent; in

---

[G] Turner's Lane General Hospital specialized in neurological injuries and became the first research center for clinical neurology in the U.S. Weir Mitchell (1824–1914), Morehouse (1825–1905), and Keen (1837–1932) had the opportunity to study numerous cases of nerve damage and coauthored the now-classic monograph, *Gunshot Wounds and Other Injuries of Nerves,* in 1864, providing original descriptions of such phenomena as phantom limb (i.e., the sense that an amputated limb is still present) and causalgia (i.e., severe burning pain, usually arising after nerve injury). Mitchell was elected the first president of the American Neurological Association when that organization was established in 1875, and is recalled by the award named after him by the American Academy of Neurology (founded in 1948) to encourage investigative work among those entering the specialty. Keen became a successful medical author and surgeon, obtaining the chair at Jefferson Medical College in Philadelphia, and, in 1893, was involved in the secret operation for cancer of the jaw performed on President Cleveland aboard the yacht *Oneida*. The Turner's Lane Hospital became The Philadelphia Orthopaedic Hospital and Infirmary for Nervous Diseases in 1867, and this, in turn, became part of the University of Pennsylvania Hospital in 1938.

twenty-seven procedures performed to remove the ball, nine patients died and four returned to duty, whereas in twenty-four operations performed to remove bone, ten patients died and seven returned to duty.[11,12] (In some of the latter cases, the injuries to the vertebral column were probably relatively mild, given the completeness of recovery.) Wounds through the chest and abdomen were invariably fatal, but the mortality rate declined from 70 percent in neck (cervical) injuries to 46 percent for lumbar injuries.[11,12] Third, it became clear that patients with spinal cord injuries required active treatment rather than benign neglect and comfort measures. It would require two world wars before the care of paraplegics was reappraised, and even more vigorous measures put into place by Sir Ludwig Guttmann in England and by others to prevent the decubitus ulcers (bedsores), kidney infections, and other devastating complications that led so often to a fatal outcome.[13]

Although Brown-Séquard was without a job, he hoped that his name and reputation would soon open up possibilities and opportunities for him, and in this regard he was not to be disappointed. It is unfortunate, however, that having secured a most prestigious appointment—no less than the first professorship of neurology (or, more specifically, of the physiology and pathology of the nervous system) in the world—he was unable to discharge the duties expected of him and eventually felt obliged to resign and return to Europe. The resulting loss to the advance of science, and especially neurology, in America is hard to estimate. The personal misfortunes that befell Brown-Séquard for the next ten years, perhaps the most painful in his life, would have been disheartening to any man but, happily, were a prelude to his eventual appointment to a chair in Paris, where he finally settled.

In and Out of the Chair at Harvard

Harvard College was founded in 1636, but its "medical institution" did not open until the latter half of the eighteenth century. The medical school expanded rapidly, and its students were able to obtain a broad clinical experience once the Massachusetts General Hospital opened in 1821. The teaching and study of physiology was within the province of anatomy and—as such—was part of the responsibility of Oliver Wendell Holmes (1809–1894),[H] the literary Parkman Professor of Anatomy and Physiology who once likened the brain to an English walnut in its shell. Holmes, who had earned his medical

---

[H] Holmes is not to be confused with his son, Oliver Wendell Holmes, Jr., (1841–1935) an eminent and much cited jurist who became an associate justice of the U.S. Supreme Court.

degree in 1836, had served as the dean of Harvard Medical School from 1847 to 1853. The time available for studying physiology was variable but usually brief. Holmes, despite his interest in the topic, lacked the expertise of an experimental investigator and was increasingly aware of the inadequacy of his teaching, which consisted primarily of remarks and asides on function during anatomy lectures and of a few more formal lectures on physiology itself at the end of the course. He therefore attempted to secure the services of an experienced and resourceful experimentalist to teach physiology, so that he could relinquish his own role in that context. The lot fell to Brown-Séquard and, at first glance, it seemed an excellent choice. He did, after all, personify the concept of experimental medicine, as formulated by François Magendie in Paris, and was the rival of the illustrious French physiologist Claude Bernard, Magendie's successor at the Collège de France.

In June 1864, the president and fellows of Harvard College had voted to elect a professor of physiology and pathology of the nervous system, with compensation to be derived from student fees. Brown-Séquard was selected and enthusiastically accepted the position.[14] Almost immediately, however, came the death, reportedly from typhoid fever,[15] of the ailing Ellen, who was buried in the Cambridge cemetery. Within three months, Brown-Séquard had become depressed, withdrawn, and too unwell with recurrent headaches to prepare for his approaching lectures, two of which he was required to deliver each week. He was preoccupied, also, with domestic problems that arose with his in-laws in Boston following Ellen's death,[16] and brooded at the way her family had behaved toward her while she was ill. And then, of course, he had to look after 8-year-old Edouard, although quite how he managed is unclear. Despite being relieved temporarily of his duties, in November, he told Dr. George Shattuck, the dean, that he intended to resign the chair. The response that he received, expressing regret that the Harvard faculty would lose the pleasure and benefits that they had hoped to gain from their association with him, must have flattered and pleased him and, within a few weeks, he had offered to deliver a lecture on the physiological effects of lesions involving the spinal cord. Over the following weeks, he wrote of his interest in assuming after all his role as Professor.[17]

His resignation was withdrawn, but instead of taking up his duties, Brown-Séquard spent much of 1865 in France and England. In February 1865, he lectured to the College of Physicians of Ireland on the importance of physiology to the practice of medicine and surgery,[18] remarking that it facilitates the interpretation of symptoms and allows many of the most complex neurological cases to be understood as easily as the simplest case of bronchitis. He emphasized the importance of experimental work on animals to the advance of clinical medicine and as an aid to diagnosing and determining the outlook of neurological disorders. (Although animal experimentation is still opposed by many, most of the major medical advances of the last century have indeed resulted from it, and Brown-Séquard's comments would need little justification to modern medical audiences.)

As his distance from Boston increased, he became swept away by increasingly grandiose notions to establish a physiological and pathological institute at Harvard that would be a model for others and grander than any of its European counterparts. With increasing excitement and enthusiasm, he offered not only to buy any necessary equipment but to pay for the building himself. Shattuck temporized, noting that "putting up a new building may be more expedient in a year's time ...."[19] Not to be delayed from the pursuit of science, Brown-Séquard asked as a temporary measure for laboratory facilities within the college, provided that there was no danger that the screaming of a few dogs would disrupt the life of his colleagues.[19] He frenziedly planned to repeat every new experiment of importance made by other physiologists or pathologists and to expand his own work in virtually every area that he had previously ventured, specifically listing some twenty topics. Within another two or three months, however, he was listless, flat, slow, and complaining of a recurrence of his headaches, and his academic plans were set aside. By September, he was again offering to resign because of ill health (see p. 133), although within a few months he was once more making plans to deliver his lectures.

The problems continued with his in-laws, so Brown-Séquard moved to New York City, commuting by train to Boston when he had to lecture. As the summer of 1866 advanced, however, the burden became too great and he decided to "forgive" Ellen's family and return to Boston.[16]

In November, Brown-Séquard gave the introductory lecture to the winter course at Harvard, entitled *Advice to Students*,[20] before a large audience that included some of the "most distinguished cultivators of natural science in our neighborhood."[21] The lecture was more than the customary exhortations to hard work and self-discipline. He encouraged the students to form small study groups, with individuals preparing talks on specific topics for discussion within the group, an approach that is still popular. As always, he emphasized the importance of an experimental and critical approach to the study of medicine, while warning against wanton cruelty to animals. Beliefs were not be accepted as facts simply because they had the support of some authority or learned society, and facts were not be denied just because they were difficult to explain. He cautioned also against the acceptance of a theory when there were facts in conflict with it, and against the drawing of erroneous conclusions by neglecting the context in which supporting evidence was obtained. It was perhaps unfortunate that, in his lecture, he chose also to make some insensitive comments concerning the United States and his belief that it lagged behind Europe in at least some respects.

> How can we learn to make scientific or practical investigations in physiology or medicine in a country like this, where the teaching of these sciences is yet only rudimentary? I do not deny that there is a great need here of an institute, where the means of prosecuting scientific researches should be taught .... I have no doubt that he who would establish such an institute ... would also do much, at the same time, to place this country on a level with Europe, for things about which the inferiority of America is notorious ....[20]

In his subsequent lectures, he covered a variety of topics in clinical neurology,[22] moving easily from the findings in patients to experimental observations in the laboratory with a facility that is remarkable even by today's standards. Brown-Séquard has been described by some as an enthusiastic lecturer, at least when he devoted his time to his teaching duties. However, he was not an eloquent speaker and refused to lecture in the didactic manner preferred by many students. Instead, he offered original concepts to his audience, expounding on his own novel beliefs that were often well ahead of their time. For example, he taught that the sensitivity of the skin to heat and cold depended on two sets of nerves some years before the publication of the definitive work on this topic by others.[23,1] On the whole, however, his interactions with his students and many of his medical school colleagues were disappointing, and he made a lasting impression on few of them, perhaps because of the swings in his enthusiasm, energy, and interest as he grappled with his own ill health and domestic problems. Certainly, little is published to suggest that he had any great influence on the subsequent careers of most of them, although to some he was perhaps able to impart an enthusiasm for experimental physiology. One such person may have been Henry Pickering Bowditch (1840–1911), who was to play an important role in the development of physiology at Harvard. In 1868, Bowditch, after graduating from Harvard Medical

---

[1] The skin contains sensory receptors and nerves (that conduct information to the spinal cord, from where it is relayed to the brain) that allow touch, pressure, vibration, hot, cold, and pain to be appreciated. Distinct receptors and sensory nerve fibers subserve these sensations. When these degenerate or malfunction, patients may be unable to feel normal sensations of, for example, light touch, hot, cold, pressure, or pain, and may experience abnormal or distorted sensations, such as spontaneous pain, pins-and-needles, or numbness. Sensory disturbances may also result from damage to the nerves between the extremities and the spinal cord or from damage to the spinal cord or brain, as discussed in an earlier chapter.

School, went to Paris expecting to work with Brown-Séquard, who had recently returned there. Unfortunately, the latter, always in great demand, was unable to accommodate the young American, who had to turn instead to Claude Bernard and Ranvier[J] for laboratory experience, and to Charcot and Broca for clinical guidance. After his return to Boston from Europe in 1871, the Parkman chair at Harvard was restricted to anatomy, and Bowditch—although an assistant professor—assumed charge of physiological instruction and initiated a course of lectures and demonstrations; in 1876, he was appointed full professor at Harvard, and from 1903 until his resignation in 1906, he held the newly established George Higginson professorship of physiology there.[24]

William James (1842–1910), the great experimental psychologist, was another medical student at Harvard whom Brown-Séquard greatly influenced by his insistence on the importance of the experimental method, including vivisection. Much of James' medical student notebook is devoted to Brown-Séquard's lectures, which correlate mental symptoms with pathology of the brain.[25,26]

Because of his concern about his salary, which was supported by the sale of admission tickets for his lectures, the college authorities agreed to raise the cost of these tickets from ten to twelve dollars each. Brown-Séquard also had no hesitation in promoting his own books, pushing for them to be included on recommended reading lists. With these academic sources of income, he decided, in January 1867, to give up the private practice that he had been conducting at Dr. Shattuck's office.[27] It was taking too much of his time and was financially unrewarding, as his fees often went unpaid. Feltus immediately wrote from Philadelphia, advising against this and suggesting instead that at the end of every consultation he present his bill for immediate payment.[28] Brown-Séquard seems initially to have ignored the advice, and instead stopped seeing patients other than friends and those who were special to him. He did, however, attend two faculty meetings, and it was surely no coincidence that the focus of these particular meetings was to allocate contingency funds to support faculty salaries, to agree on how much Brown-Séquard himself should receive for his thus-far limited participation, and to establish the fees for the following year.[29]

[J] Louis-Antoine Ranvier (1835–1922), French histopathologist and physician, one-time assistant to Claude Bernard, and professor of general anatomy at the Collège de France. His name is attached to a structural component of certain nerve fibers (nodes of Ranvier), a particular cell type (Merkel-Ranvier cells in the skin), certain sensory nerve endings in the skin (Ranvier's tactile disks), and a plexus of nerves in the cornea (Ranvier's plexus).

He also continued lecturing elsewhere. In December 1866, for example, two special meetings of the New York Academy of Medicine[K] were held to allow him to lecture on the physiology and pathology of the nervous system and, in January 1867, he was elected a corresponding member of the Academy. Still, Brown-Séquard remained dissatisfied with his lot and in early 1867—the same year that Garibaldi marched on Rome, the United States purchased Alaska from Russia for two cents an acre (some seven million dollars in total), and Alfred Nobel patented dynamite—he began negotiating with the dean for an assistant. At the same time, he continued to wander between the great cities of the developed world. In August, for example, an International Medical Congress, the first of its kind, was held in Paris and Brown-Séquard—who was a delegate of the American Medical Association and planned to talk on the early signs of cerebral disease—was one of the most eagerly awaited speakers. Unfortunately, however, the sudden death from an aneurysmal hemorrhage (i.e., bleeding from the rupture of a balloon-like swelling of an artery within the head) of P. Victor Bazire (1835–1867),[30] his friend, Mauritian compatriot, and an assistant-physician on the staff of the National Hospital for the Paralysed and Epileptic in London, who had made his name as the editor and translator of Trousseau's *Clinical Lectures*, required instead his presence in London.[31] Finally, in November, he again resigned from his chair at Harvard—for the third and last time—and insisted that it be brought to the attention of the faculty at its next meeting. This time, the faculty followed through and instructed that the resignation be transmitted to the president and fellows, who accepted it.[32,33]

Thus, Brown-Séquard ended his connection with Harvard College and returned again to France. The teaching of physiology at Harvard then passed to J. S. Lombard, an assistant professor, and was taken over by Bowditch a few years later. Lombard, whose name has since passed into obscurity, was interested in variations in temperature of different scalp regions (which were held to reflect those of the underlying brain) in relation to mental activity. He measured temperature by thermopiles placed on defined regions on both sides of the head. His findings were published in a monograph that still arouses interest among those concerned with the localization of brain function by imaging techniques but is otherwise not widely known.

[K] I am grateful to Ms. Arlene Shaner, Assistant Curator and Reference Librarian for Historical Collections at the Academy library for the following information. Founded in 1847 to advance the art and science of medicine, promote public health and medical education, and establish an outstanding medical library, the New York Academy of Medicine has been influential in advancing health-related issues at both the local and national level. Brown-Séquard was elected a corresponding fellow in 1867, shortly after his lectures; because he did not live in the New York area, he was not eligible for any other kind of fellowship.

Many learned of Brown-Séquard's decision with regret. He had received wide recognition in America, being elected a member of the American Philosophical Society[L] in 1854, a fellow of the American Academy of Arts and Sciences[M] and a corresponding member of the New York Academy of Medicine in 1867, and a member of the National Academy of Sciences[N] in the following year. Silas Weir Mitchell considered "every defection from our slim physiological ranks a great loss."[34] He wrote from Philadelphia, asking for a letter of reference in connection with the vacant chair of physiology that he sought

---

[L] The American Philosophical Society, the oldest learned organization in the United States, was founded in 1743 by Benjamin Franklin. I am grateful to Charles B. Greifenstein (the manuscripts librarian at the Society) for the following information. At the time of Brown-Séquard's election, records were not kept of the names of nominators for reasons of confidentiality, papers with their names being destroyed after balloting. At about this time, the minutes of board meetings began to use numbers to designate nominees, names being withheld until after a vote was taken to send the name to the full membership (and sometimes not even then). Names were not noted in the minutes of meetings of the full membership until after balloting was complete, when the names of those elected were recorded. During balloting, black and white balls were used (or were supposed to be used). Three-quarters of the board were required to approve a nominee before the name was presented to the general membership. There is little archival material concerning Brown-Séquard's election, except his acceptance letter, from which it is apparent that he did not hear of his election until he received his membership certificate.

[M] The American Academy of Arts and Sciences, founded in 1780 for the "cultivation and promotion of Arts and Sciences," includes among its members leaders in the academic and business worlds, the arts, and public affairs. It is unclear who nominated Brown-Séquard for membership. Elizabeth Carroll-Horrocks, Director of Archives at the Academy, has provided me with the following information, for which I am grateful. During the latter part of the nineteenth century, there were three categories of member: resident fellows (for residents of Massachusetts), associate fellows (for those living in other parts of the U.S.), and foreign honorary members (outside the U.S.). Brown-Séquard was at Harvard when he became a fellow; his status changed in 1873 to associate fellow when he was resident in New York City, and to foreign honorary member (1881) after he had returned to France.

[N] The National Academy of Sciences, established by Abraham Lincoln in 1863 to "investigate, examine, experiment, and report upon any subject of science or art" at the request of any department of the government, is made up of distinguished scholars dedicated to the advance of science and technology. Election to membership is one of the highest honors to which scientists aspire. Janice F. Goldblum, National Academies archivist, has kindly provided me with the following information. Membership of the Academy was originally limited to fifty, divided between the class of mathematics and physics (Class A) and of natural history (Class B). It is not clear who nominated Brown-Séquard for membership, but the archives indicate that the merits of the candidate were discussed by Louis Agassiz and Weir Mitchell, a ballot was then taken, and Brown-Séquard received all of the sixteen votes that were cast and was therefore elected unanimously to Class B. The class system was abolished in 1872 but in 1911, a sectional organization was reestablished and, in 1965, the classes were reintroduced. At present, the Academy is organized into six classes, which are subdivided by discipline into thirty-one sections.

unsuccessfully at Jefferson Medical College,[34] and alluded also to Brown-Séquard's recent election (which he had proposed) to the National Academy of Sciences by a vote which "was absolutely unanimous upon the first ballot."[35] Mitchell corresponded for many years with Brown-Séquard, and always acknowledged his own debt to him. When sending Brown-Séquard a copy of his book on gunshot and other nerve injuries, which was to become a medical classic, he wrote "I have always sent to you every paper I have written—my first impulse toward physiological research came to me from hearing you lecture and I have never ceased to remember you gratefully as the indirect cause of the pleasure which research has always given me."[36] In fact, each man sent manuscripts and research papers to the other for advice and comments.[37] Their last correspondence was probably in 1893, when Brown-Séquard, having previously sent Mitchell copies of several papers referring to his work on organ extracts (discussed in Chapters 12 and 13),[38] wrote to urge his colleague in Philadelphia to employ the same approach for himself.[39] Mitchell himself became a prominent literary figure later in life, writing short stories, poetry, and historical novels that became tremendously popular.

Brown-Séquard and Bipolar Disease

It is legitimate to consider the reason that Brown-Séquard's career at Harvard failed so miserably. As when his mother died during his student days in Paris, he was clearly unable to cope with the stresses of daily life in Boston after Ellen's death, with swings from profound depression, chronic headaches, and apathy to episodes in which he was energized but impulsive, unstable, distractible, even irrational, and incapable of functioning normally. The grandiosity of his thoughts as he planned for his institute, his unrealistic expectations, and his restlessness, impatience, and seemingly limited attention span are clearly beyond the bounds of normality. His constant preoccupation with money, and his anxiety about whether he could make ends meet, both in London and in Boston, are telling, and the damaged relations with his in-laws and with many of his colleagues in Boston are noteworthy. Given these factors, it is hard to escape the conclusion that he suffered with bipolar disease (or manic-depression, as it was previously called), with the first symptoms probably developing during his early adult years in France. The cause of this disorder is still unknown, although it has a strong genetic basis. The disorder is currently treated with mood-stabilizing drugs, but these were not available in the nineteenth century.

The lifestyle of his son provides some support for the belief that Brown-Séquard was unwell and is a sad epilogue to his ill-fated connection with Harvard.

Edouard was a poor student,[40] and Brown-Séquard became increasingly estranged from the moody young man who was lazy, rude, and selfish.[41] He even began to wonder whether Edouard might be an epileptic, because of several episodes in which he bit his tongue during the night and awakened late the next morning with a headache.[42] Nevertheless, it seems that the boy gained admittance to Harvard in 1873, almost certainly with the help of Louis Agassiz, the eminent scientist and a family friend,[43] but left within a year, moving to France, where he studied dentistry at Lille. He then returned to the United States but did not remain long in any one place; he supposedly married a Southern girl, worked briefly as a book seller, and avoided his classmates from Harvard, who were unable to learn much about him.[44] He achieved a certain notoriety when, while living at Cold Spring in New York, he was arrested for stealing a cat from a saloon keeper while intoxicated.[45,46] As with the older man, then, there is a pattern of restlessness, instability, constant moving about the country, and work in different fields, to suggest a similar illness, but with at least one episode of drunkenness leading to a court appearance (substance abuse is common among patients with bipolar disease). Edouard is thought by his Harvard contemporaries to have died at some point in the 1880s of unknown causes.[44]

There can be no doubt that Brown-Séquard's early departure from Harvard set back the development of neurology and the neurosciences in Boston for some years. It has been suggested that his letters reveal Brown-Séquard to be a "disarmingly 'modern' professor who avoided faculty meetings, complained constantly about lecture schedules, his salary, and the improper care of animals—and threatened to resign regularly."[19] While there is a certain truth to this, it is the extremes to which Brown-Séquard went that sets him apart and exceeds the bounds of normality, in the same way that that there is a difference between an eccentric and a lunatic.

References and Source Notes

1. Brown-Séquard CE. Undated letter to a friend, providing biographical details. MS 994/2. Royal College of Physicians, London.
2. Brown-Séquard CE. Letter to S. Weir Mitchell dated 2 February 1862. Trent Collection, Duke University, Durham, North Carolina.
3. Hawk A. An ambulating hospital: or, how the hospital train transformed army medicine. *Civil War Hist*, 48:197–219, 2002.
4. Anonymous. Notes of lecture delivered by Professor Brown-Séquard at the Smithsonian Institute, 14 June 1864. MS 991. Archives, Royal College of Physicians, London.
5. Brown-Séquard E. Recherches expérimentales sur les propriétés et les usages du sang rouge et du sang noir (quatrième mémoire). *C R Acad Sci*, 45:562–566, 1857.
6. Doan CA. The transfusion problem. *Physiol Rev*, 7:1–84, 1927.
7. Otis GA, Huntington DL. *The medical and surgical history of the war of the rebellion (1861–1865). Surgical History* (Part III, Vol. II, pp. 811–812). Washington, DC: Government Printing Office, 1883.

8. Brown-Sequard CE. *Lectures on the diagnosis and treatment of functional nervous affections* (p. 72). Cambridge: John Wilson & Son, 1868.
9. Otis GA, Huntington DL. *The medical and surgical history of the war of the rebellion (1861–1865). Surgical History* (Part II, Vol. I). Medical History (pp. 750–755). Washington, DC: Government Printing Office, 1879.
10. Brown-Séquard CE. *Course of lectures on the physiology and pathology of the central nervous system.* Philadelphia: Collins, 1860.
11. Otis GA, Huntington DL. *The medical and surgical history of the war of the rebellion (1861–1865). Surgical History* (Part III, Vol. II). Washington DC, Government Printing Office, 1870.
12. Hanigan WC, Sloffer C. Nelson's wound: treatment of spinal cord injury in 19th and early 20th century military conflicts. *Neurosurg Focus,* 16:1–13, 2004.
13. Abrams GM, Wakasa M. Chronic complications of spinal cord injury. Accessed on 1 February 2009 at www.Uptodate.com
14. Harrington TF. *The Harvard Medical School: A history, narrative and documentary* (Vol. 2, pp. 543, 544, 548, 833–835). New York: Lewis, 1905.
15. Massachusetts Archives. *1864HS6.07/Series 1411, Registers of Vital Records,* Ellen Brown Sequard, Death, Cambridge, 1864, Volume 175, p. 61.
16. Brown-Séquard CE. Letter to Dr. Shattuck dated 31 August 1866. Countway Library of Medicine, Boston.
17. Brown-Séquard CE. Letter to Dr. Shattuck dated 24 February 1865. Countway Library of Medicine, Boston.
18. Brown-Séquard CE. On the importance of the application of physiology to the practice of medicine and surgery. *Dublin Q J Med Sci,* 39:421–436, 1865.
19. Tyler HR, Tyler KL. Charles Edouard Brown-Séquard: Professor of physiology and pathology of the nervous system at Harvard Medical School. *Neurology,* 34:1231–1236, 1984.
20. Brown-Séquard CE. *Advice to students. An address delivered at the opening of the medical lectures of Harvard University.* Cambridge: John Wilson & Son, 1867.
21. Anonymous. Introductory lecture to the winter course at Harvard Medical School. *Boston Med Surg J,* 75:307–308, 1867.
22. Bowditch HP. Student notebook (1867–1868). Countway Library of Medicine, Boston.
23. Faculty, Harvard Medical School. *The Harvard Medical School 1782–1906* (p. 82). Boston, 1906.
24. Cannon WB. Henry Pickering Bowditch. *Memoirs Natl Acad Sci USA,* 17:181–196, 1922.
25. James W. Medical school notebook. Countway Library of Medicine, Boston.
26. Taylor E. New light on the origin of William James's experimental psychology. In: Johnson MG, Henley TB, eds., *Reflections on* The Principles of Psychology: *William James after a century* (pp. 33–61). Hillsdale, NJ: Lawrence Erlbaum Associates, 1990.
27. Anonymous. Retirement of Dr. Brown-Séquard from practice. *Boston Med Surg J,* 75:492, 1867.
28. Feltus HJ. Letter to Brown-Séquard dated 16 January 1867. MS 981/141. Archives, Royal College of Physicians, London.
29. Minutes and records of the Faculty of Medicine, 22 March 1867, Volume 2, p. 914. Cited by Tyler HR, Tyler KL. Charles Edouard Brown-Séquard: Professor of physiology and pathology of the nervous system at Harvard Medical School. *Neurology,* 34:1231–1236, 1984.
30. Anonymous. Obituary: P. Victor Bazire, M.D. *Br Med J,* 2:141, 1867.
31. McMenemey WH. International Congress of Medicine 1867 and some of the personalities involved. *Br Med J,* 3:487–489, 1967.

32. Minutes of the meeting of the president and fellows of Harvard College, 28 December 1867. Harvard Archives. Cited by Tyler HR, Tyler KL. Charles Edouard Brown-Séquard: Professor of physiology and pathology of the nervous system at Harvard Medical School. *Neurology*, 34:1231–1236, 1984.
33. Minutes and records of the Faculty of Medicine, 1868, Volume 2, p. 21. Cited by Tyler HR, Tyler KL. Charles Edouard Brown-Séquard: Professor of physiology and pathology of the nervous system at Harvard Medical School. *Neurology*, 34:1231–1236, 1984.
34. Weir Mitchell S. Letter to Brown-Séquard dated 14 April 1868. MS 980/28. Archives, Royal College of Physicians, London.
35. Weir Mitchell S. Letter to Brown-Séquard dated 27 January 1868 MS 980/26. Archives, Royal College of Physicians, London.
36. Weir Mitchell S. Undated letter to Brown-Séquard. MS 980/90. Archives, Royal College of Physicians, London.
37. Goetz CG, Aminoff MJ. The Brown-Séquard and S. Weir Mitchell letters. *Neurology*, 57:2100–2104, 2001.
38. Brown-Séquard CE. Letter to S. Weir Mitchell dated 27 December 1890. College of Physicians of Philadelphia (Historical Library & Wood Institute) MSS 2/0134-01.
39. Brown-Séquard CE. Letter to S. Weir Mitchell dated 5 November 1893. Trent Collection, Duke University, Durham, North Carolina.
40. Brown-Séquard CE. Undated letter to his wife Maria. MS 978/9. Archives, Royal College of Physicians, London.
41. Brown-Séquard CE. Letter to Emma Dakin dated 7 September 1876. MS 979/27. Archives, Royal College of Physicians, London.
42. Brown-Séquard CE. Letter to Emma Dakin dated 12 October 1876. MS 979/39. Archives, Royal College of Physicians, London.
43. Agassiz JLR [Louis]. Letter to Brown-Séquard dated 24 August 1973. MS 981/10. Archives, Royal College of Physicians, London.
44. Harvard College. *Seventh report of the class of '77* (pp. 39–40). Privately printed for the class by the Plimpton Press, Norwood, Massachusetts, 1917.
45. Anonymous. Who stole Kelly's cat? A well-known doctor arrested for the offense. *New York Times*, 21 January 1881.
46 Anonymous. Dr. Brown-Sequard and the cat. The animal restored to Mr. Kelly and the prisoner released. *New York Times*, 22 January 1881.

9

Musical Chairs

WHEN BROWN-SÉQUARD left Boston at the end of 1867, he made his way back to Paris and the academic life there that he loved. Almost immediately, he joined forces with Jean-Martin Charcot, the leading clinical neurologist in France, and Edmé-Félix Alfred Vulpian, now professor of pathological anatomy, to establish a new periodical, the *Archives de Physiologie Normale et Pathologique*, with the first volume appearing in 1868.[A] Brown-Séquard himself hoped to be appointed to a newly created chair (in experimental and comparative pathology) at the Sorbonne. In November 1868, his friend Louis Agassiz, the naturalist, wrote on his behalf to the Emperor Napoleon regarding a different appointment—the chair of experimental physiology (at the Jardin des Plantes). Brown-Séquard, he suggested, was the most capable man for the job but refused to compete with (and perhaps lose to) those he considered his inferiors.[1] Although Brown-Séquard failed to gain that chair,[B] he was summoned

---

[A] The *Archives de Physiologie Normale et Pathologique* continued until 1898 and then became the *Journal de Physiologie*, which continues to this day as the *Journal of Physiology (Paris)*. Brown-Séquard remained as editor (initially with Vulpian and Charcot, subsequently just with Charcot, and finally alone) until his death in 1894.

[B] Joseph Schiller indicates that Brown-Séquard's qualifications as a scientist were questioned by some, including Agassiz, Claude Bernard, and Vulpian. These beliefs are summarized elsewhere (Schiller J. Claude Bernard and Brown-Séquard: the chair of general physiology and the experimental method. *J Hist Med*, 21: 260–270, 1966.). Schiller's conclusions are almost certainly incorrect. Agassiz was a strong supporter and friend who pushed hard for his appointment (see pp. 142–144), Bernard singled him out for special commendation in a report on the state of physiological research in France (which assisted him in eventually obtaining

shortly thereafter to the Ministry of Education with regard to the new one. It soon became apparent, however, that it might take a year for him to become a naturalized French citizen—he was a British subject by virtue of his birth in Mauritius after it had become a crown colony—and thus become eligible for the position.[2,3] Accordingly, in early 1869, Brown-Séquard—armed with an imperial decree permitting him to establish permanent residence in France and enjoy full civil rights—agreed to serve in the lesser role of *chargé du cours* while the nationality issue was resolved.[4]

The *British Medical Journal* hailed the appointment of "such a master mind."[5] Within a few months, however, his lectures were temporarily halted because his demand for animals could not be met by the budget of the Faculty[6] and—just as in Boston—he became increasingly despondent and again spoke of resigning. In July 1870, Augustus Waller,[C] his friend and an eminent neuroscientist, wrote from England to urge him to take a break, perhaps at a resort on the south coast of England, and otherwise take things more gently, reduce the running costs of his laboratory (or get them approved by the government, like other professors), and "hold at least another year before deciding [about resigning] and stepping 'out into space again.'"[7]

His social life blossomed uneasily in Paris, despite his increasing melancholia. He was invited to dine with Napoleon at the Palais Royal[8] and to many other social functions, because of his intellectual prominence. His return to Europe had also allowed him to renew certain longstanding friendships established during his many visits to England. Thomas Huxley, who—as mentioned earlier—was an ardent advocate of Darwinism and had worsted Bishop Wilberforce at Oxford, was now President of the Royal Society and was very influential in a wide range of areas. He wrote to Brown-Séquard in 1870 about the forthcoming annual meeting of the British Association for the Advancement of Science, at which he was to preside:

> I am naturally very anxious that the meeting should be scientifically, as well as numerically, distinguished, and such papers as those you propose to communicate are alone sufficient to give it the desired character ....[9]

Bernard's own chair at the Collège de France; see p. 151), and Vulpian reported very favorably on his work to the Académie des Sciences, as a result of which he won several major prizes in the 1880s (see Chapter 12).

[C] Augustus Volney Waller (1816–1870), distinguished physiologist and histologist, is remembered for the technique that he developed for studying neuroanatomical pathways by tracing the degenerative changes (Wallerian degeneration) that follow a lesion interrupting fiber tracts.

The meeting was held in September, in Liverpool, and included papers by Brown-Séquard on the hereditary transmission of acquired characters (relating to his work on experimentally induced epilepsy in guinea pigs) that were singled out by Huxley for especial praise.

One of the persons at the Liverpool meeting was a formidable Irish woman, Frances Power Cobbe, who became one of the founders of an organized antivivisection movement in Great Britain.[10,11] There was increasing agitation among a certain influential segment of the lay public, which included the queen, peers, leaders of the clergy, and the poets Tennyson and Browning, about alleged cruelties to animals at academic institutions. Even in America, it was believed by some that, "Out of all these multiplied torments of Richet and Mantegazza, of Chauveau and Castex, of Magendie and Brown-Séquard, Science has found not one single remedy to disease, not one discovery of the slightest value to mankind!"[12] This led the British Association to appoint a committee to consider the topic of physiological experimentation, and ultimately led the British government to establish, in 1875, a Royal Commission of Enquiry on Vivisection.

Huxley's support for Brown-Séquard's work at Liverpool[13] aroused the antivivisectionists. For some years thereafter, Huxley himself was subjected to personal attacks and became the recipient of abusive letters that he attributed to his defense of Brown-Séquard at the meeting. In fact, as late as 1876, he advised the experimental physiologist against appearing at a scientific meeting in England:

> A not uninfluential section of the public here is, at present perfectly mad on the vivisection question and I am afraid that your appearance would have the effect of a red rag upon a bull, on the fanatics who would be among your audience .... There is nothing to it but to wait until the violence of the storm has exhausted itself ....[13]

Huxley wrote also to his friend Sir John Donnelly[D] on the issue:

> It will be the best course, perhaps, if I set down in writing what I have to say respecting the vivisections for physiological purposes which have been performed here .... I have always felt it my duty to defend those physiologists who, like Brown-Séquard, by making experiments on living animals, have added immensely not only to scientific physiology, but to the means of alleviating

---

[D] Sir John Donnelly (1834–1902), one-time controller of the Royal School of Mines in London, played a major role in the development of the South Kensington Museum, now the Victoria and Albert Museum.

human suffering, against the often ignorant and sometimes malicious clamour which has been raised against them.

But personally, indeed I may say constitutionally, the performance of experiments upon living and conscious animals is extremely disagreeable to me, and I have never followed any line of investigation in which such experiments are required .... It was no less clear from what had happened to me when, as President of the British Association, I had defended Brown-Séquard, that I might expect to meet with every description of abuse and misrepresentation if such [experimental] demonstrations [in physiology] were given.[15]

Such hostility from the antivivisectionists did not seem to bother Brown-Séquard, who performed experimental studies in animals throughout his entire professional life, even before anesthetic agents became available. He considered such studies to be essential for expanding knowledge about the functioning of the body and the changes that are the cause or consequence of disease, as well as for gaining knowledge that, while of no immediate application, sometimes led to unforeseeable fundamental advances in the biological sciences. He also believed that experimental demonstrations in animals provided the best means of teaching students certain facts that were not always appreciated simply by reading about them.[16] Thus, he faced the hostility of those opposed to vivisection for much of his professional life, even when in later life he took up permanent residence in France. An English woman, Anna Kingsford,[E] successfully established an Antivivisection Society in Paris in the early 1880s, and gained the support of such notables as Victor Hugo.[17] She targeted many of the leading scientists in France, including Brown-Séquard. Indeed, one of his demonstrations (in 1883) was interrupted when he was attacked by an angry woman[F] with a parasol as he prepared to experiment on a monkey without any anesthesia; she had to be escorted from the premises, even as she complained about the "barbarous methods of vivisection."[18–21]

Brown-Séquard's personal situation was, however, affected by the crisis developing in Europe. During 1869 and 1870, the authorities in Spain had been seeking to fill the throne vacated by the deposed Queen Isabella. Eventually, Prince Leopold of Hohenzollern Sigmaringen—a relative of King William of

---

[E] Anna Kingsford (1846–1888) was an ardent proponent of women's rights and an advocate of vegetarianism. She was one of the leaders of the antivivisection movement, becoming a physician (in Paris) in the belief that this would better empower her to improve animal (rather than human) welfare.

[F] The woman is said to have been the poet and antivivisection activist Marie Huot, who also disrupted lectures by Pasteur.

Prussia—agreed to accept it. Concerned at the prospect of potentially hostile neighbors linked by family ties on two of its frontiers, the French government insisted that Leopold withdraw his candidacy and—when this was agreed—demanded a guarantee from William that the candidacy would not be renewed, thereby implying that he was not dealing in good faith. The King broke off further discussion with the French ambassador, considering the matter at an end, and telegraphed a report to his minister. Otto von Bismarck subtly revised the royal telegram to make it appear that the French had been snubbed and then made it public (the Ems dispatch). Smarting under the perceived humiliation, the French—in a moment of madness and believing in their military superiority—declared war on Prussia in July 1870. Within a few weeks, the great armies of France had been defeated, Napoleon III capitulated at Sedan, and a Republic—the third since the Revolution—replaced the Second French Empire. Paris was encircled, besieged, and surrendered. Léon Gambetta, one of the leaders of the new republic, escaped from the capital in a dramatic flight by balloon—the *Armand Barbès*—to take control of the country in the provinces. In January 1871, an armistice was signed, and the German states proclaimed their union in the German Empire—with William as Emperor—in the Hall of Mirrors at Versailles. Unrest followed as the radical members of the Paris commune rose against the new republic and held the city for several weeks, doing more damage than the Prussians; the revolt was savagely crushed and many of the communards were executed by the new government, the number exceeding those killed in the recent war.

Brown-Séquard was away from home when war broke out and stayed away for its duration, although he sent his earnings from lectures to support the wounded and the French war effort, and then to those in need in the defeated land. In 1871, for example, he lectured in Boston on behalf of the "suffering poor in France, made destitute by the war," being introduced in such terms by Agassiz.[22] With peace eventually restored and the communards crushed, he returned to Paris in 1872, worrying as before about the expenses involved in running his laboratory, even though the Ministry of Education was able to put 2,000 francs at his disposal to cover laboratory costs.[23] Paris, however, was not the city that he had left, repressive laws having been passed to ensure the stability of the new administration against any further experiments in social revolution. With these financial and political issues in mind, Brown-Séquard finally decided to resign his faculty appointment in Paris and, later in 1872, he returned to New York. Vulpian was appointed to the chair of experimental pathology that became vacant with the resignation of Brown-Séquard, and Charcot—in turn—was nominated professor of pathologic anatomy, the position previously held by Vulpian.

On March 13, 1872, Brown-Séquard, now in New York, married Maria Rebecca Carlisle, a woman some thirteen years his junior, the daughter of Sarah Blossom Loring and George Carlisle, a wealthy businessman, of Cincinnati. It is not known how they met. It was not to be a happy union.

Louis Agassiz

While Brown-Séquard was at Harvard in the mid-1860s, he had become especially close to the Swiss-born Louis Agassiz (1807–1873). Agassiz had studied in France and Germany, and eventually settled in America where—in 1848—he was appointed professor of zoology and geology at Harvard College. In that same year, 1848, his unhappy first marriage to the once-attractive Cecile, a talented artist, ended with her premature death from consumption, leaving him with a son and two younger daughters. Within two years, he had married again, this time to Elizabeth Cabot Cary, a well-connected Bostonian. She made him a home and—although herself childless—cared for the children of his earlier marriage. Indeed, she became "my mother, my sister, my companion and friend, all in one," as Agassiz's son (who became a marine zoologist) later recalled with tenderness. In addition to the comfortably ordered domestic life that she created, Lizzie opened a school for girls in Boston and became Agassiz's intellectual partner, sharing his interest in science, helping to arrange (and accompanying him on) several of his field trips, and creating for him a rich social life. Agassiz established the first great research museum in the United States (the Harvard Museum of Comparative Zoology), and did much to promote science by serving as its popular symbol although, curiously, he was a creationist and opposed Darwin's theory of evolution. He studied fossil fishes and glaciers, suggested that ice had covered large parts of the earth's surface in an earlier age, and believed that drastic events such as the Ice Age had led to the extinction of animals and plants, with the subsequent creation of more advanced species. He proposed that the change from primitive to more advanced forms among a group of organisms paralleled the order that these forms appear in the fossil record, with the most primitive forms found lowest (earliest) in the rock record.

When, in 1869, Agassiz was paralyzed by a stroke that also affected his speech, Brown-Séquard cared for him and supervised his remarkable recovery. The naturalist had suffered with headaches for many years, perhaps from hypertension, and Brown-Séquard insisted on a long period of bedrest and that he give up cigar smoking, one of his greatest pleasures. Despite this heavy burden, the two men became close friends and wrote to each other frequently.

In the year following his illness, Agassiz was able to write that "I have not deviated in the least from your directions on what I have to do to recover strength and a little liveliness."[24] At the same time, he was able to report on geological excursions that he had undertaken, referring to glaciers in the White Mountains! As Lizzie wrote to Brown-Séquard, "the mere fact of your presence here is so cheering to him that I think it does him more good than any remedy."[25]

During the 1870 Franco-Prussian War, Agassiz tried to organize another chair for Brown-Séquard at Harvard, but one "which would permit you to follow your researches without interruptions."[24] Late in 1871, Agassiz wrote to Brown-Séquard in Paris that, "I think every day of you, not only with affection but with the highest admiration ...."[26] One year later, Agassiz wrote urging Brown-Séquard to come to a meeting that he was planning in Cambridge.[27] This may have been the occasion in April 1873 when Brown-Séquard lectured in Boston to a large and enthusiastic audience that included Agassiz, Oliver Wendell Holmes, Putnam, and others. Brown-Séquard's account to his wife reveals the warmth of his relationship with Agassiz:

> The people laughed when they saw Agassiz and myself after the lecture, throw each of us in the arms of the other and kiss as if one of us was a woman. Agassiz is in most excellent spirits and good health. He received yesterday a letter from Mr. Anderson [a prosperous merchant, landowner, and sponsor] telling him that he can employ at once the $50,000 to organize laboratories. He will go to work at once, building not only a natural history museum, but also a Physiological Laboratory.[28]

It seems that Agassiz was hoping to establish for Brown-Séquard a well-paid chair of physiology at the School of Natural History that he was setting up on Penekese Island in Buzzard's Bay, on land deeded to him by John Anderson, a wealthy New York cigar merchant. The island was made up of more than one hundred acres and included a splendid mansion house. The school was to be the educational core of the Museum of Comparative Zoology at Harvard, but was to be financially independent. Agassiz, who first visited the island in April 1873, intended to erect a two-storey building, the lower level for laboratories and work and lecture space, and the upper for living quarters. He planned to enroll as students those who were already teaching natural history and to charge them nothing for tuition.[29] It was an ambitious plan, but Agassiz died a few months later and the school (the forerunner of the Marine Biological Laboratory in Woods Hole, Massachusetts) closed in 1875, after a fire and because of problems related to its location, even though it had attracted a large number of students,[30] some of whom were to achieve considerable prominence in their fields.

It was Brown-Séquard who cared for the 66-year-old Agassiz when he became terminally ill and died in December 1873, after another stroke that occurred the day after a birthday celebration for Lizzie at which—neglecting medical advice—he yielded to the temptations of a cigar.[31] As his friend, Brown-Séquard was invited to the funeral service in the college chapel. The family had appreciated his friendship with and care for the older man, and accepted with gratitude that the ailing scientist had "passed away at the height of his powers and in the midst of his labours."[32] Agassiz was buried at Mount Auburn, where his grave is marked by a massive granite boulder transported from the Alpine glacial moraine near his former home in Switzerland. For Lizzie, Agassiz's death left an intellectual emptiness that the love and comfort of her family could not entirely counter,[33] although she remained active in society, busy with educational endeavors, and was much involved in establishing a college where women could be instructed by Harvard faculty (Radcliffe College).

Clinical Practice and Publishing Ventures

In 1873, Brown-Séquard planned to settle permanently in practice in New York. After having negotiated for the preceding three or four years with the publishing house of Lippincott (in Philadelphia),[34] he finally started a new English-language journal, the *Archives of Scientific and Practical Medicine*, co-edited by Dr. Edward Constant Seguin (1843–1898). Seguin had studied neurology under Brown-Séquard and Charcot in Paris in the winter of 1869–1870, and then returned to New York to become professor of diseases of the nervous system at the College of Physicians and Surgeons. In addition to his neurological bent and his flair for teaching, he was interested in the measurement of temperature, introducing this into American clinical practice and devising the first form used in the United States to chart graphically the vital signs of temperature, pulse, and respiration.[G]

The new monthly *Archives* was intended to appeal to medical practitioners by its content of clinical papers or scientific papers of clinical relevance, and was to be available for an annual subscription of four dollars.[35] Part of the

---

[G] Dr. Seguin's later years were marked by a dreadful tragedy: in 1882, while he was out, his wife, who suffered from episodes of mild depression, blindfolded and tied the hands of their three children—aged 4, 5, and 6—before shooting them in the head and then turning the gun on herself. It is ironic that just a few years earlier, Seguin had written about the treatment at home of mild cases of melancholia.

reason for founding it was to provide an impetus for Brown-Séquard to complete "a good many papers which are half written and which I would most likely never finish,"[36] although he was still editing his French-language physiology journal. The first issue appeared in January 1873, but the new journal was short-lived. By March, Brown-Séquard had concluded that his publisher was paying him less that he deserved, and he determined to merge the journal with another in Boston or New York, or to give it up altogether if Lippincott were unwilling to part with it.[37] His relations with Lippincott became increasingly sour, to the extent that he came to believe that they had deliberately deceived the public by giving the publication date of one of his books as 1873 instead of 1860,[38] an unlikely explanation for what was surely an unfortunate mistake. In any event, he took the journal to Putnam's, another publisher, but it was beyond redemption and only five issues ever appeared.[39] This led to problems, as seven additional issues were due to those who had paid for an annual subscription. Correspondence between angry subscribers and the embarrassed publisher were particularly awkward because Brown-Séquard "flitted southward" and for several months could not be contacted.[40]

About one year later, he wrote from Paris and sent funds to reimburse subscribers for six of the issues that they had not received. Subscribers were promised that the remaining issue would be sent to them shortly, but the publisher never received any material for the missing number and eventually had to remit thirty-five cents to each of about a thousand dissatisfied subscribers.[40] Such heavy-handed dealings contrast with his sensitive approach to Baillière, his Paris publisher, when he wrote as a young man about a tardy submission on May 19, 1856: "I am convinced that you and I have much to gain thanks to the delay in my delivering the manuscript to you. As you know I have recently been awarded the prize for experimental physiology and, moreover, all the principal journals in Europe and the United States have taken an interest in my work and have given me high praise. Thanks to this ... the sales of my book will be increased considerably."[41]

Clinical practice in New York—like his new publishing venture—did not go as well as he had hoped. He had previously run from the oppressive hordes of patients seeking his care, but now found that he could not build up a successful practice. He lacked the easy manner and sympathetic nature of the society physician, but failed to recognize that the problem lay with himself. Instead, he preferred to believe that rich Americans were too busy to need his attention and their women used their "nerves" simply as a means to a prolonged visit to Europe, whereas poorer Americans were too ignorant or too patriotic to distinguish between an expert and an ignoramus.[42] He wrote of settling down, but was unsure whether this should be in Cincinnati, for Maria's sake, or in

Cambridge or Boston, which he preferred.[43] Regardless, he spent much of 1873 in traveling between various East Coast cities and in returning again to London and Paris. His letters to Maria are affectionate, but—as with his first wife—are focused on his own health and the heavy demands on his time.[44] He told her also about the oddities and eccentric personalities that he encountered, such as the physician who considered that, because young ladies had to study so hard just as they were reaching puberty, all but the best of them were out-of-sorts thereafter.[45] And he mused how one of his patients could complain about the size of his bill even as she expressed her boundless gratitude to him.[46]

Nevertheless, influential patients did come by appointment to consult him, regardless of whether he was in the United States or, as later, in Paris: archbishops and cardinals such as Charles Lavigerie[47]; the wealthy such as Leland Stanford[H] and his wife[48]; the well-placed such as Pedro d'Alcantara[I] (Emperor of Brazil)[49]; and the intelligentsia, such as his friend Louis Agassiz and the writer Alphonse Daudet. In most instances, details of the medical problems for which they sought out Brown-Séquard have been lost in the quicksands of time. The case of Senator Sumner is an interesting exception.

Senator Sumner

Charles Sumner (1811–1874) was one of Brown-Séquard's longstanding patients and one to whom he felt an especially close friendship. The Massachusetts statesman was renowned for his antislavery beliefs (which must have had an especial appeal to Brown-Séquard) and was a leader of the Republicans in the U.S. Senate during and after the American Civil War, when he fought for equal civil and voting rights for the freedmen and to block ex-Confederates from power. In May 1856, he was unexpectedly attacked with a heavy cane in the Senate by Preston "Bully" Brooks, congressman for South Carolina, apparently in retaliation for his wounding criticism of South Carolina

---

[H] Leland Stanford (1824–1893) was a railroad baron, business leader, governor of California, and U.S. senator. He endowed a private university in California in memory of his son (Leland Stanford Jr.), who died of typhoid fever in Italy while still a teenager.

[I] Dom Pedro d'Alcantara (1825–1891), the second and last Emperor of Brazil, was related to many of the royal houses of Europe. An enlightened patron of the arts and sciences, he made many reforms in Brazil and ultimately was successful in abolishing slavery. He was deposed by a military coup d'état in 1889, and spent his last years in exile in Europe. His ill health seems to have been attributed by the many physicians whom he consulted to diabetes, overwork, and the consequences of a malarial infection.

and its senator a few days earlier. The injuries were serious but not fatal. As he recovered, he developed headaches, back and leg pain, chest pains, weakness in the legs, fatigue, lassitude, and a variety of other nonspecific complaints. Some wondered whether his symptoms were feigned, despite a public announcement that he was suffering with "softening of the brain." His symptoms were worsened by mental strain, and his illness was punctuated by relapses ands remissions that were not helped by consultations with a number of medical specialists. In 1858, he finally consulted Brown-Séquard, who was then back in Paris after his brief sojourn in Virginia, and he was treated by cauterization some seven times, his back being burned by the application of *moxa* or red-hot irons (depending on the account)[50,51]; Sumner refused any anesthetic in the belief that he would get a better response to treatment, and his suffering must have been intense. Whether as a result of this counterirritant treatment or the baths and douches that he afterward took at Aix-les-Bains,[52,53] he was temporarily cured and returned to the Senate. The basis of his symptoms remains obscure and, certainly, many of them probably did not have a physical basis. Brown-Séquard believed that Sumner "... had no disease of the brain and no paralysis. He had only an irritation of the vasomotor nerves, at their exit from the spine."[50] His symptoms recurred episodically, however, and he remained in close contact with the peripatetic Brown-Séquard, sometimes corresponding with him daily.[52] The end came in March 1874, when he developed especially severe chest pain of cardiac origin and his physicians gave up any hope for his survival. Brown-Séquard, then in New York and familiar for years with Sumner's condition, was summoned to Washington, but arrived by train too late to be of any service.[51]

In February 1874, Brown-Séquard had begun a course of six lectures at Boston's Lowell Institute, as a tribute to Agassiz. He spoke on "nervous force," of the physical correlates of mental activity, based on clinical cases that he had observed. He devoted part of the fifth lecture to an account of his clinical experience with Sumner,[50] and at one point became so distressed that he could barely continue. Within a few weeks, however, he suffered a more personal loss.

Domestic and Professional Ups and Downs

In May 1874, two years after their marriage and a week after giving birth to a baby girl, Maria—who seems to have been mentally ill[54]—died, leaving Brown-Séquard a widower once more. The little girl was named Charlotte, despite the fact that an earlier daughter, born in 1860 and similarly named after Brown-Séquard's mother, had survived for only seven weeks. Over the following months, he kept himself busy with lectures in New York, Boston, Dublin, and London on a variety of neurological and physiological topics. Despite the professional insecurity of having no permanent appointment, he declined the offer of a chair of physiology at the University of Glasgow because of the harsh Scottish climate.

During the summer of 1875, he began experiments on rejuvenation, working with the family's permission at the private laboratory that Agassiz had used in his summer cottage at Nahant, a small coastal town a few miles north of Boston. These experiments were to lead to the work that he announced to the world in 1889, bringing on himself much derision and scorn even as he initiated modern hormone replacement therapy. He then returned to Europe, to make his home in Paris, but the next two or three years were to be the most difficult in his professional life.

In 1876, he began spending more and more time in the company of Emma Dakin—the English widow of an obscure painter, Thomas Doherty—and they became so close that, during enforced absences, they would often write to each other several times daily. Emma also took to caring for little Charlotte, thereby helping to keep from others their developing intimacy.[55]

They were apart for much of the time, however, with Brown-Séquard in Paris and Emma in England. Their letters emphasize Brown-Séquard's financial difficulties and the uncertainties of his life. He wanted to live in Paris, but worried about the cost. If he were to depend on clinical earnings, he might not cover the rent for a consulting room if only a few patients were referred to him. He was involved in a lawsuit concerning money owed him by a woman occupying his New York house, and success in the courts, together with money to be earned in England by lecturing, would give him some financial security. If he lost the case, however, he would have to move to London, where the cost of living was cheaper.[56,57] He mused about seeing patients for two days a week in a London hotel and spending the rest of the week in practice in Paris, traveling between the two cities by the night train.[55,57] It was apparent even to him, however, that family illness, delay of the cross-Channel ferry, or any medical emergency among his patients would disrupt such a plan.[58] He regretted not having rented (because of the cost) an apartment at the corner of the rue de Rivoli and the rue Castiglione in the heart of fashionable Paris "… as I have no doubt the place would have given me patients, as the Americans are stupid enough to look upon such things as a fine house and fine rooms as a sign of merit—and so are the French—but it is too late now …."[59]

As he ruminated about the future, he spent much of his time at the library of the Paris Faculty of Medicine, in Vulpian's laboratory, and at Masson's (his French publishers).[60] He accepted and then resigned from the chair of physiology at the

University of Geneva,[61] and became increasingly isolated in his views as a neurologist. In particular, he argued eloquently—but with ill-considered speculations and limited evidence—against the developing doctrine of functional localization within the brain, despite the mounting clinical and experimental evidence that certain portions of the cerebral cortex (the outer mantle of the brain) did indeed have specific functions.

Although he tried to set up in practice in Paris, he was disappointed at the small number of patients referred to him. He then tried his luck in London, but this led to difficulties with certain prominent physicians and especially with Dr. Radcliffe, who had succeeded him on the staff of the National Hospital and had taken over his house in Cavendish Square. An announcement was to be published in *The Lancet* that Brown-Séquard intended to resume practice in London, but Radcliffe considered this unethical and feared that the resulting competition would be detrimental to his own practice.[62] Brown-Séquard was distressed enough by his response to discuss the matter with both Dr. Wakley (the powerful editor of *The Lancet*) and Dr. Quain,[J,63] who agreed that no valid reason existed to withhold publication of such a notice, especially since Brown-Séquard had not sold his practice to Radcliffe or been paid by him for vacating the Cavendish Square property. In any event, Brown-Séquard's attempt to reclaim his position as a leading specialist in diseases of the nervous system was not an immediate success[64] for times had changed, others had seized the opportunities that he had cast aside, and a fading reputation alone was insufficient to attract patients. Indeed, he could not earn enough even to cover the office rent. He briefly wondered about some sort of professional association with his old assistant, the now-renowned Dr. Hughlings Jackson, but was too embarrassed to proceed.[65,66] Matters looked so bleak that he wrote to Emma, "I dread immensely the fast approaching moment when I will have to beg the help of friends ...."[67]

When friends did try to help, Brown-Séquard could not bring himself to accept. Thomas Huxley wrote from Edinburgh, "... if you will let me know how I can serve you, it will be a pleasure to me ..."[68] Brown-Séquard's only consolation was in Emma and his daughter. He doted on Charlotte and found evidence of great intellect in all that she did, writing with delight of her evident originality to Emma.[69] As for Emma herself, she was acquiescent, thoughtful, and sensible, a kindly and affectionate soul who was content to

---

[J] Sir Richard Quain (1816–1898), an Irish physician who practiced in London, held influential offices in various professional (medical) societies and edited a widely respected textbook, *The Dictionary of Medicine,* to which Brown-Séquard contributed chapters on epilepsy and spinal irritation.

leave all major decisions to him. She wrote to him at least daily, often writing between seven and ten pages at a time, and her trust sometimes worried Brown-Séquard. In October he wrote to her from Paris, "I prefer blame, I prefer criticism to eulogy. I don't ask you to blame me unless you find cause for that, but I pray you to express more moderately, if at all, your appreciation of any merit I may have .... To take an instance, it reads like a sarcasm (certainly not intended) that I am brave—while, alas! I am a great coward and constantly suffer for my cowardice. I am all the time in dread of this or that thing. I create dangers to tremble about them ...."[70]

In November 1876, Brown-Séquard—unhappy, infirm with arthritis, and on the verge of despair—made his way to Dublin and its medical community. Here, at last, he met again with success in the lecture hall, and the patients flocked back to him during his brief visit.[71-73] His visit to Ireland seemed to herald a change in his fortunes. Although he traveled frequently between London and Paris over the following weeks, he was able to spend more time with Emma and Charlotte, and his professional earnings in London began to increase. In one encouraging fortnight, he was able to earn eighty pounds, despite the fact that one of his patients was himself a professional colleague from whom Brown-Séquard—despite his own recent problems—refused to accept any payment.

In 1877, he married Emma at the British Embassy in Paris, then returned to the United States, to lecture in Cambridge, New York, and elsewhere while his wife and Charlotte remained in Boston. The litigation concerning his New York house was finally settled, but the verdict went against him. The woman who owed him money claimed that the house was unhealthy. Although she swayed the jury, no damages were allowed against Brown-Séquard.[74]

On 10 February 1878, Claude Bernard died. The noted scientist, professor of medicine at the Collège de France, had served France well, and the government accorded him the state funeral generally reserved for royalty, military leaders, and statesmen. The ceremony at the Church of St. Sulpice was followed by a funeral procession across Paris to the famed Père Lachaise Cemetery, where he was buried with honor on Saturday, 16 February. Brown-Séquard was in the United States when he heard about the death of his old rival (see Chapter 5) and the vacancy thus created at the Collège de France. That venerable institution, founded in 1530 by François I and located close to the Sorbonne in the Latin quarter of Paris, is a center of advanced education that functions independently of the university and does not need to tailor its courses to satisfy examination requirements. The vacant chair of medicine represented a wonderful opportunity—a prestigious appointment in the city where he wished to live and had himself studied medicine, an appointment that offered financial stability and permitted him to follow his own interests without the usual burden of didactic teaching required of professors. He returned immediately to the French capital to promote his own candidacy. To avoid any problems that his British nationality might pose, he became a French citizen.[75] In support of his application for the chair, he published an account of his scientific writings, which numbered more than three hundred original papers, listing these by subject and briefly summarizing the significance of the findings that they reported.[76] One hundred eight-two publications dealt with the physiology and pathology of the nervous system, twenty-two with experimental epilepsy, twelve related to vision, nine to the regulation of body temperature, sixty-two focused on a variety of other physiological topics, and fourteen were on miscellaneous subjects.

His candidacy was probably helped by a report—authored by Claude Bernard at the request of Napoleon III and published some ten years earlier—on the status and achievements of physiology in France.[77-79] The report referred to the work of some forty scientists, and repeatedly singled out Brown-Séquard for special mention.[79] He also received strong support from Marcelin Berthelot (1827–1907),[K] the renown organic chemist who had been appointed inspector-general of higher education in 1876, and thus had a strong influence on the selection process.[80] He was ranked highly by the Section of Medicine and Surgery of the Académie des Sciences,[81] but was their second choice for the chair.[L] However, the professors at the Collège voted by a large majority to put him at the top of the list, according to a report by Edouard Laboulaye (1811–1883; administrator and president of the Assembly of Professors) and Leon Renier (1809–1885; vice president and professor of Roman antiquities). Their choice was based on his record and in the belief that he would maintain the experimental tradition of Magendie and Claude Bernard, thereby ensuring that the field would continue to advance.[82]

[K] Berthelot was professor of chemistry at the Collège de France for more than forty years and was a pioneer in the synthesis of organic (i.e., carbon-containing) compounds. He subsequently became interested in thermochemistry (chemical reactions that absorb or produce heat) and then in explosives, which gave him an important national role during the Franco-Prussian war. His other interests included the history of science. Toward the end of his career, he became involved increasingly with the government and served as minister of public instruction (education) and later as foreign minister.

[L] The top-rated candidate is referred to only as Dareste, but is almost certainly Gabriel Madeleine Camille (Camille) Dareste (1822–1899), a French physician and experimental embryologist who held various chairs before becoming director of a laboratory of teratology, where he worked on the artificial production of developmental monstrosities in chicks in order to understand the mechanisms that lead to their occurrence in nature.

On August 3, 1878, Brown-Séquard was appointed to the chair.[83] His traveling days were over, his academic dignity restored, his home finally established in France.

References and Source Notes

1. Agassiz JLR [Louis]. Letter to the Emperor Napoleon in Paris dated 3 November 1868. MS 981/3. Archives, Royal College of Physicians, London.
2. Brown-Séquard CE. Letter to Victor Duruy, Minister of Education, dated 25 December 1868. MS 980/31. Archives, Royal College of Physicians, London.
3. Duruy V. Letter to Brown-Séquard dated 26 December 1868. MS 980/32. Archives, Royal College of Physicians, London.
4. Imperial Decree dated 6 February 1869, granting Brown (sic) the right to live in France with full civil rights. MS 987/7. Archives, Royal College of Physicians, London.
5. Announcement. Dr. Brown-Séquard. *Br Med J*, 1:52, 1869.
6. Medical Miscellany. *Boston Med Surg J*, 80:444, 1869.
7. Waller A. Letter to Brown-Séquard dated 17 July 1870. MS 980/35. Archives, Royal College of Physicians, London.
8. Invitation to Brown-Séquard to dine with Prince and Princess Napoleon on 3 April 1869. MS 980/34. Archives, Royal College of Physicians, London.
9. Huxley TH. Letter to Brown-Séquard dated 3 August 1870. MS 981/63. Archives, Royal College of Physicians, London.
10. Westacott E. *A century of vivisection and anti-vivisection* (p. 25). Ashingdon (England): CW Daniel Co., 1949.
11. Mitchell S. *Frances Power Cobbe: Victorian journalist, feminist, reformer*. Charlottesville: University of Virginia Press, 2004.
12. Leffingwell A. *Vivisection in America*. London: Macmillan, 1894.
13. Editorial. British Association for the Advancement of Science. *Lancet*, 2:436–438, 1870.
14. Huxley TH. Letter to Brown-Séquard dated 12 March, 1876. MS 981/64. Archives, Royal College of Physicians, London.
15. Huxley L. *The life and letters of Thomas Henry Huxley* (Vol. 2, pp. 463–464). New York: Appleton, 1901.
16. Brown-Séquard CE. Notes on vivisection (undated). MS 993. Royal College of Physicians, London.
17. Westacott E. *A century of vivisection and anti-vivisection* (pp. 170–173). Ashingdon (England): CW Daniel Co., 1949.
18. Anonymous. A l'Académie. *Le Gaulois*, 2 July 1885.
19. Rouget FA. *Brown-Séquard et son oeuvre. Esquisse biographique* (p. 61). Ile Maurice: General Printing & Stationery Co., 1930.
20. Anonymous. Détails biographiques sur M. Brown-Séquard. *Le Moniteur Universel*, July 1, 1885.
21. Anonymous. Vivisection in France. *Med Record*, 14 July 1883.
22. Anonymous. Agassiz on France. *New York Times*, 10 February 1871.
23. Minister of Education (France). Letter to Brown-Séquard dated 16 April 1872. MS 980/39. Archives, Royal College of Physicians, London.
24. Agassiz JLR [Louis]. Letter to Brown-Séquard dated 25 July 1870. MS 981/2. Archives, Royal College of Physicians, London.
25. Agassiz EC [Elizabeth]. Letter to Brown-Séquard dated 11 February (? year). MS 981/5. Archives, Royal College of Physicians, London.

26. Agassiz JLR [Louis]. Letter to Brown-Séquard dated 7 November 1871. MS 981/7. Archives, Royal College of Physicians, London.
27. Agassiz JLR [Louis]. Letter to Brown-Séquard dated 3 November 1872. MS 981/8. Archives, Royal College of Physicians, London.
28. Brown-Séquard CE. Letter to his wife Maria dated 6 April 1873(?). MS 978/6. Archives, Royal College of Physicians, London.
29. Anonymous. Penekese Island. Transfer of the island by Mr. Anderson to Prof. Agassiz—provisions of the deed. *New York Times*, 23 April 1873.
30. Anonymous. The Anderson School of Natural History. *Nature*, 11:167–168, 1874.
31. Lurie E. *Louis Agassiz: A life in science*. Chicago: University of Chicago Press, 1960.
32. Agassiz A. Letter to Brown-Séquard dated 15 December 1873. MS981/12. Archives, Royal College of Physicians, London.
33. Agassiz EC [Elizabeth]. Letter to Brown-Séquard dated 19 December 1873(?). MS 981/13. Archives, Royal College of Physicians, London.
34. Lippincott JB. Letters to Brown-Séquard dated 21 October and 12 December 1868. MSS 989/1, 989/2. Archives, Royal College of Physicians, London.
35. Brown-Séquard CE, Seguin EC. Prospectus. *Archives of scientific and practical medicine*. MS 999/7 (12a). Archives, Royal College of Physicians, London.
36. Brown-Séquard CE. Undated letter to his publishers (unnamed). MS 989/6. Archives, Royal College of Physicians, London.
37. Brown-Séquard CE. Letters to his wife Maria dated 2 April, 3 April, 10 April, 12 April, 16 April, 19 April 1873. MSS 978/4, 978/5, 978/10, 978/12, 978/17, 978/19. Archives, Royal College of Physicians, London.
38. Brown-Séquard CE. Letter to his wife Maria dated 20 April 1873. MS 978/20. Archives, Royal College of Physicians, London.
39. Putnam GH. Letters to Brown-Séquard dated 22 May and 20 September 1873. MSS 989/4 and 989/5. Archives, Royal College of Physicians, London.
40. Putnam GH. *George Palmer Putnam: A memoir together with a record of the earlier years of the publishing house founded by him* (pp. 436–437). New York: GP Putnam's Sons, 1912.
41. Régnier C. Jean-Baptiste Baillière (1797–1885): the pioneering publisher who promoted French medicine throughout the world. *Medicographia*, 27:87–96, 2005.
42. Anonymous. Death of Dr. Brown-Séquard. *The Standard (London)*, 3 April 1894.
43. Brown-Séquard CE. Undated letter to his wife Maria. MS 978/13. Archives, Royal College of Physicians, London.
44. Brown-Séquard CE. Correspondence with his wife Maria dated 1872–1873. MSS 978/1–22 Archives, Royal College of Physicians, London.
45. Brown-Séquard CE. Letter to his wife Maria dated 7 April 1873. MS 978/7. Archives, Royal College of Physicians, London.
46. Brown-Séquard CE. Letter to his wife Maria dated 15 April 1873. MS 978/15. Archives, Royal College of Physicians, London.
47. Lavigerie CMA. Telegram to Brown-Séquard regarding his symptoms and asking his advice, dated 28 September 1892. MS 980/74. Archives, Royal College of Physicians, London.
48. Stanford L. Letter to Brown-Séquard dated 31 August 1883. MS 980/50. Archives, Royal College of Physicians, London.
49. Pedro d'Alcantara. Letters to Brown-Séquard dated 24 February and 29 June 1876, concerning health matters. MSS 981/21 and 22. Archives, Royal College of Physicians, London.
50. Chaplin J, Chaplin JD. *Life of Charles Sumner* (pp. 313–320). Dover, NH: Lothrop, H., 1874.

51. Anonymous. Death of Senator Sumner; last hours of the great statesman. Charles Sumner. *New York Times*, 12 March 1874.
52. Sumner C. Letters to Brown-Séquard, reporting on his health, 1858–1874. MSS 981/179–203. Archives, Royal College of Physicians, London.
53. Stearns FP. *Cambridge sketches*. Philadelphia: Lippincott, 1905.
54. Holmes G. The National Hospital, Queen Square, 1860–1948. Edinburgh: Livingstone, 1954.
55. Brown-Séquard CE. Letter to Emma Dakin dated 6 September 1876. MS 979/26. Archives, Royal College of Physicians, London.
56. Brown-Séquard CE. Letter to Emma Dakin dated 3 September 1876. MS 979/21. Archives, Royal College of Physicians, London.
57. Brown-Séquard CE. Letter to Emma Dakin dated 5 September 1876 (morning). MS 979/24. Archives, Royal College of Physicians, London.
58. Brown-Séquard CE. Letter to Emma Dakin dated 7 September 1876. MS 979/27. Archives, Royal College of Physicians, London.
59. Brown-Séquard CE. Letter to Emma Dakin, undated but probably written in October 1876. MS 979/109. Archives, Royal College of Physicians, London.
60. Brown-Séquard CE. Correspondence with Emma Dakin. MSS 979/1–162. Archives, Royal College of Physicians, London.
61. République et Canton de Genève. Extrait des Registres du Conseil d'État du 21 Mars 1876. [Official acceptance of Brown-Séquard's resignation from the position of professor of physiology in the Faculty of Medicine at the University of Geneva.]
62. Brown-Séquard CE. Letter to Emma Dakin dated 3 November 1876. MSS 979/48. Archives, Royal College of Physicians, London.
63. Brown-Séquard CE. Undated letter to Emma Dakin. MS 979/107. Archives, Royal College of Physicians, London.
64. Brown-Séquard CE. Letters to Emma Dakin dated 8 November 1876. MS 979/57 and MS 979/58. Archives, Royal College of Physicians, London.
65. Brown-Séquard CE. Letter to Emma Dakin dated 7 November 1876. MS 979/54. Archives, Royal College of Physicians, London.
66. Brown-Séquard CE. Letter to Emma Dakin dated 8 November 1876. MS 979/60. Archives, Royal College of Physicians, London.
67. Brown-Séquard CE. Letter to Emma Dakin dated 16 November 1876. MS 979/65. Archives, Royal College of Physicians, London.
68. Huxley TH. Letter to Brown-Séquard dated 30 June 1876. MS 981/66. Archives, Royal College of Physicians, London.
69. Brown-Séquard CE. Letter to Emma Dakin dated 19 October 1876. MS 979/45. Archives, Royal College of Physicians, London.
70. Brown-Séquard CE. Letter to Emma Dakin dated 18 October 1876. MS 979/44. Archives, Royal College of Physicians, London.
71. Brown-Séquard CE. Letter to Emma Dakin dated 23 November 1876. MS 979/80. Archives, Royal College of Physicians, London.
72. Brown-Séquard CE. Letter to Emma Dakin dated 24 November 1876. MS 979/83. Archives, Royal College of Physicians, London.
73. Brown-Séquard CE. Letter to Emma Dakin dated 25 November 1876. MS 979/84. Archives, Royal College of Physicians, London.
74. Brown-Séquard CE. Letter to his wife Emma dated 16 November 1877. MS 979/114. Archives, Royal College of Physicians, London.
75. Presidential Decree dated 21 May 1878, granting French citizenship to Brown (sic). MS 987/6. Archives, Royal College of Physicians, London.

76. Brown-Séquard CE. *Notice sur les travaux scientifiques de M.C.-E. Brown-Séquard.* Paris: Masson, 1878.
77. Olmsted JMD, Olmsted EH. *Claude Bernard and the experimental method in medicine.* New York: Schuman, 1952.
78. Tarshis J. *Claude Bernard: Father of experimental medicine.* New York: Dial Press, 1968.
79. Bernard C. *Rapport sur les Progrès et la Marche de la Physiologie Générale en France.* Paris: L'Imprimerie Impériale, 1867.
80. Delhoume L. *De Claude Bernard à d'Arsonval* (p. 251). Paris: Baillière, 1939.
81. Vulpian E. Rapport de M. Vulpian—sur les travaux de M. Brown-Séquard. Archives, Académie des Sciences, Institut de France, Paris.
82. Laboulaye E, Renier L. Rapport sur les travaux et les titres scientifique de M. C. E. Brown-Séquard. Archives, Académie des Sciences, Institut de France, Paris.
83. Le Président de la République Française. Décret, 3 August 1878 [appointing Brown-Séquard to the Chair of Medicine at the Collège de France]. MS c-XII-1A. Archives, Collège de France, Paris.

10

Thoughts About the Brain

THE MOST OBVIOUS parts of the human brain are the large, paired cerebral hemispheres; these are connected to the spinal cord by the brainstem, which is composed of the midbrain and hindbrain, and by the cerebellum (or "little brain") and its two hemispheres, which covers the hindbrain and fills the back of the head. On casual inspection, then, the brain appears physically duplicated, with the right and left cerebral and cerebellar hemispheres overlying the midline brainstem, which is also duplicated. Such duality, commented upon even by Hippocrates, still troubles many neurologists, even as they remain unconcerned that we have, for example, two lungs and two kidneys.[1] This duality and the specific relationship of each hemisphere to the rest of the body puzzled many biologists and philosophers in the nineteenth century as well. Neurologists now accept that the nervous system is crossed in its functional organization, so that the right hemisphere is concerned with motor and sensory phenomena primarily involving the left side of the body, and vice versa, but the reason for such complexity is not clear. The cerebral hemispheres are divided into lobes: the frontal lobe is at the front of the brain, the occipital lobe is at the back, and the parietal lobe is between them; the temporal lobe is below and on the outer side of the frontal and parietal lobes.

In Chapter 3, it was remarked that the gray, outer mantle of the brain is formed of nerve cell bodies, and the white inside of the brain is largely composed of nerve fibers (*axons*) running between different parts of the brain or between the brain and spinal cord. Gray masses of nerve cells exist within the white matter of the brain, where they make up various nuclei or relay stations.

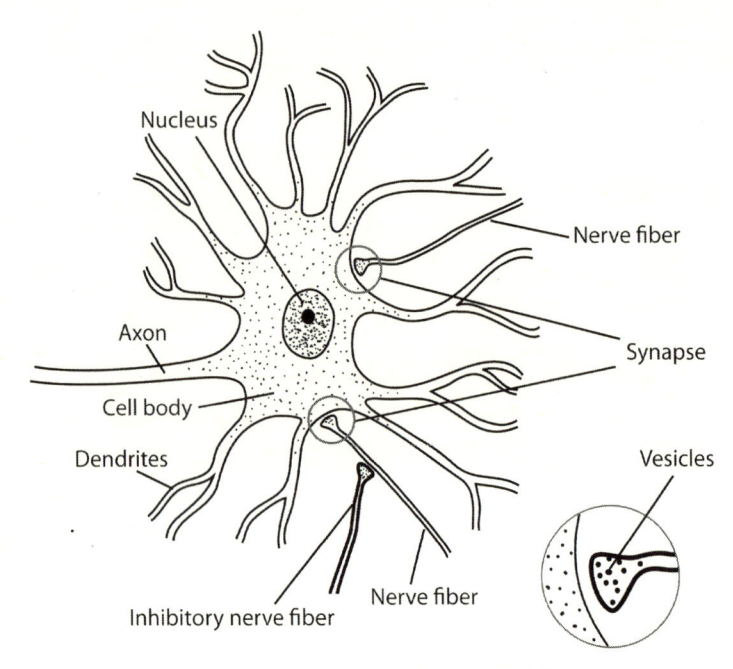

FIGURE 10.1 The cell body, axon, and dendrites of a nerve cell. The inset figure shows a magnified view of one of the many synapses on the cell body or dendrites.

The nerve cell body has numerous projections (*dendrites*) from it that resemble the branches of a tree and enlarge its surface area; it also gives rise to the longer *axon* that passes to another nerve cell, often in other parts of the nervous system (Figure 10.1). A slight space exists between the end of the axon and the neuron to which it connects; at this *synapse*, a chemical neurotransmitter is released from the presynaptic nerve endings and excites the postsynaptic neuron. This neuron receives inputs from many sources, some of which are excitatory and others inhibitory, and whether it discharges depends on the sum of these inputs. The outcome—whether the postsynaptic neuron discharges—also depends on where the input is received: in other words, on the geometry of the neuron and its dendrites. Input on dendrites may be less effective in exciting the neuron that input direct to the cell body, and the shape and location of dendritic branching may also be important. The excitability of different neurons varies, and the excitability of the same neuron varies with time and preceding activity. Further, the input to a nerve cell may be altered before it actually reaches the cell by a process called *presynaptic inhibition* or *excitation*; nerve fibers act on the endings of other axons, inhibiting or exciting them before they can affect the target postsynaptic neuron. Neurons do not respond in a graded manner but either discharge or do not discharge in an "all-or-none" manner once they are excited beyond a certain threshold; the character of the response (whether a sustained or single discharge, for example) varies with the neuron.

The notion that the brain is arranged in a hierarchical manner, that is, in various "levels," depending on when certain parts evolved, became popular during the nineteenth century. The more primitive animals were supposed to have only the lowest (least organized) level of the central nervous system (the spinal cord and hindbrain, i.e., pons and medulla—see p. 35), where all parts of the body were represented, as were vital control functions such as of the circulation and respiration; a middle level was present in the cerebral hemispheres, where representation was more complex, and a highest (most organized) level in the front of the cerebral hemispheres was supposed to relate to consciousness and the mind itself. It was envisioned that the higher centers exerted a chronic suppressive effect on the lower centers and that this inhibitory effect was released by disease. Such concepts are still regarded as valid today.[A]

Nerve fibers within the spinal cord or brainstem are said to be *ascending* when they transmit impulses up toward higher levels of the central nervous system, or *descending* when the reverse is true. Ascending fibers or pathways are generally sensory or afferent, conveying information to the brain, whereas descending fibers or paths are typically motor or efferent, leading to activation of muscles, glands, or other effector structures. The more direct the pathway, the less modification is possible of the information that it conveys. Some pathways that involve the central nervous system involve only two neurons and thus a single synapse, whereas others involve many synapses (i.e., are polysynaptic), convey information more slowly, and allow it to be modified. An analogy can be made with airplane travel: on direct nonstop flights from San Francisco to New York, the passengers disembarking are the same ones who boarded the plane some six hours earlier; there are also longer flights that go

---

[A] Patients who are in coma with, for example, an expanding brain tumor in the cerebral hemisphere have disturbances of function that initially reflect involvement of "high" and then progressively "lower" levels of the central nervous system. Thus, the pupillary responses to light are initially preserved but come to be lost, reflex eye movements come to be disturbed, and painful stimulation leads to responses that vary from purposive (the arms reach toward the painful stimulus), to decorticate posturing (the arms flex purposelessly at the elbows), and then decerebrate posturing (arms extend), until finally no response occurs as brain function is increasingly impaired. See also: Hughlings Jackson J. Evolution and dissolution of the nervous system. In Taylor J, ed., *Selected writings of John Hughlings Jackson* (Vol. 2, pp. 45–75). London: Hodder & Stoughton, 1932.

to New York via Chicago, and on these less-direct flights the passengers who arrive at the final destination some eight or nine hours later are not necessarily all of those who boarded originally in San Francisco, for some will have remained in Chicago whereas others may have first joined the flight there.

The basic unit of neural function is the *reflex*. The simplest reflexes, such as the spinal stretch reflex (which occurs when a muscle is suddenly stretched and restores the muscle to its original length), involve an afferent (sensory) neuron whose axon conveys information to the central nervous system and an efferent (motor) neuron whose axon goes to an effector structure, such as a muscle (Figure 10.2). Such simple reflexes do not allow the sophisticated activities exhibited by many animals. More complex reflexes involve one or more neurons between the afferent and efferent arcs (intermediate neurons) in the spinal cord; with even greater complexity, the afferent or efferent loop comes to involve several neurons at different levels of the central nervous system. This arrangement permits the reflex to be modified, and allows for a variety of responses and for the production of more coordinated, complex responses. Some very complicated reflex responses are organized at a purely spinal level.

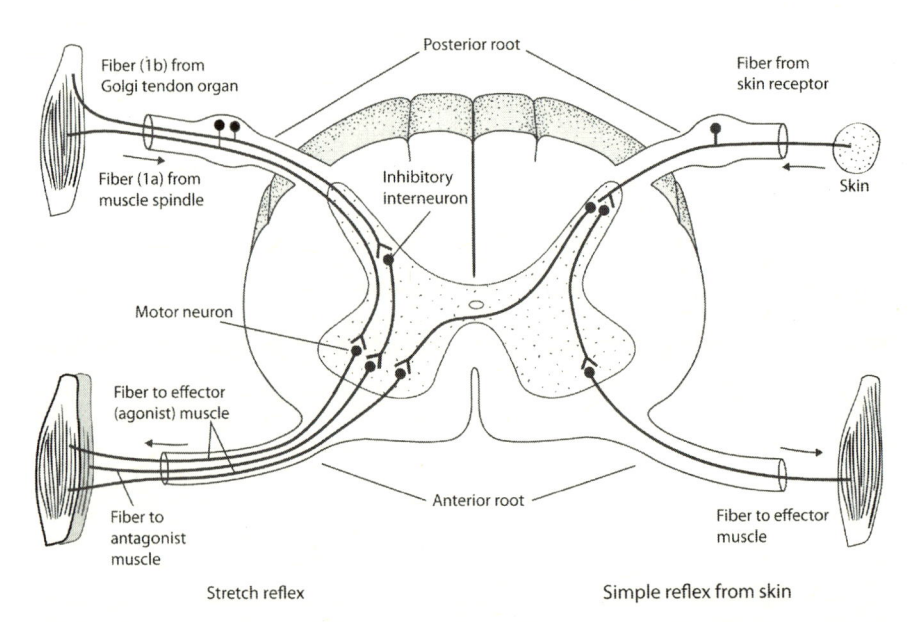

FIGURE 10.2 The stretch reflex (*left side of illustration*) involves a sensory neuron conveying information to the spinal cord and an efferent (motor) neuron whose axon goes to the stretched muscle. More complex reflexes involve one or more interneurons, that is, neurons interposed between the sensory and motor neurons. A simple reflex from the skin is shown on the right side of the illustration and involves just one interneuron.

A good example is the scratch reflex of animals such as cats and dogs: an irritant on the skin is localized and the animal then adopts a stable posture involving just two or three limbs, allowing the remaining limb to be brought to the site of irritation and scratch repetitively until the source of irritation has been removed. Other complicated responses involve the brain.

How does the brain work? How does it organize and control movement or behavior? How does it make use of the information coming to it through the senses and enable us to understand the environment in which we live? The ability of the brain or spinal cord to coordinate sensory information with motor performance indicates that it has the ability to activate or excite some parts of the nervous system (and its related effector structures, such as the muscles) while, at the same time, turning off or inhibiting other parts. Even the simplest movement requires both excitatory and inhibitory influences. When the elbow is to be bent (flexed), for example, the central nervous system excites those of its contained nerve cells that activate the muscles bending the elbow (flexors) and inhibits those opposing this movement (extensor muscles).

Functional Processes

In 1845, the Weber brothers[B] reported that the contraction of the heart could be inhibited (so that the heart was slowed or arrested) by stimulation of the so-called vagus nerve, which passes to the heart from the base of the brain. This was a remarkable finding, as it was widely believed then that positive—rather than negative—effects followed nerve stimulation, and it strongly influenced the young Brown-Séquard, who repeated the experiments himself. The inhibition in this instance actually occurs peripherally (i.e., beyond the confines of the brain), but in 1863, experimental evidence was obtained by a Russian, Ivan Sechenov, that inhibition also occurred within the central nervous system. He sectioned the brain of frogs at different levels and found that limb reflexes (the withdrawal of the leg from the painful stimulus of a dilute acid) could be depressed by stimulation of the exposed midbrain.[2] From this and related work, Sechenov concluded that reflexes may be either excitatory or inhibitory and that they could themselves be augmented or inhibited; this led him to believe that mental and voluntary activity were simply the

---

[B] The physicist Eduard Friedrich Weber (1806–1871) and the physiologist Ernst Heinrich Weber (1795–1878) stopped the heart by connecting the nostril and spinal cord of a frog with an electromagnetic apparatus. They presented their findings to the Congress of Italian Naturalists in 1845.

expression of modulated reflexes, a view that was not popular with the Russian government and religious authorities of the day.[C]

These inhibitory phenomena[D] intrigued Brown-Séquard, who had been fascinated for several years by the depressor effect on cardiac and respiratory movements of transecting the base of the brain, a point that he discussed in his 1860 book.[3] He returned to the subject later in his career, publishing a number of reports concerning the occurrence and significance of such phenomena.[4-14] Indeed, it was Brown-Séquard who really introduced the term "inhibition" into the French scientific literature. He also attempted to integrate physiology with pathology, with especial regard to the influences of one part of the central nervous system on other parts.[15]

First referring specifically in 1873 to the phenomenon as the basis of symptoms of cerebral disease, he wrote in his short-lived American journal that "all the parts of the brain ... [are] able, under irritation, to act on any other of its parts, modifying their activity, so as to destroy, or diminish, or to increase and to morbidly alter it."[4] It is not entirely clear what he meant by "irritation" (was it the stimulation or destruction of a focal cerebral region?), but clearly Brown-Séquard is describing effects that occur at sites distant to the involved region and that differ in character at different sites. In a subsequent flood of papers or communications to learned societies, he reported that lesions in a variety of locations in the brain or spinal cord could affect the excitability of other regions of the central nervous system,[9] and even that cutting the sciatic nerve (a major nerve in the leg) or spinal cord on one side in various animals was followed immediately by diminished excitability of the opposite side of the brain,[7,9] including the so-called motor centers (discussed later), whereas excitability was sometimes increased on the same side as the nerve or spinal cord lesion.[10,12] In these reports, Brown-Séquard generally focused more on inhibitory phenomena (i.e., the reduction of excitability) than on excitatory effects, and he failed to account for the basis or cause of the phenomena that he described.[15]

Nevertheless, Brown-Séquard reached several important conclusions from such work, probably more from intuition than reasoned judgment. First, lesions

---

[C] Ivan Sechenov (1829–1905), Russian physiologist, championed the concept of inhibitory influences of the brain on spinal reflexes. He showed that external stimuli could elicit brain reflexes, and believed that reflexes were the basis of mental activity.

[D] In psychology, ill-defined concepts of inhibition had been popular for many years—centuries—as a means of explaining aspects of mental activity and the control of impulsive behavior. This is discussed further by Smith R. *Inhibition: History and meaning in the sciences of mind and brain.* Berkeley: University of California Press, 1992. See also MacMillan M. The concept of inhibition in some nineteenth century theories of thinking. *Brain Cogn*, 30: 4–19, 1996.

localized to one part of the brain could influence the responses of other cerebral regions and of the spinal cord, on either the same or opposite side. Second, such localized lesions could excite some regions of the nervous system even as they inhibited other areas. These two conclusions suggested a level of interaction and dynamic interplay within the central nervous system that seemed to conflict with the growing belief of contemporary scientists that localized areas of the brain had discrete and specific functions. He also concluded that lesions of the spinal cord or a peripheral nerve could inhibit regions of the opposite side of the brain; in other words, that, contrary to the beliefs of his colleagues, there was peripheral modulation of the function of the central nervous system, as well as the converse. Finally, he believed that spinal lesions could inhibit the reflex properties of other spinal areas, both proximal and distal to the lesion, implying a greater degree of spinal integration than had previously been recognized. Such concepts were correct, but his failure to gain their acceptance surely related to the sloppy manner in which he conducted his experiments or reported them to his contemporaries. Most reports involved extrapolation from ambiguous clinical case descriptions or related to poorly designed experiments so lacking in the detail that makes up the substance of any scientific study that they were hard to take seriously. His reasoning was convoluted and opaque, his hypotheses poorly substantiated, his publications nonsubstantive and unconvincing. Indeed, his continuing opposition to the concept of discrete localization of function in the brain left him on the fringe of science as something of an outdated and irrelevant crank.

For all his failings, Brown-Séquard suggested answers to questions that were yet to be formulated about issues of fundamental importance. He also revealed inconvenient weaknesses in theories that others found attractive and that perhaps were not receiving the critical scrutiny to which they should have been subjected. But his greatest contribution was to emphasize that the activity of the nervous system should be considered in terms of processes rather than anatomical structures, a major step for which he has never received proper credit. He had conceived intuitively that one part of the central nervous system can exert inhibitory or excitatory ("dynamogenic") influences on distant parts, and that these opposing forces have a major operational role in ensuring the modulation, coordination, and integration of different functions.

Brown-Séquard was selected by an advisory committee consisting of Charcot, Vulpian, Gosselin, Richet, and Paul Bert[E] to receive the 1884 Prix

---

[E] Paul Bert (1833–1886), who chaired the committee that nominated Brown-Séquard for the Prix Lallemand, was a French physiologist, anticlerical politician, and diplomat. Appointed governor-general of what is now Vietnam, he died there of dysentery. He studied the effects

Lallemand of the Académie des Sciences (established for work on the nervous system).[16] They singled out for particular commendation his demonstration that two fundamental processes (inhibition and excitation) regulated the operation of the nervous system. They accepted that the manner in which he had interpreted his experimental observations had led him to oppose the now-accepted doctrine of the cerebral localization of motor function, but recognized that he had opened up a new chapter in the story concerning the properties and functions of the nervous system. Given this recognition by such an influential body, it may seem surprising that his beliefs were so disregarded by others. In addition to the reasons given earlier, this was partly because he seemed to extravagantly attribute virtually every aspect of neurological dysfunction to the distant effects of a lesion of the nervous system, and because he used this concept as an alternative explanation for the phenomena ascribed by others to the increasingly popular notion of localized function in the central nervous system.

The concept of two central regulatory processes governing the activity of the nervous system subsequently gained wide acceptance, largely as a result of the meticulous and elegant experimental work of an English physiologist, Charles Sherrington,[F] especially in the early part of the twentieth century. Brown-Séquard's concepts clearly influenced him for, in a brief paper published in 1893, when he first became involved with studying inhibitory phenomena, Sherrington wrote, "It is interesting for the study of the functions of the cerebral cortex to find experimentally that it has not only an excitatory but also an inhibitory action .... M. Brown-Séquard has for a long time emphasized this dual action, and in his writings he refers to dynamogenic and also inhibitory activities of the cortex."[17] He went on to report how he had shown in monkeys that stimulation of the frontal cortex so as to cause deviation of the eyes to the opposite side is accompanied by an inhibition of muscles

---

of barometric pressure on the body, including the phenomenon of altitude sickness (which affects people at high altitudes—and thus low air pressure—such as mountain climbers and aviators). He also studied decompression sickness ("the bends") that occurs in subjects under high pressure (such as divers), determined that this was due to the formation of bubbles of nitrogen in the circulation, and indicated how it could be avoided (slow decompression with stops; recompression; and oxygen therapy). His work made possible the later exploration of space, as well as the depths of the oceans.

[F] Sir Charles Scott Sherrington (1857–1952), British scientist, received the Nobel Prize in Physiology or Medicine in 1932. He was professor of physiology at the University of Liverpool and then at Oxford. His book, *The Integrative Action of the Nervous System*, remains a classic in the field. He had a major role in showing the presence and importance of reciprocal innervation, by which the activation of a muscle leads to the inhibition of its antagonist (opposing) muscles.

opposing the movement. Over the following years, he provided the experimental evidence that inhibition was an important coordinating factor in the operation of the central nervous system by its interaction with excitatory processes.[2] He was to receive the Nobel Prize for Physiology or Medicine for this work.

The Anatomy of Brain Function

It has been debated for years whether the brain operates as a single unit or with specific functions localized to discrete cerebral regions.[18–21] The concept of cerebral localization had a remarkable and somewhat shaky beginning. In the latter half of the eighteenth century, the functions of the brain were poorly understood, although it was known that some parts looked and felt different than others. In this context, the Austrian anatomist Franz Josef Gall (1758–1828) achieved considerable notoriety by suggesting that different mental functions originated in different and discrete parts of the brain. The opposition he faced was considerable, not least because religious doctrine held that mental activity and the "mind" itself to be distinct from the operation of the brain. Despite this, the discipline that resulted—phrenology (from *phrenos*, mind; *logos*, study)—flourished and initially had quite a following. Gall and his disciple Johann Gaspar Spurzheim (1776–1832) believed—without a shred of evidence—that each aspect of mental function related to a specific cerebral region in a one-to-one manner. They believed also that the shape of the head depended on the brain contained within it and that overdevelopment of specific parts of the brain, which influenced the mental faculties of the individual, were reflected by characteristic features of the head. For example, Gall had noticed as a child that certain of his friends with an especially good memory had rather protuberant eyes. This suggested to him that bulging of the eyes was caused by overdevelopment of the subjacent brain, which he took to be responsible for verbal memory. By analogous means, then, he constructed a system in which specific mental faculties, character traits, and moral attributes were correlated with the shape or size of the head and with irregularities (protuberances and depressions) on its surface, supposedly reflecting regional variation in the size of the brain. Complex topographic maps were produced to facilitate the application of this system by individual practitioners and helped to give an air of scientific precision where none existed. The reader who potters around antique shops may still find the occasional chart of the head or brain, or even a china head on which is written such characteristics as "intuition," "wit," and the like—reminders of the age of phrenology.

Such propositions were based simply on fantasy, but they gained for a period a certain fashionable following. At one time, almost thirty societies were devoted to phrenology, and those sympathetic to its approach included many who were well-placed in English society, including members of the royal family itself. An exponent was even summoned by Queen Victoria to examine the royal children and advise on the aptitude of the Prince of Wales.[22]

The popularity of the new cult was short-lived. Faced with the opposition of both the Catholic church and Austrian emperor, Gall left Vienna and eventually settled in Paris, where his reception was equally mixed. It is said that Napoleon himself came to oppose the approach when the shape of his own head revealed certain failings. Scientists were only too ready to turn to any work that appeared to repudiate the views of the phrenologists, perhaps encouraged by political and religious expediency. The experimental studies of Pierre Flourens[G] were pivotal in discrediting phrenology. Working on a variety of different animals, but especially on pigeons and dogs, Flourens studied cerebral function by examining the effect of *sectioning* or removing different parts of the brain, and he concluded that the cerebral cortex acted as a functional unit, without any regional specialization of function. His conclusions were widely accepted in the first half of the nineteenth century, if only because they accorded conveniently with what people wanted to believe. There are, however, scientific objections to Flourens' approach: slicing successively through the hemispheres, as he did, would fail to disclose localized functions within them.[23]

Although it was soon discredited, phrenology helped to advance concepts concerning cerebral function. It focused attention on the brain and implied that the convolutions of the brain have a certain consistency of form and function; it stimulated physicians to correlate clinical and pathological abnormalities (i.e., to relate the clinical problems of patients to the findings at autopsy)[22]; and it led to renewed efforts to relate mental processes to cerebral activity[24] because it suggested that the mind relates to the operation of the brain. Ironically, if the phrenologists had directed their attention to such functions as language, vision, hearing, and movement, their views would have been corroborated with time. The advances that occurred over the following years

---

[G] Pierre Flourens (1794–1867), French physiologist and politician, one of the pioneers in ablating (removing) parts of the nervous system to examine its function. He showed that certain functions were indeed localized in a general way in the brain, such as cognitive functions to the cerebral hemispheres and the control of the circulation and respiration to the medulla, but he did not believe that specific cognitive functions had a more discrete localization within the cerebral hemispheres. One of his many pupils was Vulpian (considered elsewhere in this work).

were related to clinical–pathological correlations and electrical stimulation of the nervous system in humans and animals in the laboratory.

In 1861, Broca showed that certain cerebral regions have specialized functions. He reported in Paris at a meeting of the Société d'Anthropologie, and later to the Société Anatomique, his findings at postmortem examination of a fifty-one-year-old epileptic who had been unable to speak for more than twenty years. The poor man had developed increasing weakness of the right arm and leg in his later years, was admitted to hospital under Broca's care with an infected leg, died shortly thereafter, and was found to have softening and destruction of parts of the second and especially the third frontal convolution of the left cerebral hemisphere, as well as more diffuse cerebral atrophy. Broca attributed the speech disturbance to the destruction of this convolution (the so-called inferior frontal gyrus), where pathological changes were maximal, because the abnormality of speech was the first and major clinical symptom.[25,26] He subsequently encountered a second patient with a similar disorder of speech due to a stroke, in whom the autopsy showed similar findings.[27] Over the following months, he collected other cases and reports of similar speech disturbances, which he called "aphemia" (now termed *aphasia*), and noted that the lesion was always confined to the same circumscribed region and always involved the left cerebral hemisphere.[28] Thus it was that he identified a distinct functional center for speech in the human brain (Figure 10.3). In 1865, three major papers were published—two by Marc and Gustave Dax[H] and the other by Broca—all showing that the left and right hemispheres of the brain are not functionally equivalent, based on disturbances of language with disease.[29]

After Broca's original reports, it came to be realized that disturbances of language may take a variety of forms, and these led to the development of convoluted terminologies that are difficult for the nonspecialist to understand. The aphasia described by Broca is characterized by paucity of conversational speech, difficulty in naming objects and repetition, and impaired ability to write or read aloud, but a relatively preserved comprehension of language. The Prussian physician and pathologist Carl Wernicke (1848–1905) subsequently found a region primarily in the left temporal lobe (Figure 10.3) to be important in the comprehension of language. Damage to this area was

---

[H] Marc Dax, an obscure country doctor from southern France, had earlier noted a relationship between certain speech disturbances and pathology involving the left cerebral hemisphere, but Broca had heard of neither the physician nor his work when he formulated his own thesis; furthermore, he localized the underlying pathology not simply to the left hemisphere but to a localized area within it. Nevertheless, Dax deserves credit for his original observation that functional differences existed between the two hemispheres, as does his son Gustave, who extended his work.

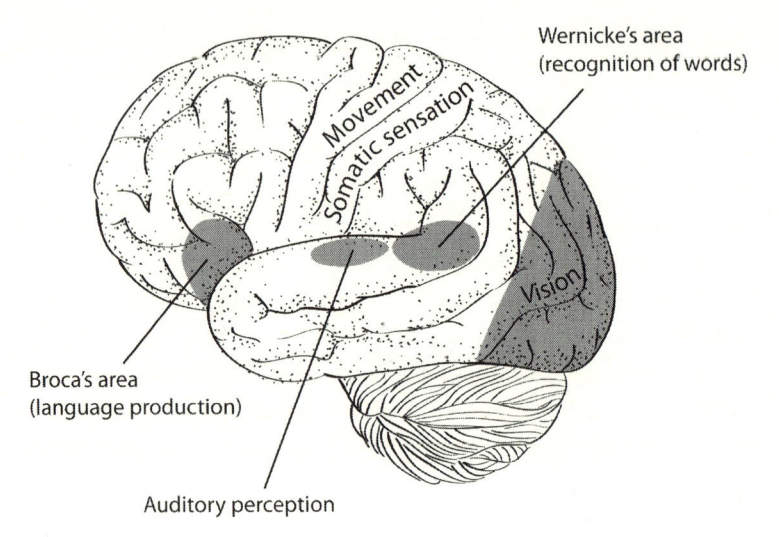

FIGURE 10.3 The surface of the left hemisphere showing several regions of localized cortical function.

associated with profuse but meaningless speech and a failure of language comprehension. Other regions came also to be recognized as playing a substantial role related to language.

The recognition that the two sides of the brain were not identical but differed in certain functional respects had major implications that were variously interpreted by different physicians and neuroscientists. For example, Hughlings Jackson—Brown-Séquard's former assistant—accepted that there were lateralized differences of function concerning speech, but held that the left side served the automatic and voluntary use of words, whereas the right was concerned with the more automatic use of words.[30-32] He was also careful to point out that, "to locate the damage which destroys speech and to locate speech are two different things."[31]

Brown-Séquard and Broca had been friends as young men, and each had attempted to further the other's career. Broca had helped Brown-Séquard when first he moved to America and had chaired the committee of the Société de Biologie that investigated and confirmed, in 1855, his then-revolutionary views on sensory physiology. Brown-Séquard, in turn, had published some of Broca's controversial theories in his own journal and had joined Broca when—against all opposition—he established the Société d'Anthropologie in Paris, becoming a founder-member. Nevertheless, putting aside any personal feelings, Brown-Séquard was unable to accept Broca's conclusion about a center for speech and did not believe that specific functions were localized to discrete areas of the brain. He reported a disparity between focal cerebral pathology and the occurrence of aphasia, noting that some aphasic patients did not have lesions in Broca's area (the third left frontal convolution) or had lesions elsewhere, and that lesions in Broca's area sometimes occurred without any associated major deficit of language. He found that many aphasic patients have pathology situated rather posteriorly in the left hemisphere, and stressed the occurrence of aphasia in certain right-handed patients with disease of the right (rather than the left) hemisphere, a disturbance called "crossed aphasia." He also pointed out that some aphasic patients retain the ability to speak when confused, delirious, asleep, or singing.

All of his observations were correct. Crossed aphasia may occur because speech is represented on the "wrong" side or on both sides of the brain in certain people; that is, there is a mirror representation in the right hemisphere of that in the left hemisphere. Other explanations have also been invoked. Word-finding difficulties, a rather nonspecific abnormality, may occur with lesions in many different areas on either side of the brain, and posteriorly situated lesions are indeed associated with certain types of aphasia. Furthermore, in some patients with aphasia resembling that described by Broca, the pathology spares the third frontal convolution in favor of neighboring areas (as in what is now called a mixed transcortical aphasia or transcortical motor aphasia, in which Broca's area is disconnected from other brain regions that are important for speech); in Broca's aphasia, the lesion is usually more extensive than originally suggested; and in patients with lesions restricted to Broca's area, the disturbance of language may be short-lived.

Brown-Séquard believed that the clinical accompaniments of a focal lesion of the brain reflect neither the normal function of that region nor the opposite of that function. In connection with speech, he famously wrote:

> Concluding that, because aphasia comes from an irritation of those organs, that they are the centres of the faculty of speech, is doing just the same thing as we would do if we concluded that the soles of the feet are the centre for the emotional power of laughter, because we laugh when the soles of the feet are tickled.[33]

Instead, he believed that various specialized activities of the brain—such as speech production or the use of language—were carried out by cells that formed a functional rather than an anatomical unit, being arranged in a diffuse interconnected network rather than in a discrete localized mass.

> My own view ... is that each function of the brain is carried on by special organs, but that those organs, instead of being composed of cells forming a

cluster or mass in one part, are composed of scattered cells diffused in many parts of the brain, in communication, of course, one with the other by fibres, and forming a whole by this union of fibres, but still so diffused that a great many parts of the brain—I would not be bold enough to say all parts—contain the elements endowed with each of the various functions that we know to exist in the brain.[33]

He accepted—indeed, he emphasized—that the two hemispheres differed in certain functions, especially with regard to speech, but suggested that the right hemisphere has in some individuals the ability of the left, and that in all individuals it has the *potential* for communicative functions.[34] His views were derided and ignored, for the emerging new concepts of localized functions within the cerebral hemispheres were seductive.

Broca's clinicopathological studies on speech led neurologists and physiologists to localize other functions to different regions of the cerebral hemispheres. Many scientists believed, based on the work of Flourens and other prominent physiologists, that the cerebral cortex had sensory and psychic functions, and that movement was controlled by subjacent structures (in particular, the so-called corpus striatum). During the 1860s, however, Hughlings Jackson studied the clinical manifestations and underlying pathology of patients with seizures, and he related convulsive motor activity involving one side of the body to pathology affecting the opposite cerebral hemisphere, thereby coming to the concept of cerebral localization of movement.[35,36] His work stimulated interest in cerebral localization, and this concept received more direct support from studies involving experimental stimulation of the brain. Such studies had been performed earlier, with little impact. Indeed, the cerebral cortex itself was thought to be inexcitable. Then, in 1870, two German neuroscientists—the physiologist Gustav Theodor Fritsch (1838–1927) and neuropsychiatrist Eduard Hitzig (1838–1907)—reported on studies that they had performed on dogs. Working on the dressing table in Hitzig's Berlin home, as they were without adequate university facilities, they found that muscle contractions of the limbs on one side were elicited by stimulation of specific regions of the opposite frontal cortex.[37] Low-intensity stimuli produced very discrete responses, and excision of the cerebral areas from which these responses could be obtained led to weakness of the opposite limbs. Thus, it seemed that the cerebral cortex was excitable and that function was localized within the brain, so that only certain parts of the hemispheres were concerned with movement.

Similar studies in monkeys, particularly by David Ferrier (1843–1928) in England, supported the concept of motor centers and suggested that sensory centers could also be localized in the cerebral cortex.[38] It is of interest that Ferrier's original paper, submitted for publication to the Royal Society of London, reported his work on both monkeys and dogs. The manuscript had a difficult time with the scientific reviewers, experts who were asked to determine whether it justified publication, and a third reviewer (T.H. Huxley) was needed to adjudicate; it was felt that sufficient credit had not been given to the earlier work of Fritsch and Hitzig, and the paper therefore had to be revised. The reviewers remained dissatisfied with the revisions, Hitzig was angered, and eventually Ferrier decided to omit all reference to dogs, limiting his report to work on monkeys to avoid making the requested changes.[39]

The work in animals stimulated interest in the human brain. In Cincinnati, Roberts Bartholow (1831–1904) undertook a series of analogous studies in a terminally ill Irish housemaid—Mary Rafferty—with a cancerous defect in her skull. He was able to focally stimulate localized regions of the cerebral hemisphere using needle electrodes that were inserted directly into her brain,[40] thereby inducing muscle contractions or sensory phenomena in the limbs on the opposite side. He thus confirmed the findings obtained in animals, but his publication aroused the disapproval of a public concerned especially with the ethics of such invasive experiments on human subjects. Their concern was not misplaced: Mary had a seizure shortly after one of his experiments, became comatose, and died shortly thereafter, although whether this can be attributed to Bartholow's manipulations seems doubtful.[41]

Taken together, these various experiments confirmed that the cerebral cortex is excitable, showed that the results obtained in animals were relevant to humans, and indicated that the regions from which motor responses can be elicited are anterior to sensory regions (Figure 10.3). They also had clinical relevance in suggesting the basis of various neurological symptoms and thus in helping to localize the causal lesion in patients with such symptoms or signs. Just a few years later, the brain tumor of a patient was successfully removed for the first time by the British surgeon Rickman Godlee after it had been localized by such means.[42] The success of the operation was marred by the death of the unfortunate patient from infection, a fact that led to a considerable but brief public outcry that the surgery had been unjustified. The obstacle to such surgery had not been technical factors, but the difficulty in knowing where to operate, that is, to localize the tumor before operation. The new doctrine of cortical localization provided a means of doing just that.

Dispute continued concerning the issue of cerebral localization, leading to a dramatic confrontation between Ferrier and Friedrich Goltz (1834–1902) at the lavish International Medical Congress of 1881, held in London under the patronage of Queen Victoria and widely attended by the leading clinicians and scientists of the period.[43] Goltz, who was professor of physiology at Strasbourg and an opponent of the concept of localization, considered the stimulation experiments inconclusive because of uncertainty regarding what was being stimulated and where, and especially because the stimuli may have spread to other (lower) regions of the brain that were responsible for the observed effects. He also pointed out that the plasticity of the brain, that is, the ability of surviving brain regions to take over the functions of ablated areas, conflicted with the concept of specialized cortical regions. He then displayed a dog from which a large area of cortex had been removed without producing the loss of function to be expected if the localizers were correct. Ferrier (and his colleague, Gerald Yeo) then described a monkey from which part of the motor cortex had been removed, leading to paralysis of the opposite limbs precisely as they had predicted, and subsequently demonstrated the animal at the King's College laboratory. Following this exchange, the two animals were sacrificed under chloroform and their brains examined by three eminent scientists, who concluded that the lesion in the dog's brain was not as extensive as Goltz had believed, whereas that in the monkey was in the intended site.[44] This was taken as an endorsement of the views advanced by Ferrier.[I]

Attention was focused initially on motor phenomena, as these are easier to study in the laboratory than sensory or cognitive phenomena, but, with time, these also came under scrutiny. For the next half-century, men of science focused on defining the function of different areas of the cerebral cortex based on the activities elicited by electrical stimulation and on the microscopic appearance of different parts of the cortex. Complicated maps were constructed showing the division of the cortex into many different areas, to which different functions were ascribed. In the 1930 and 1940s, neurosurgeons created similar maps of the motor and sensory cortex in conscious patients undergoing brain surgery, usually for epilepsy or to remove tumors. Electrical stimulation was used to determine where different parts of the body were represented. For example, when different parts of the motor cortex were

---

[I] Later in 1881, Ferrier was charged before a London magistrate with a violation of the Vivisection Act because of the events that occurred at the Congress, and in particular because—while not possessing the requisite governmental license—he performed an operation that was likely to cause pain and then failed to destroy the animal. The charges were dismissed when it was shown that the experiments were actually performed (at King's College) by his collaborator, Professor Yeo, who did possess the necessary license and conducted the study in strict accordance with the law, using anesthetics as appropriate and having the necessary certificate for maintaining the animal alive thereafter. A detailed report of the proceedings can be found in the *British Medical Journal*, 2: 836–842, 1881.

stimulated, movement occurred in various parts of the body, and motor maps were created showing the cortical representation of the body. Similarly, stimulation of the sensory part of the brain elicited sensations perceived by the patient on different parts of the body surface, and sensory maps were thereby constructed. The maps showed a topographical representation of the body in the brain, that is, a representation that reflects the organization of the body, so that adjacent parts of the body are represented next to each other in the brain. Some parts—such as the hand—were much larger than others where motor function is less skilled or demanding. For years, it was held that such maps are fixed and unchanging, implying a strict localization of function within the brain. This is now known to be incorrect. The cortical representation of motor and sensory function varies with time and preceding brain activity, and between individuals, to a far greater extent than envisioned by those subscribing to a strict localization of function. Such variability implies that the brain is much more plastic in its functional abilities than would be expected if it is a hard-wired system. It has the potential to change, to adapt to the prevailing circumstances.

Most neuroscientists, including Ferrier, originally related the neural events associated with electrically evoked motor and sensory responses to the natural occurrence of voluntary motor activity or sensory perceptions in response to mental events. For example, they came to believe that the motor center was the site responsible for the initiation and execution of voluntary activity, because the activity generated by electrical stimulation sometimes seemed so coordinated and purposeful. Brown-Séquard took particular objection to such a position, stating in a lecture at the Boston Society of Natural History in 1875:

> There are several decided obstacles to admitting the conclusions which have been drawn from these experiments; one of these is that the parts, through the galvanization of which these movements are caused, are the will-centres for such movements.[45]

He was disturbed by the localization of complex functions to discrete and isolated cerebral regions simply because responses resembling such functions could be obtained from these regions by focal electrical stimulation. Even "simple" functions depended on the complex interactions of several neurological systems. The voluntary movement of a finger, for example, likely involved systems concerned with initiating a decision to move, planning the intended movement, limiting the movement to the selected finger, executing correctly the intended movement, and other related factors. With regard to the production of volitional movement, he himself proposed that two distinct systems are involved.

> On set of them [cells], used in the mental part of such an action, are chiefly, if not exclusively, disseminated through the cerebrum; and the other set, used in putting in play nerves and muscles for a movement, are located in the base of the brain and the spinal cord.[46]

He also distinguished between the "will" or volition on the one hand and volitional motor activity on the other, believing that separate neurological substrates existed for these two processes. Clinical distinction between the two processes was probably not possible in most instances because they were likely to be lost together, but "in certain cases of hysterical paralysis there is nothing but a paralysis of volition—that is, a loss of the faculty of *willing* to make certain movements."[47]

He believed, then, that specialized function depended upon elements scattered diffusely throughout the brain, rather than collected in discrete areas within the hemisphere,[11,46,48] but accepted that these elements could be influenced by the activity of localized cerebral regions. Stimulation of the same area of the brain, however, could induce different movements at different times, suggesting a more dynamic control system than others were prepared to accept. Indeed, he emphasized that the weakness produced by focal lesions results from a dynamic inhibitory influence exerted on parts directly involved in executing motor activity. The cerebral mechanisms regulating movement were diffuse, he argued, because motor responses on the same (ipsilateral) or opposite (contralateral) side could be elicited by the electrical or mechanical stimulation of several different regions of the brain; because fibers from the supposed motor centers in the brain reached the spinal cord by pathways descending from them but also by passing from one hemisphere to the other (in the corpus callosum) before descending; and because lesions of the so-called cortical motor area sometimes failed to cause (both in patients and animals) significant weakness of the contralateral limbs.[48-52] He recalled also that lateralized convulsions in humans could occur on the same or opposite side as underlying abnormalities of the brain. Despite his observations that limb movements on one side of the body could be generated from either side of the brain, he nevertheless accepted that the opposite hemisphere had a predominant role in this regard.[34]

Brown-Séquard's observations suggested concepts of functional localization that lacked the disarming simplicity of the increasingly popular theories of anatomical localization then prevalent and were based on poorly supported beliefs concerning the remote effects of one part of the nervous system

Brown-Séquard's birth certificate. His maternal grandfather, Pierre Paul Séquard, is one of the official witnesses. With permission from The Royal College of Physicians of London Heritage Centre.

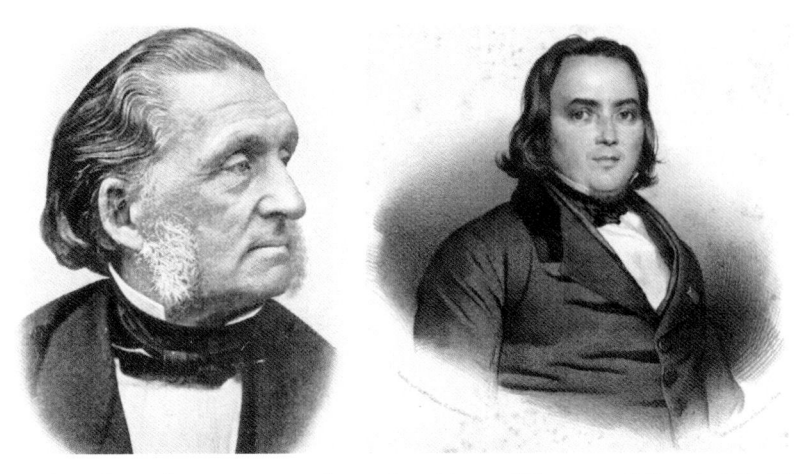

Brown-Séquard served as an extern on the service of Armand Trousseau (*left*) at the Hôtel-Dieu Hospital and Pierre Rayer (*right*) at the Charité Hospital in Paris. Both men were much loved and respected by their students. Trousseau authored a classic textbook of medicine and—among his many other accomplishments—described a sign of malignancy. Curiously, it later occurred in him, signaling a cancer of the stomach that proved fatal. Rayer, another eminent clinician, investigator, and medical politician, was one of the founders, with Brown-Séquard and several other young physician-scientists, of the Société de Biologie and served as its first president. Courtesy of the National Library of Medicine.

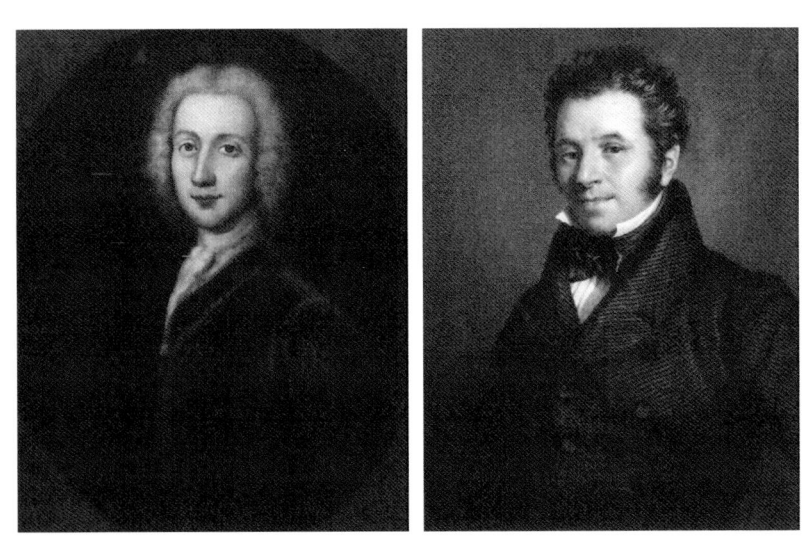

Early investigators of spinal cord function. Robert Whytt (pronounced White; *left panel*) described the muscle stretch and cutaneous reflexes and the phenomenon of spinal shock. The brilliant but abrasive Marshall Hall (*right*) established the importance and broadened the concept of reflexes in the operation of the nervous system. His achievements have been equated (notably by Hall himself but also by others) with those of William Harvey, who demonstrated the circulation of the blood. Courtesy of the National Library of Medicine.

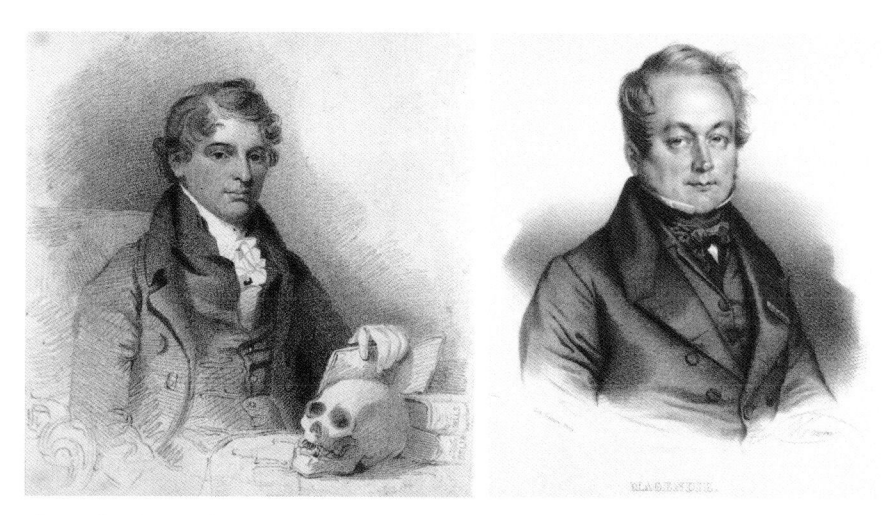

The rivals. The British anatomist-surgeon Sir Charles Bell (*left*) and French physiologist François Magendie (*right*) showed that the anterior and posterior nerve roots have different functions, but argued bitterly over priority and credit for the discovery. Courtesy of the National Library of Medicine.

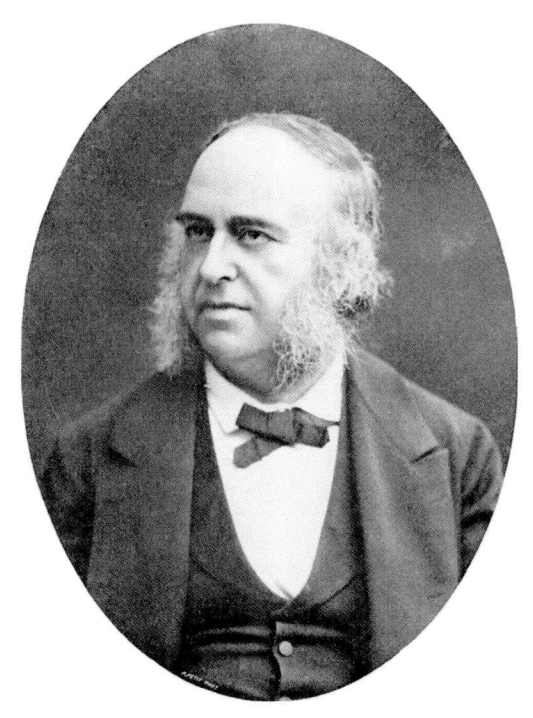

Pierre Paul Broca. Broca wrote a letter introducing Brown-Séquard to colleagues in the United States and chaired the committee that examined and vindicated his claims concerning the sensory pathways in the spinal cord. Brown-Séquard, in turn, supported and admired his younger colleague, although he could not accept Broca's views on cerebral localization. Courtesy of the Wellcome Library, London.

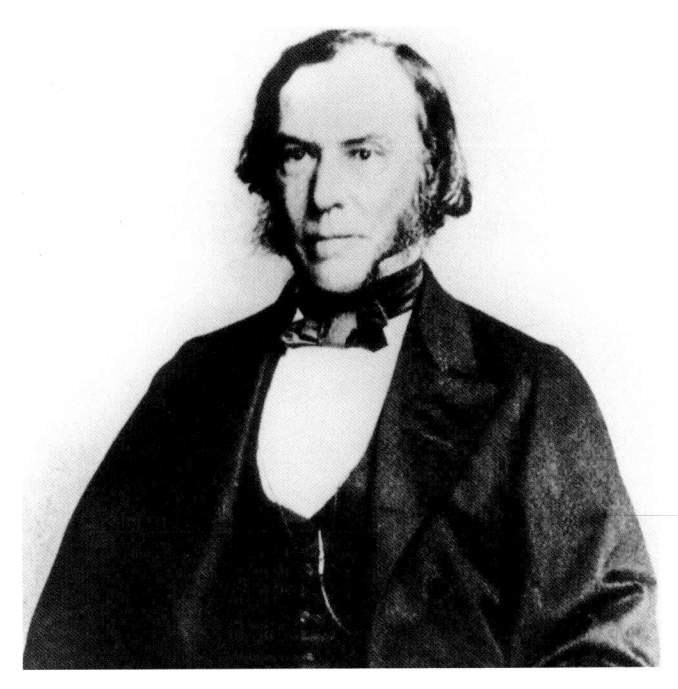

Portrait of Brown-Séquard at about the age of 40. No other photographs of the young man are known to exist. Courtesy of the Royal College of Physicians of London Heritage Centre.

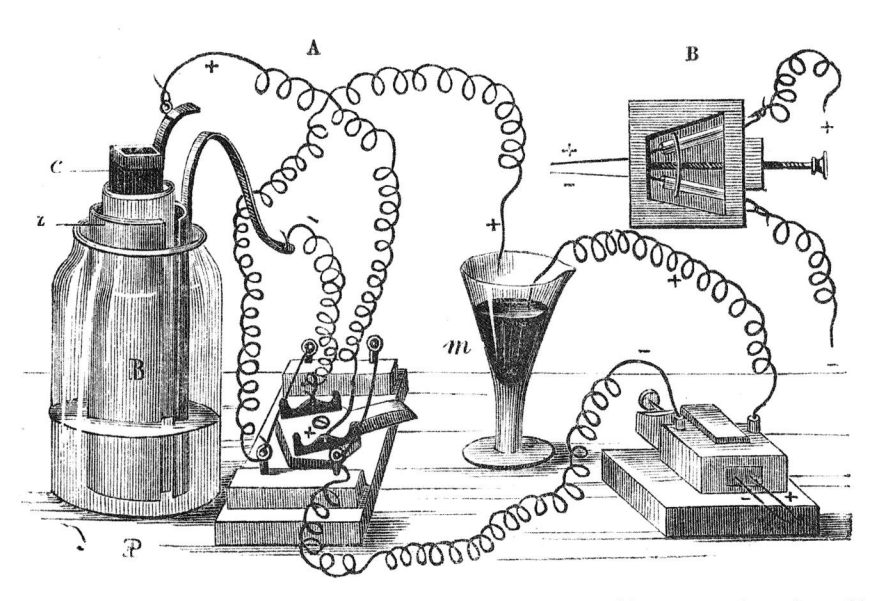

Apparatus for electrical stimulation of nerves. The apparatus used by Brown-Séquard would have been similar. From Bernard C. *Leçons sur la physiologie et la pathologie de la système nerveux*. Figure 19, p. 156. Paris: J B Ballière, 1858. Courtesy of the Wellcome Library, London.

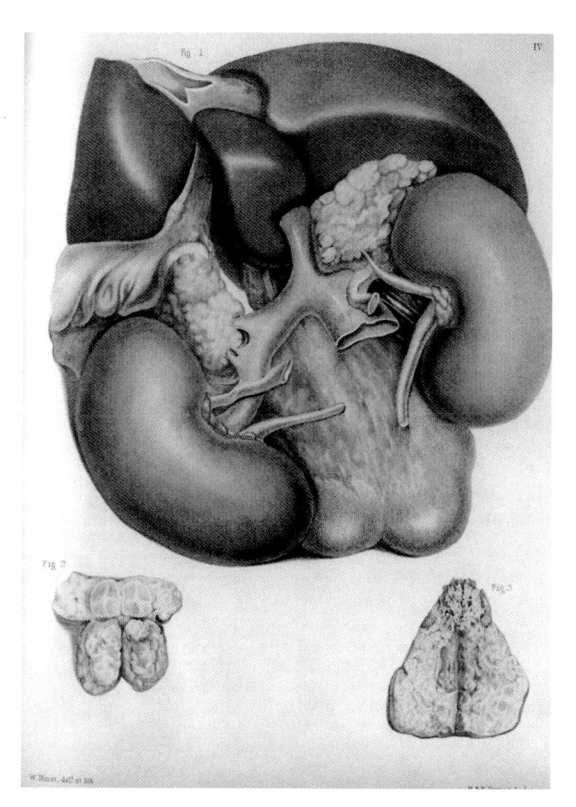

The liver and adrenal (suprarenal) glands from one of the patients described by Thomas Addison in his monograph. In the bottom corners of the plate (Figs. 2 and 3) are sections through the diseased adrenal glands. From Addison T. *On the constitutional and local effects of disease of the suprarenal capsules.* Case III, Plate IV. London: Highley, 1855.

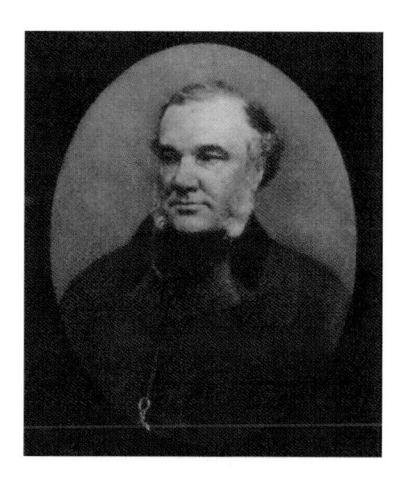

Thomas Addison. Addison, an Edinburgh graduate, was physician to Guy's Hospital, London, when he described an obscure clinical disorder (named after him by Armand Trousseau) associated with disease of the adrenal glands, as determined at autopsy. This led Brown-Séquard to study the effects of removing these glands in animals, showing thereby that they were essential to life. The brilliant but charmless Addison suffered with recurrent depression and leaped to his death "whilst of unsound mind" five years after publishing his famous monograph. Neither *The Lancet* nor the *British Medical Journal* chose to publish an obituary of him. Courtesy of the National Library of Medicine.

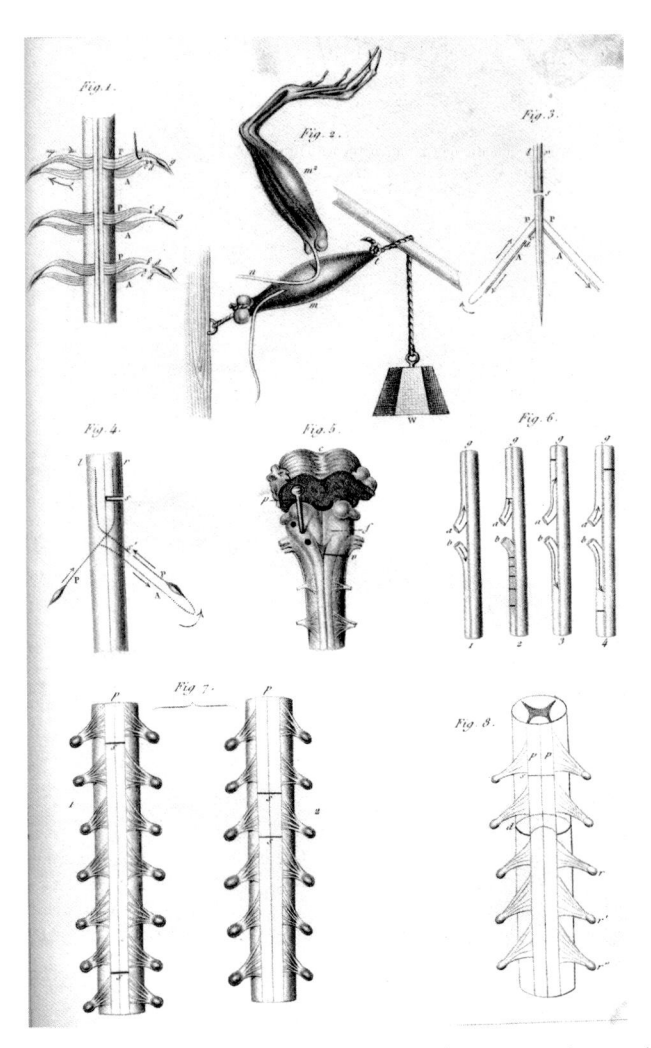

Plate 1 from Brown-Séquard's published lectures, delivered in 1858 at the Royal College of Surgeons of England. There are eight figures. They depict various experiments that he conducted primarily to determine the course of the sensory pathways in the spinal cord. Figure 1, the anatomy of the nerve roots; Figure 2, an arrangement for an experiment on muscle contraction; Figure 3, the anterior and posterior nerve roots and spinal cord of a frog, illustrating the direction of nerve impulses following a stimulus to sensory fibers that results in muscle contraction; Figure 4, mammalian spinal cord showing sensory fibers crossing from one side to the other, and a lateral hemisection of one side of the cord; Figure 5, part of the brainstem and cerebellum, showing the region of the so-called "vital knot," which was thought to contain the center controlling respiratory movements; Figure 6, various sections of the posterior columns; Figure 7, two illustrations showing a double section of the posterior columns, in one instance (*left panel*) several segment apart and in the other just separated by a single segment; Figure 8, transverse section of the posterior columns (*p*) of the spinal cord (*s*) and of the entire spinal cord except for the posterior columns (*d*). From Brown-Séquard CE. *Course of lectures on the physiology and pathology of the central nervous system.* Philadelphia: Collins, 1860.

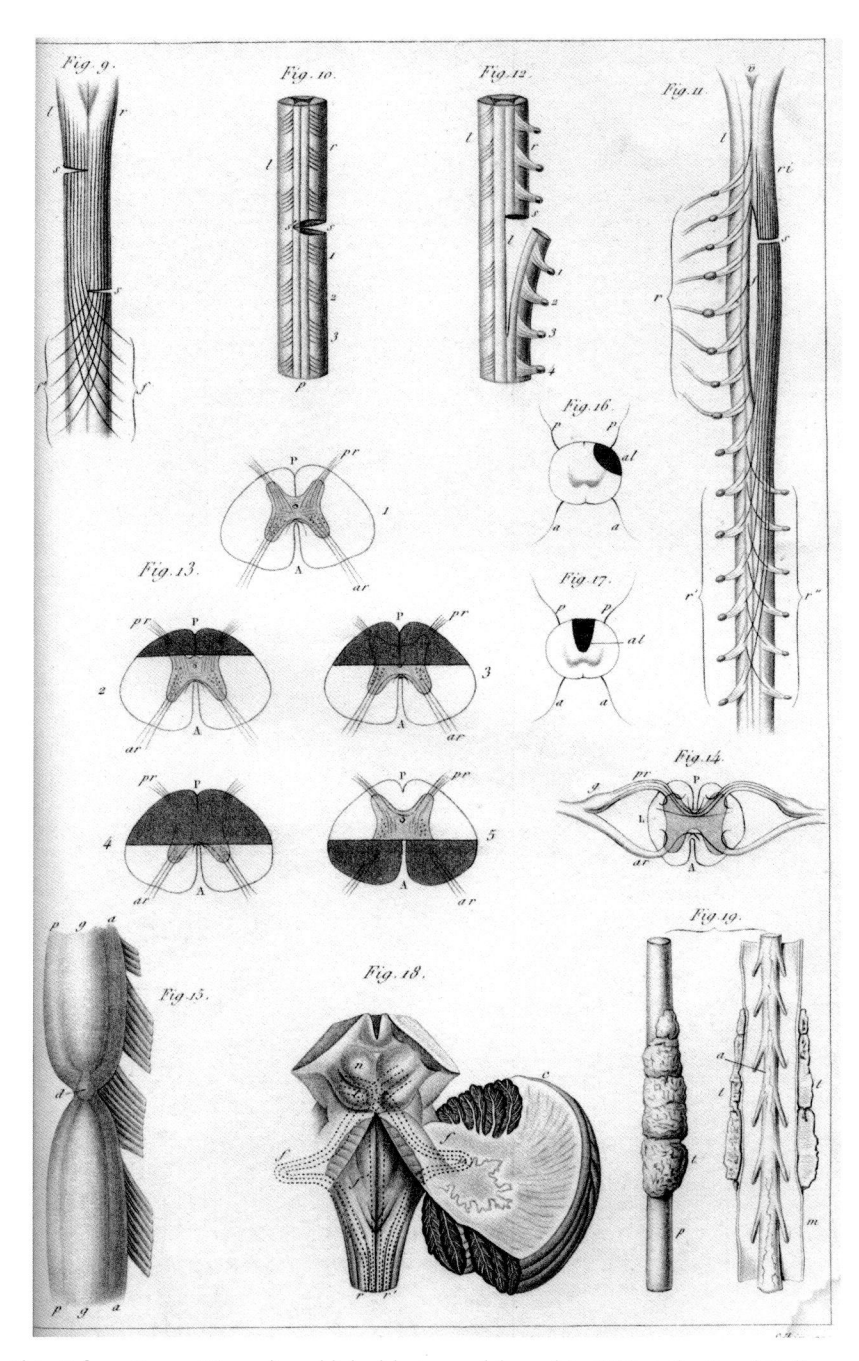

Plate 2 from Brown-Séquard's published lectures, delivered in 1858 at the Royal College of Surgeons of England. Figures 9–17 show lesions in various parts of the spinal cord in various animals and in humans (Figs. 16 and 17) to determine the effect on sensation. Figure 18 shows the course (*dotted line*) of the sensory pathways in the brainstem and cerebellum. Figure 19 represents a tumor in the spinal cord. From Brown-Séquard CE. *Course of lectures on the physiology and pathology of the central nervous system*. Philadelphia: Collins, 1860.

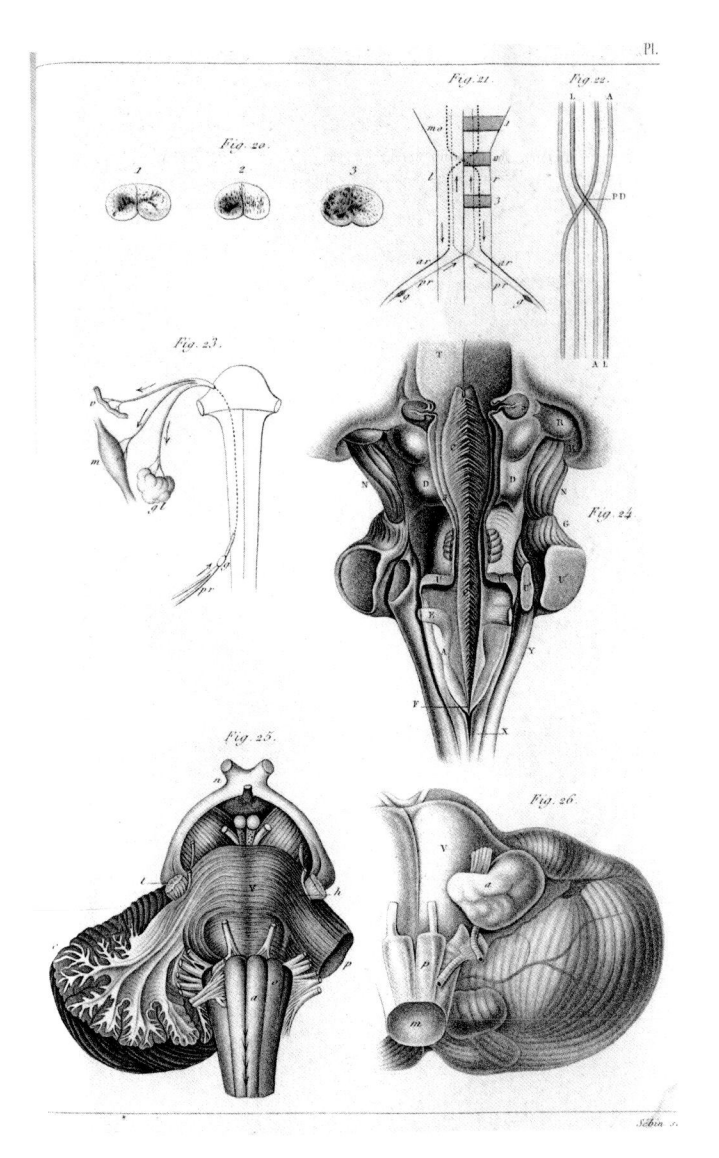

Plate 3 from Brown-Séquard's published lectures, delivered in 1858 at the Royal College of Surgeons of England. Figure 20, hemorrhage into the spinal cord of a patient. Figure 21, the crossing of motor (*arrows pointing down*) and sensory fibers in the spinal cord or lower brainstem. It can be seen that fibers cross at different levels, the sensory fibers soon after entering the spinal cord to ascend to the brain, the descending motor fibers at the junction of the spinal cord and brainstem. Figure 22, the crossing of the motor fibers in the lower brainstem: some cross, whereas others do not do so but pass straight into the spinal cord. Figure 23, sensory fibers enter the spinal cord to reflexly activate muscle, glandular tissue, and blood vessels. Figures 24–26, different views of the anatomy of the brainstem and cerebellum, showing in one a tumor (Fig. 26). From Brown-Séquard CE. *Course of lectures on the physiology and pathology of the central nervous system.* Philadelphia: Collins, 1860.

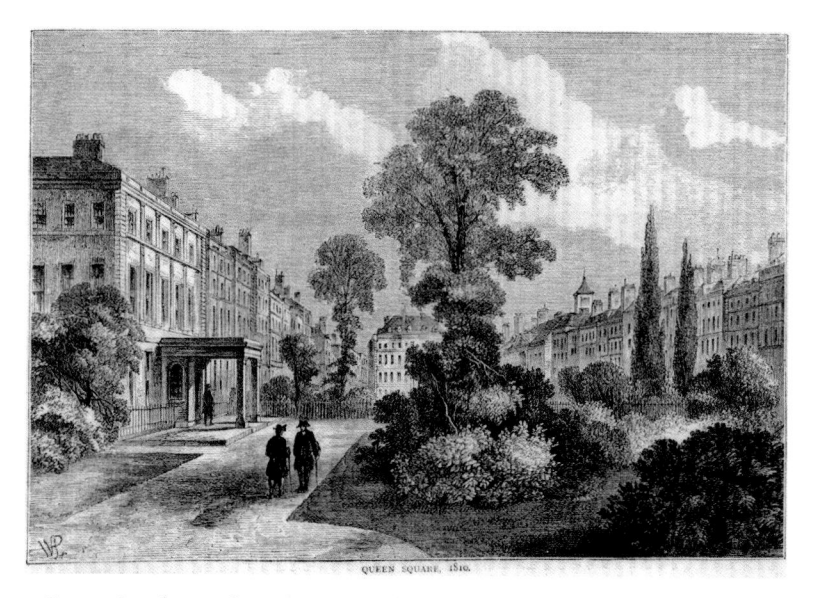

Queen Square, London, in the early nineteenth century. It was here that the National Hospital for the Paralysed and Epileptic was founded, with Brown-Séquard as one of the founder-physicians. Courtesy of the Wellcome Library, London.

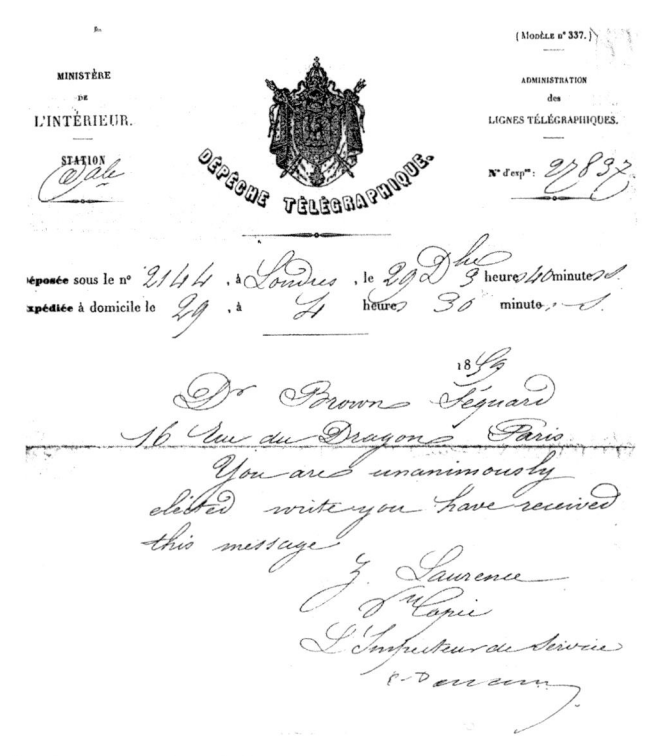

Telegram informing Brown-Séquard, then in Paris, that he had been elected unanimously to the staff of the National Hospital for the Paralysed and Epileptic in London as a founder-physician. Courtesy of the Royal College of Physicians of London Heritage Centre.

> Cambridge, June 16, 1864
>
> Sir;
>
> I have the honor to inform you that at a meeting of the Overseers of Harvard College held in Cambridge this day they unanimously confirmed the vote of the Corporation appointing you professor of the Physiology & Pathology of the Nervous System in the Medical School.
>
> Hoping that your connection with our University may prove as pleasant to you as it must prove advantageous to us, I am
>
> With the greatest respect
> Yours
> Thomas Hill.
>
> Dr E. Brown Séquard.

Letter dated 16 June 1864, appointing Brown-Séquard a professor at Harvard College. Courtesy of the Royal College of Physicians of London Heritage Centre.

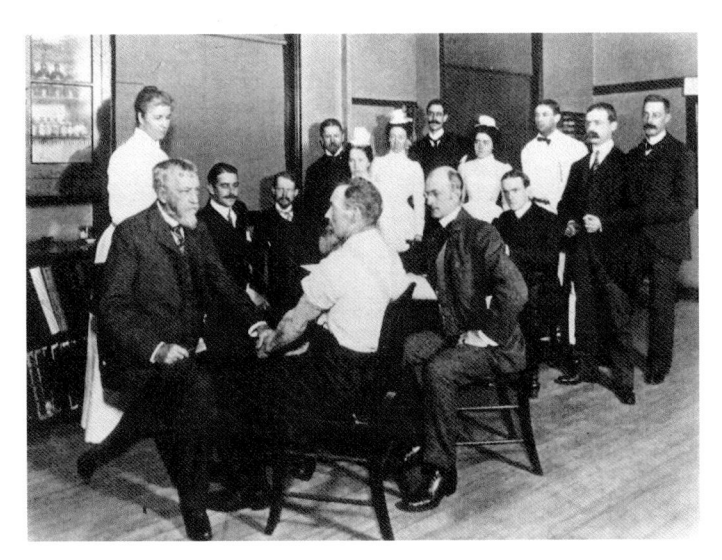

Silas Weir Mitchell. Brown-Séquard made a number of friends while a professor at Harvard, including Dr. Silas Weir Mitchell, seen here (*seated*) taking the pulse of a patient at his clinic at the Infirmary for Nervous Diseases in Philadelphia. Courtesy of the National Library of Medicine.

The *Archives de Physiologie Normale et Pathologique*. The journal was founded in 1868 by Brown-Séquard on his return to Paris, together with Charcot (*left*) and Vulpian (*right*). Brown-Séquard remained editor until his death. The *Archives* continued under the same title until 1898. Brown-Séquard also founded and edited two other journals, both of which were short-lived. Charcot photograph used courtesy of the Wellcome Library, London. Vulpian photograph courtesy of the National Library of Medicine.

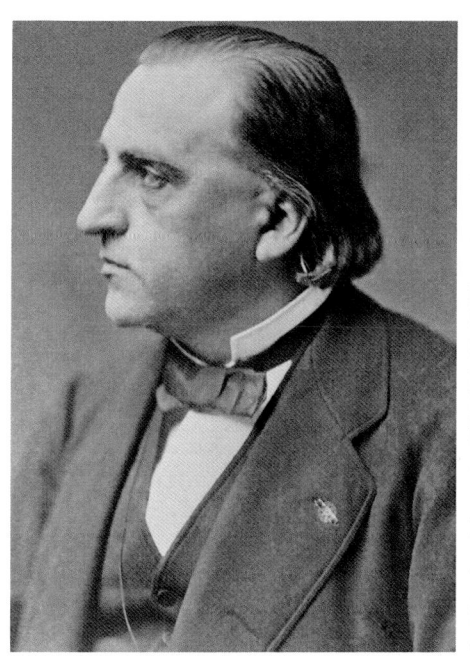

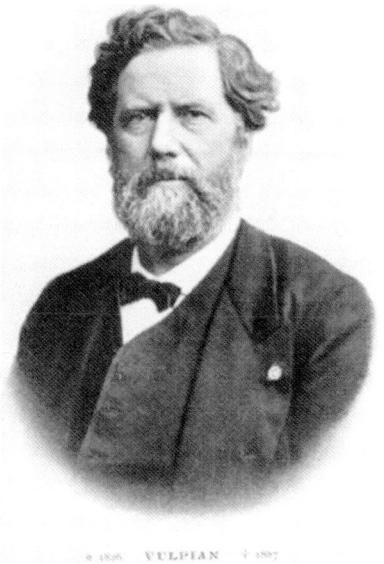

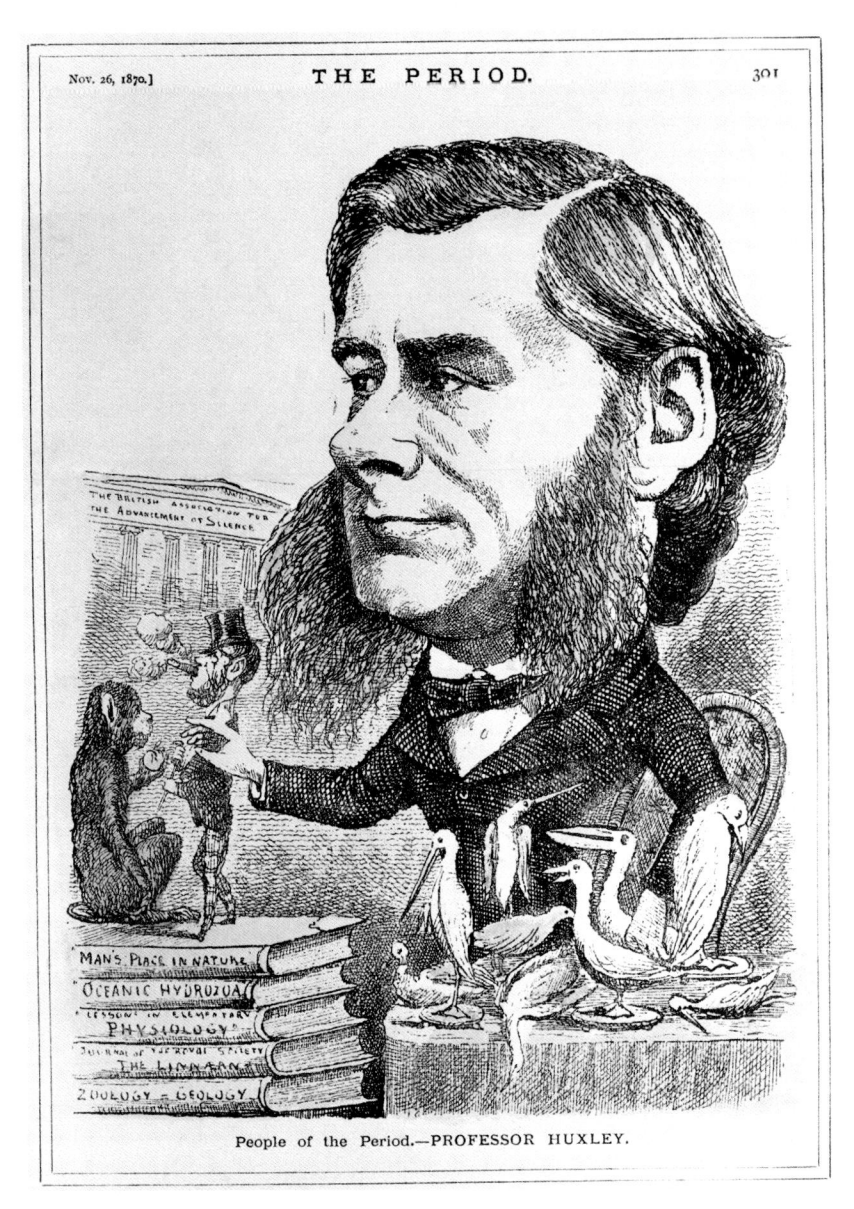

Thomas Henry Huxley (wood engraving 1870). Huxley is shown surrounded by books reflecting his writings and by animals reflecting his interest in evolution and comparative anatomy. Huxley was an influential champion of Darwinism and of the need to improve scientific education. He was an ardent supporter of Brown-Séquard and defended the need to undertake experiments in animals to advance human understanding of biology and disease. Courtesy of the Wellcome Library, London.

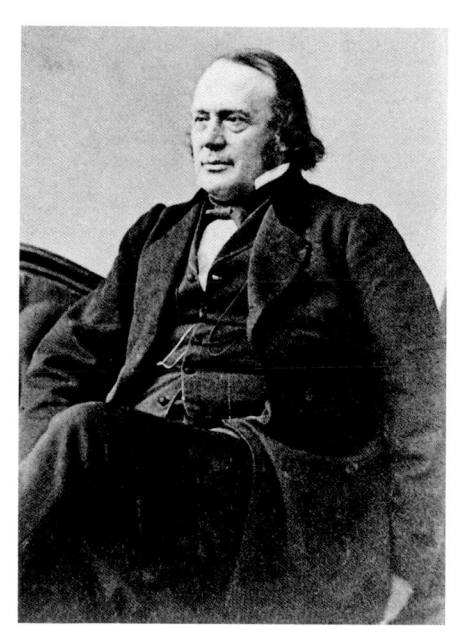

The naturalist Louis Agassiz, a professor at Harvard, befriended Brown-Séquard when he was in Boston, helped him to secure an academic appointment in France, and later tried to induce him to accept a chair of physiology at the School of Natural History he was establishing on Penekese Island. Brown-Séquard, in turn, looked after Agassiz when he suffered a stroke in later life and during his terminal illness. Courtesy of the Wellcome Library, London.

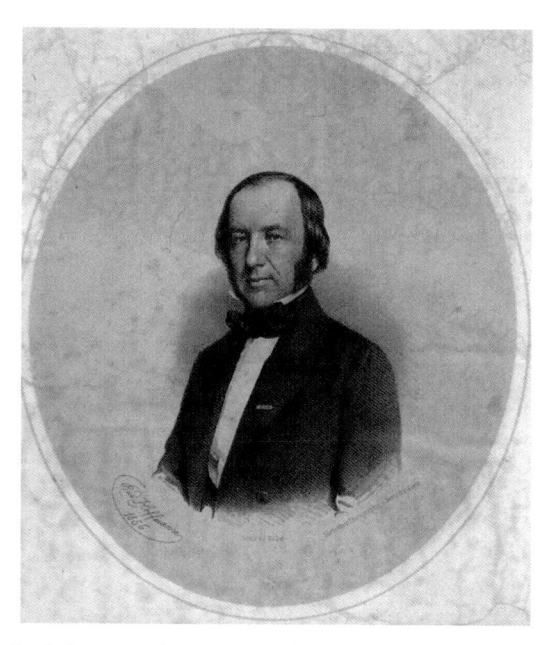

Claude Bernard, the lofty man of science to whose chair Brown-Séquard succeeded at the Collège de France. Courtesy of the National Library of Medicine.

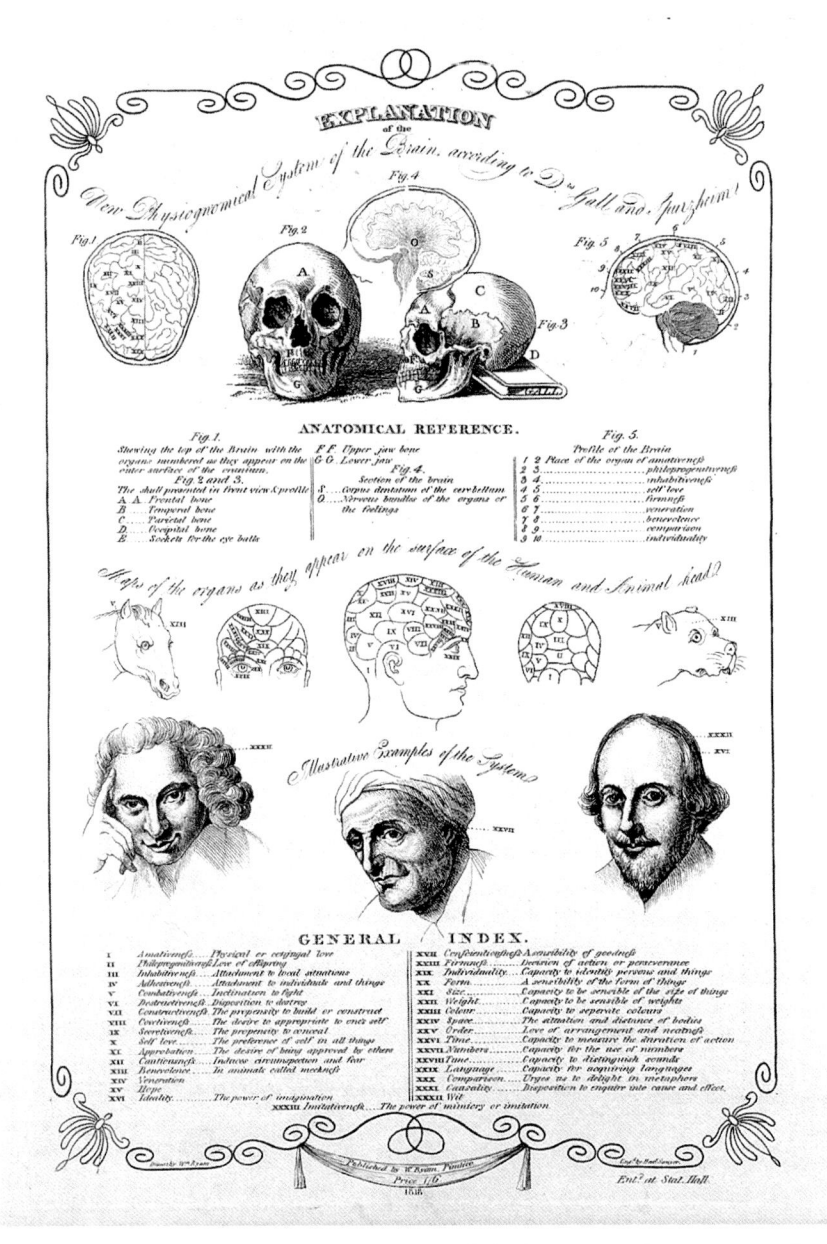

Explanation of the new physiognomical system of the brain, according to Drs. Gall and Spurzheim. Engraving with etching by Henry Sawyer, after William Byam. From Byam W. *Phrenological diagrams of the skull and brain, with three portraits: Laurence Sterne, a mathematician, and Shakespeare; exemplifying the faculties of wit, number, and imagination respectively.* London: William Byam, 1818. Courtesy of the Wellcome Library, London.

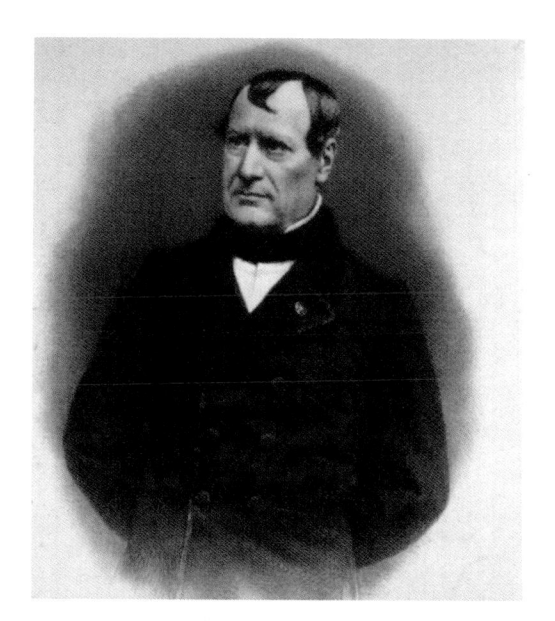

The physiologist Pierre Flourens believed that regional specialization of function did not occur in the cerebral cortex, and he had a major role in discrediting phrenology. He was active in politics and is remembered also for having been elected to membership of the Académie française in preference to the writer Victor Hugo in 1840. His seat (no. 29) passed to the magisterial Claude Bernard in 1868, and then to Ernest Renan in 1878. Courtesy of the National Library of Medicine.

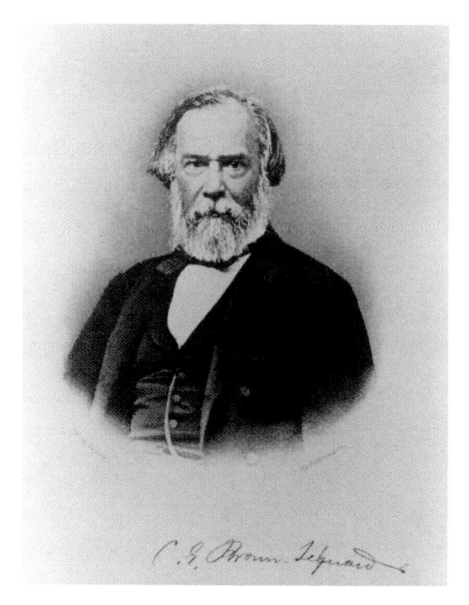

Brown-Séquard, professor of medicine at the Collège de France. The atmosphere in the laboratories that he took over from Claude Bernard soon changed from calm deliberation to restless excitement under his leadership.

Institut de France.

Académie des Sciences.

Paris, le 16 février 1885

Les Secrétaires perpétuels de l'Académie à Monsieur le Professeur Brown Séquard

Monsieur,

Nous avons l'honneur de vous informer que l'Académie des Sciences vous a décerné le Prix Lallemand de l'année 1884.

Nous vous invitons, Monsieur, à assister à la séance publique qui aura lieu le 23 février à 2 heures précises, pour y entendre proclamer le résultat des concours, nous saisissons avec empressement cette occasion de vous offrir nos félicitations personnelles et de vous témoigner l'intérêt que l'Académie prend à vos travaux et à vos succès.

Veuillez agréer, Monsieur, l'assurance de notre considération la plus distinguée.

Formal notification from the Académie des Sciences of the award to Brown-Séquard of the 1884 Prix Lallemand. Courtesy of the Royal College of Physicians of London Heritage Centre.

Letter to Brown-Séquard from Vulpian informing him that he had been selected for the prize with a large majority and enclosing the tally of the two rounds of voting. It is unclear from the letter itself to what Vulpian was referring, but it was probably the vote in the Académie des Sciences concerning the nomination for the 1885 Prix Biennal, which was then confirmed by vote of the entire Institut. Courtesy of the Royal College of Physicians of London Heritage Centre.

List of candidates and votes they obtained in the nomination process of the Académie des Sciences for the 1885 Prix Biennal of the Institut de France. Brown-Séquard was the candidate of the Section of Medicine and Surgery. The African explorer, de Brazza, was his main rival and the candidate of the Section of Geography and Navigation. Courtesy of the Royal College of Physicians of London Heritage Centre.

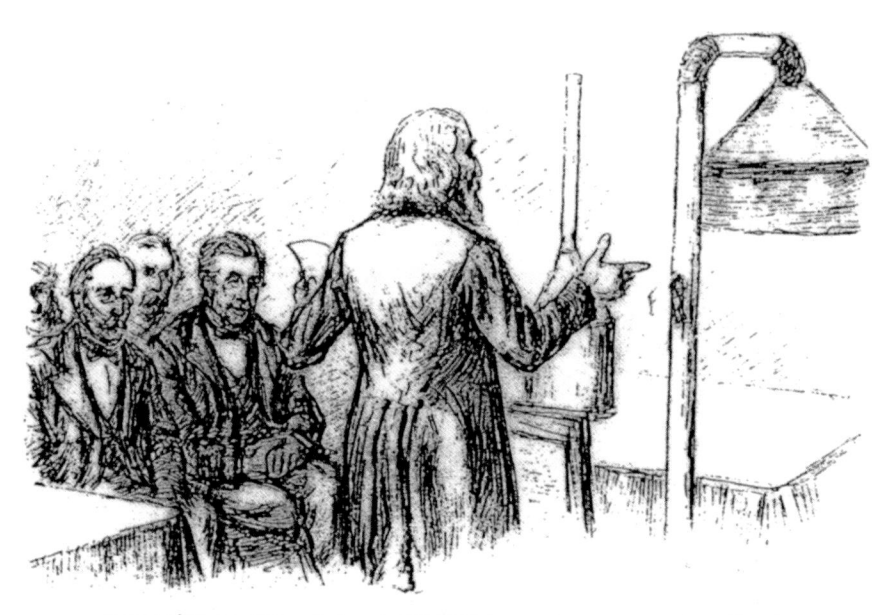

Brown-Séquard explaining an experiment at the Académie des Sciences in Paris. From Child T. The Institute of France. In *Harper's New Monthly Magazine,* 78:501–520, 1889.

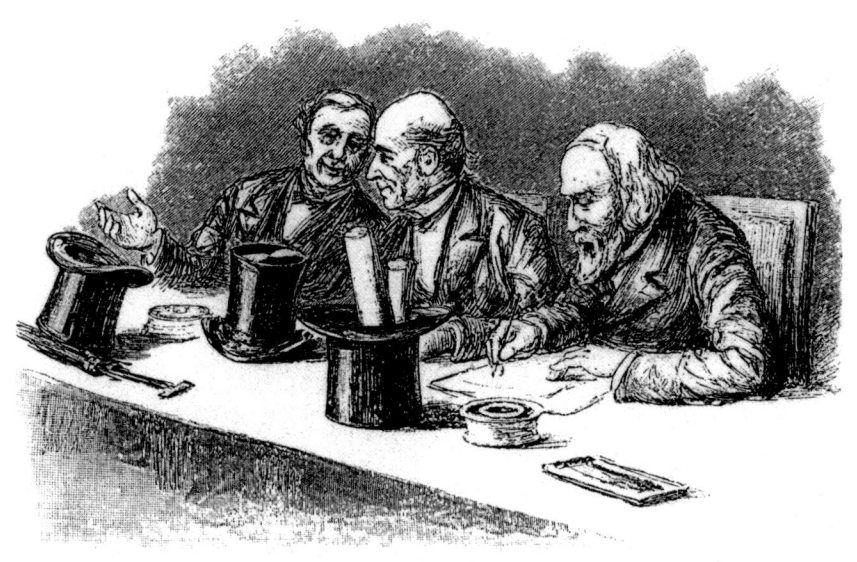

Brown-Séquard preparing a speech at the Académie des Sciences in Paris. From Child T. The Institute of France. In *Harper's New Monthly Magazine,* 78:501–520, 1889.

TOUT
A
BROWN-SÉQUARD!...

MONOLOGUE FANTAISIST

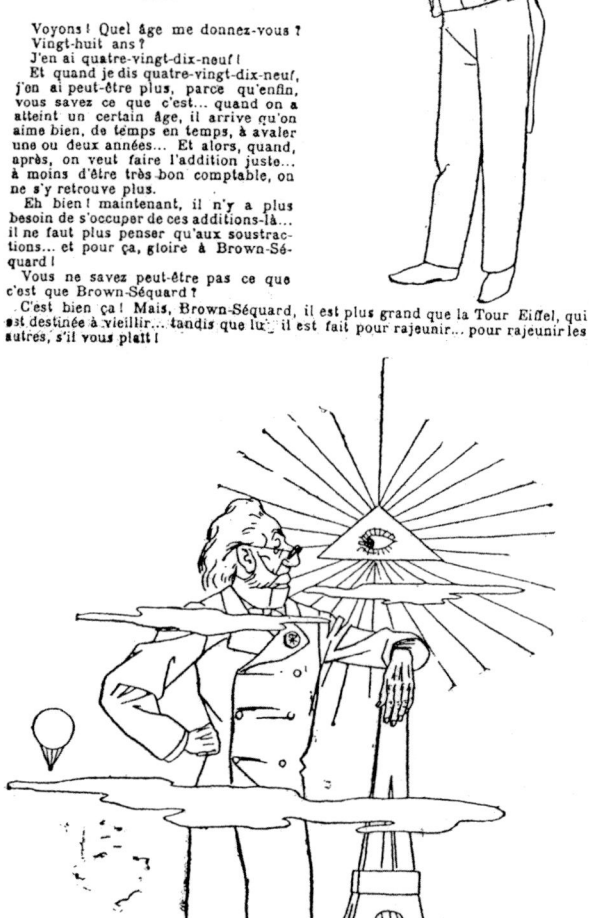

Voyons! Quel âge me donnez-vous?
Vingt-huit ans?
J'en ai quatre-vingt-dix-neuf!
Et quand je dis quatre-vingt-dix-neuf, j'en ai peut-être plus, parce qu'enfin, vous savez ce que c'est... quand on a atteint un certain âge, il arrive qu'on aime bien, de temps en temps, à avaler une ou deux années... Et alors, quand, après, on veut faire l'addition juste... à moins d'être très bon comptable, on ne s'y retrouve plus.

Eh bien! maintenant, il n'y a plus besoin de s'occuper de ces additions-là... il ne faut plus penser qu'aux soustractions... et pour ça, gloire à Brown-Séquard!

Vous ne savez peut-être pas ce que c'est que Brown-Séquard?

C'est bien ça! Mais, Brown-Séquard, il est plus grand que la Tour Eiffel, qui est destinée à vieillir... tandis que lui, il est fait pour rajeunir... pour rajeunir les autres, s'il vous plaît!

Portion of the front page of the literary supplement of *Le Figaro* dated 12 October 1889. The entire page pokes fun at Brown-Séquard, who is shown standing taller than the Eiffel Tower, a structure that—despite being the tallest building in the world—was destined to age.

SEQUARINE

THE MEDICINE OF THE FUTURE.

THE one great remedy of the future will undoubtedly be the Serum. The mere fact that Scientists are now able to transfer energy from one animal body to another is sufficient to arouse enthusiasm among Doctors.

The perfection of the Sequarine Serum (which embodies the very essence of animal energy) in a form for everyday use, places animal therapy far in advance of other branches of medical science. This Serum is being used with astonishing success in treating:—

Nervousness,	Kidney Disease,	Paralysis,
Neurasthenia,	Diabetes,	Locomotor Ataxy,
Anæmia,	Dropsy,	General Weakness,
Rheumatism,	Dyspepsia,	Influenza,
Gout,	Liver Complaints,	Pulmonary
Sciatica,	Indigestion,	Troubles.

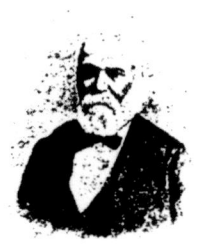

BROWN-SEQUARD, F.R.S., F.R.C.P. (London), who discovered the vital principle which is the basis of natural immunity from disease.

Advertisement for organ extracts published in *The Strand Magazine* (London) in 1912. The death of Brown-Séquard some years earlier clearly failed to deter speculators from making extravagant claims based on his work.

PROFESSOR

BROWN SEQUARD'S
METHOD.

EXTRACTS OF ANIMAL ORGANS.
Testicle Extract,
Grey Matter Extract,
Thyroid Gland Extract, &c., &c.

Concentrated Solutions at 30%.

These preparations, completely aseptic, are mailed to any distance on receipt of a money order. Directions sent with the fluids:

Price for 25 Injections, $2.50.
Syringe Specially Gauged, (3 cubic c.,) $2.50.

Used in the Hospitals of Paris, New York, Boston, etc.
Circular Sent on Application.

New York Biological and Vaccinal Institute,
Laboratory of Bovine Vaccine and of Biological Products.

Portion of another advertisement for organ extracts that made use—without his consent—of Brown-Séquard's name. It appeared in the *New York Therapeutic Review* of 1893.

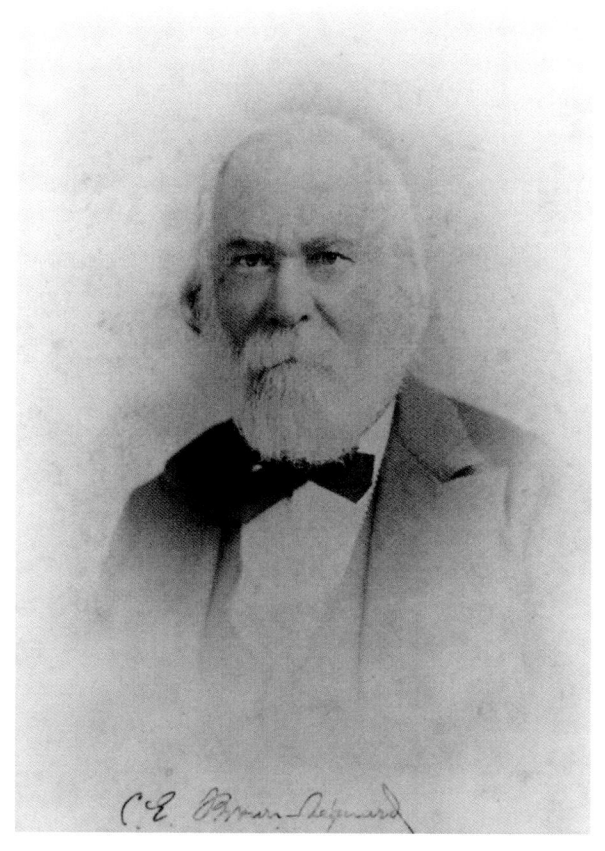

A rare photograph of the elderly Brown-Séquard. Many thought that his organotherapy was an attempt to recapture his youth. Courtesy of the Royal College of Physicians of London Heritage Centre.

Organ extracts were prepared at the Collège de France and sent by Brown-Séquard and d'Arsonval without charge to medical practitioners for the purposes of scientific experimentation, as stated on the label of the extracts. Courtesy of the Royal College of Physicians of London Heritage Centre.

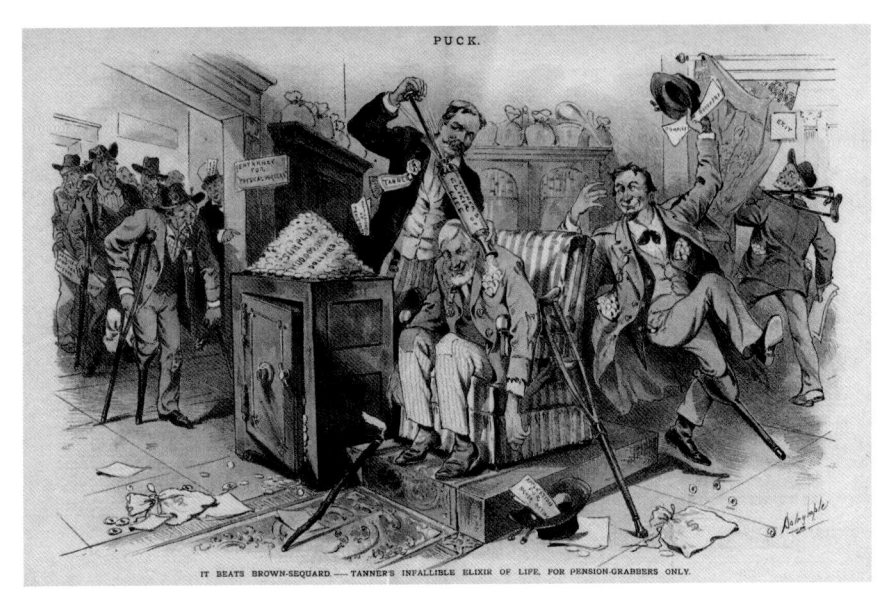

Center spread from *Puck*, 28 August 1889, entitled "It beats Brown-Séquard—Tanner's infallible elixir of life for pension-grabbers only." Organotherapy was used as a means of attacking the Republican's proposed policy of expanding pension benefits for Civil War veterans and their families. Tanner was the commissioner of pensions. Chromolithograph by Louis Darymple. Courtesy of the Bert Hansen Collection, New York City.

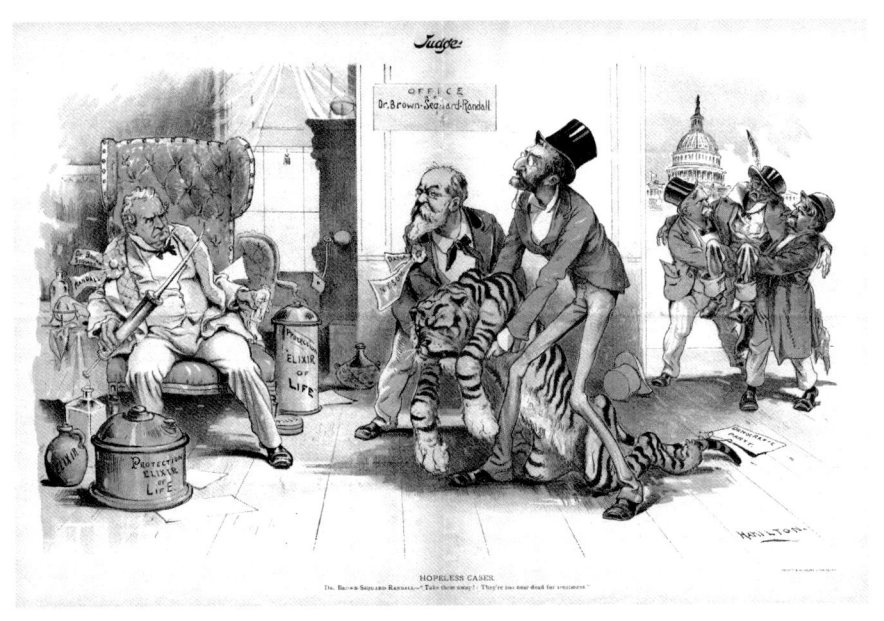

"Hopeless cases." Center spread from *Judge*, 31 August 1889. Another satirical cartoon using organotherapy as a means of political ridicule. The illustration depicts a Democrat congressman, Samuel J. Randall ("Brown-Séquard Randall"), a protectionist despite his party's position on the issue, who considers it too late to revive his party and its free-trade policy with the Elixir of Life. Chromolithograph by Grant Hamilton. Courtesy of the Bert Hansen Collection, New York City.

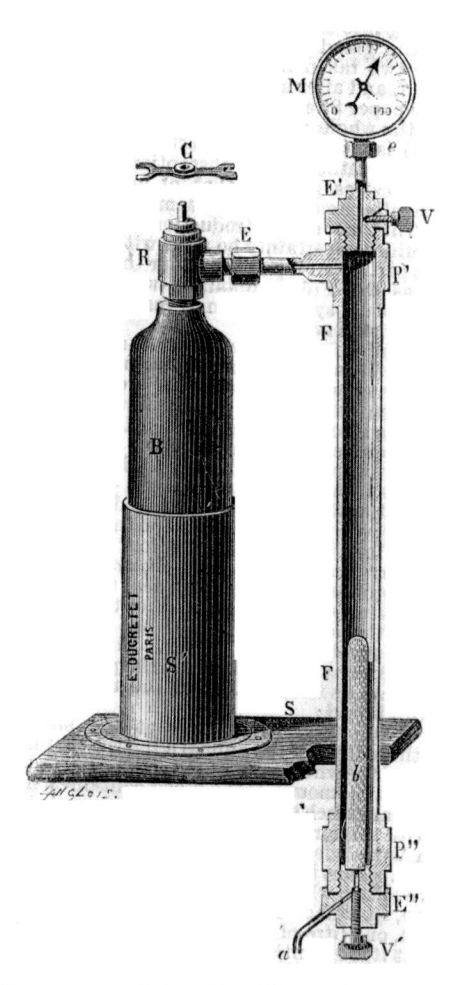

Filtration apparatus. The apparatus designed by d'Arsonval to act as a filter when preparing liquid organic extracts. A hollow metallic cylinder (S') keeps immovable a thick steel bottle (B) filled with liquid carbonic acid. A metal tube (F, F'), which can bear a pressure of 200 atmospheres, has screwed into its lower end a metallic stopper that carries the filtration bougie (b), a rubber tube containing a "kind of clay in which kaolin is replaced by pure alumina." A screw top (v') attached to the metallic stopper allows the apparatus to be opened or closed at will. When open, liquid that has passed through the filter runs out through a tube (a). The top of the tube (F) is closed by a metal stopper (V) and connected with a manometer and a screw that allows for the escape of carbon dioxide gas when required. A side tube (E) allows communication between the filter and liquid carbonic acid in B. A stopper (R), opened or closed by a key (C), allows communication between B and F. To sterilize the liquid, it is first introduced into the tube F, and carbonic acid is allowed to enter and presses over it. A pressure of 50–60 atmospheres is maintained for about an hour, "during which all the microbes that may be present are crushed or killed." The tap v' is then opened and the liquid filters rapidly through b. From Brown-Séquard CE. On a new therapeutic method consisting in the use of organic liquids extracted from glands and other organs. *Br Med J*, 1:1145–1147 and 1212–1214, 1893.

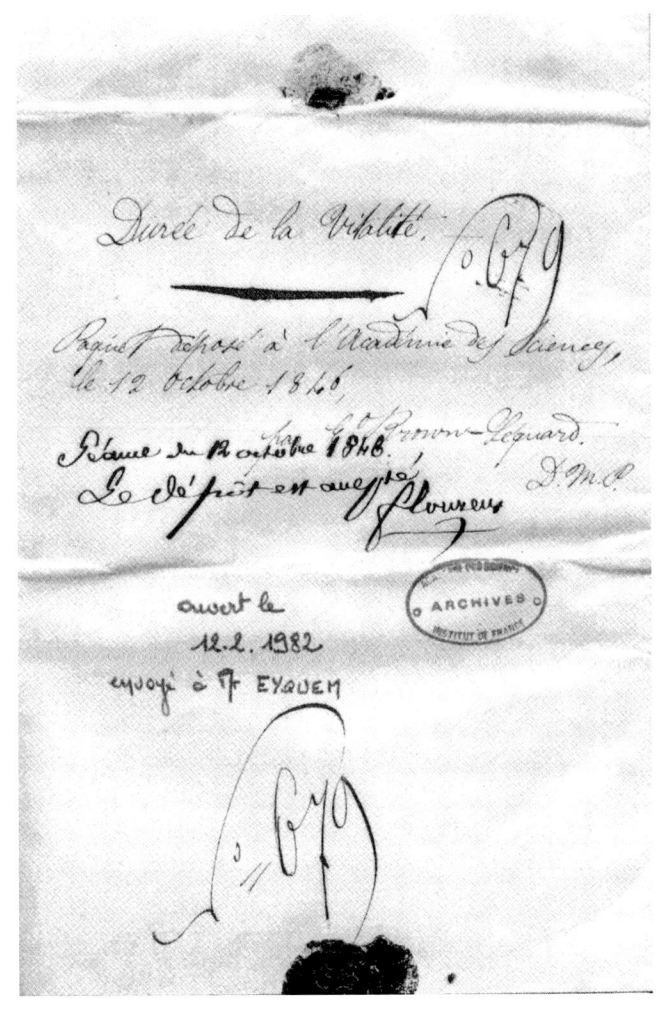

Sealed report packet. Front sheet of a report on postmortem rigidity deposited unopened at the meeting of 12 October 1846 at the Académie des Sciences in Paris by Brown-Séquard, where it was to be opened in case of any dispute about priority. Such packets were typically deposited by members reporting an important but incompletely delineated discovery that was not yet ready for publication. The document was accepted by Flourens, the permanent secretary, who sealed and signed it on the cover. Sealed packets were only to be opened at the request of the submitting member or by vote of the Académie. Brown-Séquard's was opened in 1982 (as also noted on the document) for historical reasons. Courtesy of the Académie des Sciences, Institut de France.

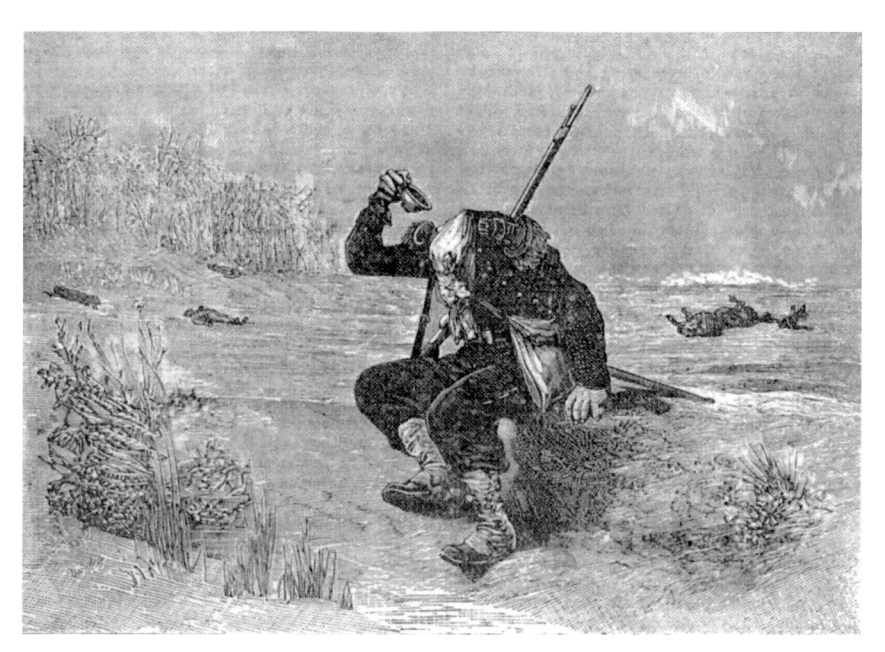

A case of instantaneous death on the battlefield at Sedan in 1870. The corpse of a headless soldier is seated with the right arm raised, holding a tin cup directed at the mouth that is no longer present. The soldier had been decapitated by a cannonball while about to take a drink, and his body developed an instantaneous rigidity that maintained its position at the moment of death. The illustration is taken from a paper by Brown-Séquard. From *Knowledge*, 6: 115–117, 1884.

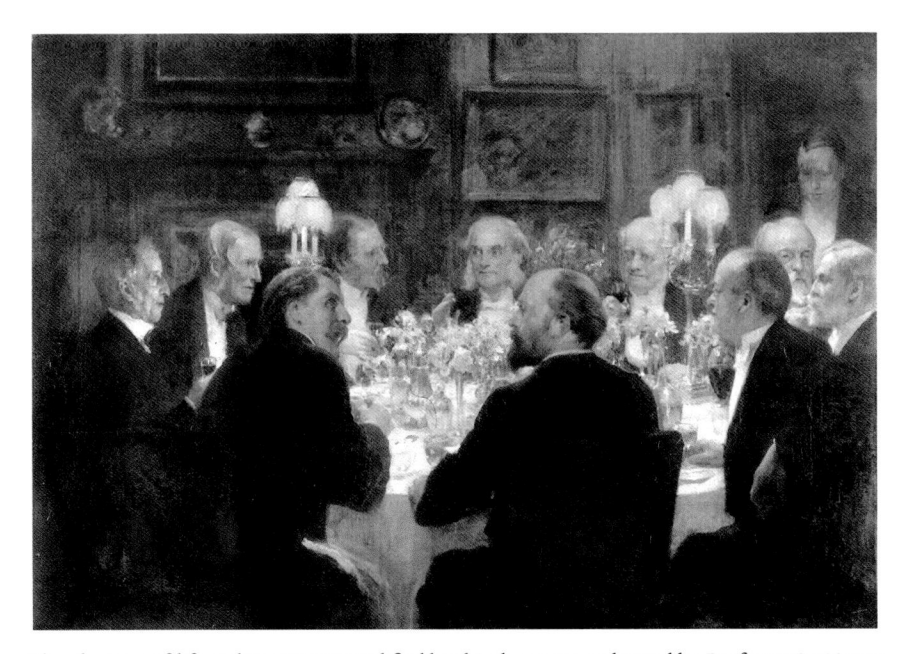

The glamour of life at the top is exemplified by this dinner party hosted by Professor Sir Henry Thompson to honor Ernest Hart, editor of the *British Medical Journal* (at back, to right of mantelpiece). Clockwise from Hart are Sir Thomas Spencer Wells, gynecological surgeon, after whom is named a type of forceps; Sir Joseph Fayrer, President of the Medical Board at the India Office in London and an international authority on snakes and their venoms; Newman, Thompson's butler; Sir Thomas Lauder Brunton, physician and pharmacologist, who helped to introduce amyl nitrite for the treatment of angina; Sir William Broadbent, physician to Queen Victoria and later King Edward VII; Sir George Anderson Critchett, ophthalmic surgeon; Sir Victor Horsley, pioneer neurosurgeon and physiologist (p. 244); Sir Richard Quain, physician (p. 149); Sir James Paget, surgeon (p. 50); and Sir Henry Thompson, urological surgeon, sketcher, astronomer, and founder of the first cremation society in England. Brown-Séquard was on good terms with Paget and Quain, and corresponded with Horsley, who was familiar with his work on cerebral localization and tried out some of his testicular extracts. He had also corresponded and spoken at length with Thompson about his organ extracts (p. 211). Thompson's dinner parties were famous. Known as "octaves," they involved eight courses accompanied by eight wines served at eight o'clock to eight guests plus the guest of honor. Brown-Séquard would have had no patience with such dinner parties. He had little charm, no small talk, disliked alcohol and tobacco, had severe flatulence and merycism (from his self-experimentation while a student), and preferred to go to bed at about eight o'clock (rather than dine) so as to arise in the early hours of the morning to work undisturbed. (Oil painting by Solomon Solomon, circa 1897). Courtesy of the Wellcome Library, London.

> M
>
> Vous êtes prié d'assister aux Convoi et Enterrement de
>
> **Monsieur le Docteur C. E. Brown-Séquard,**
>
> Membre de l'Institut,
> Professeur au Collège de France,
>
> décédé le 1er Avril 1894, en son domicile, rue François 1er, N° 19, dans sa 77ème année ;
> Qui se feront le Mercredi 4 courant, à 11 heures très précises.
>
> On se réunira à la maison mortuaire.
>
> De la part du Docteur Edouard Brown-Séquard, son fils ; de Mademoiselle Charlotte Brown-Séquard, sa fille ; de Mesdemoiselles Caroline et Grace Fletcher ; de Monsieur Fletcher ; de Monsieur et Madame John Carlisle ; de Monsieur William Carlisle ; de Monsieur et Madame Mendenhall ; de Monsieur et Madame Ford ; de Madame Murdoch, ses beaux-frères et belles-sœurs ; de Monsieur et Madame Aristide Séquard ; de Monsieur et Madame Arnould, des Familles Coe et Waterhouse, ses cousins, cousines et alliés ;
> Et de ses amis.
>
> L'Inhumation aura lieu au Cimetière Montparnasse.
>
> Administration Spéciale des Funérailles. 2. Rue d'Anjou. Maison Henri de Borniol.

Invitation to the burial of Brown-Séquard at the cemetery of Montparnasse in Paris. Note that his son Edouard is listed as among the mourners, even though he was estranged from his father and evidence suggests that he had died some years earlier, as discussed in the text. Courtesy of the Royal College of Physicians of London Heritage Centre.

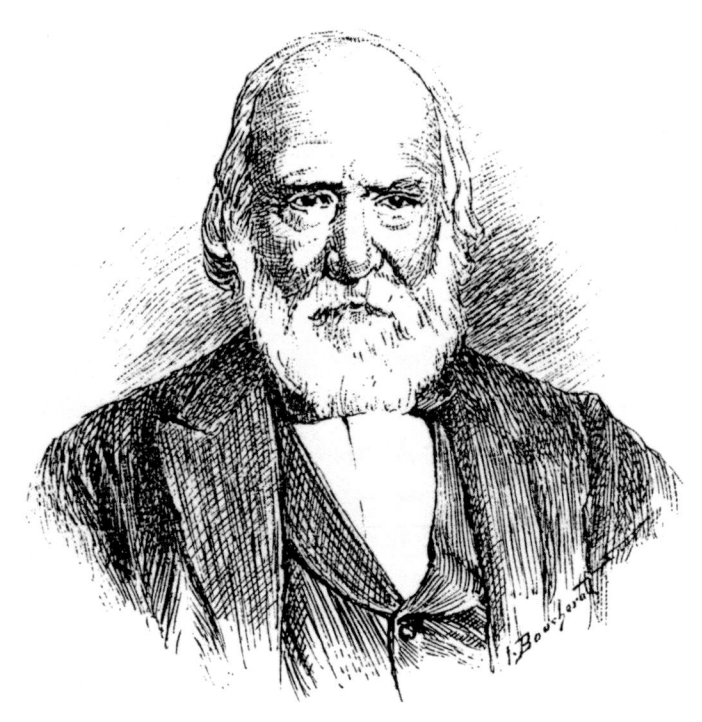

Obituaries of Brown-Séquard were often accomplished by an artist's impression of his likeness because no photographs of him were available. This particular drawing was the frontispiece of a booklet of tributes to him published in Mauritius in 1898. Courtesy of the Royal College of Physicians of London Heritage Centre.

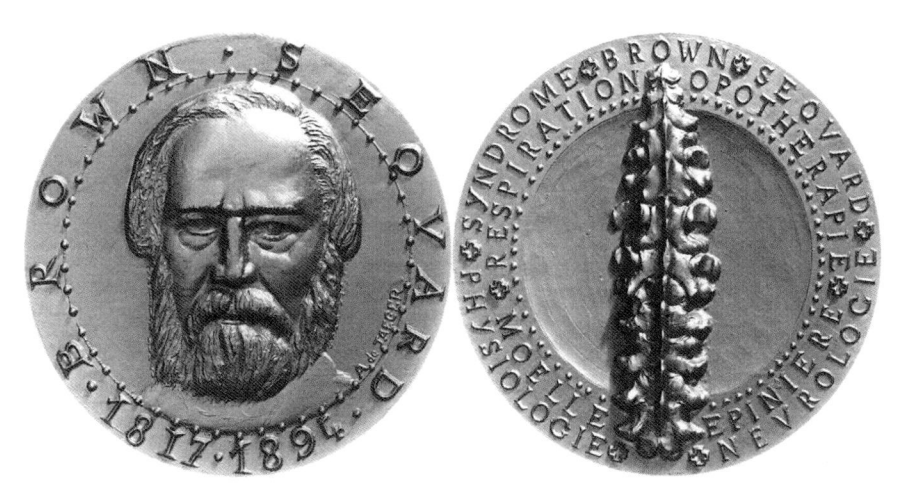

Commemorative bronze medal of Brown-Séquard. The 68-mm medal by Albert de Jaeger, issued in 1972 by the Monnaie de Paris (the Paris or French Mint), bears his likeness and lifespan on the obverse. The reverse side commemorates his syndrome, depicts the vertebrae, and lists some of his areas of expertise [physiology, neurology, respiration, opotherapy (organotherapy), and the spinal cord]. ©Monnaie de Paris. Reproduced with permission.

on another. His views were therefore cast aside by most neuroscientists. Nevertheless, subsequent experimental studies revealed a greater complexity of cerebral function than initially was appreciated, indicating for the motor system, for example, that there are both primary and secondary motor cortical areas and motor association areas in the cortex that receive inputs from wide areas of the brain. Stimulation of these diverse cortical areas leads to movement (although at higher intensities of stimulation in some areas than others). Moreover, depending on the cortical area under consideration and its projection pathways, stimulation may induce movements ipsilaterally as well as contralaterally. In fact, considerable individual variation exists in the extent that the descending corticospinal tract (that passes directly from the motor or motor-sensory cortex to the spinal cord) crosses from one side to the other in the brainstem, and there are also indirect pathways from the motor cortex to the cord that are bilateral.

In any event, the relevance of these phenomena to normal motor function is unclear. The early, unrestrained enthusiasm of the cerebral cartographers has given way to a less-confident realism, and simplicity and certainty have been replaced by complexity and ambiguity. The motor cortex, perceived by some as the "will-centres" for movement, may, after all, simply constitute the gateway from the cerebral cortex of motor traffic that—having drifted along the maze of highways and byways interconnecting different parts of the brain—passes either directly or indirectly to a rendezvous in the spinal cord. There also remains uncertainty concerning the precise effect on motor function of discrete lesions in these different regions. The clinical consequences in humans even of lesions directly affecting (and restricted to) the region that physicians and neuroscientists have elected misleadingly to designate the primary motor cortex are still debatable.

The scientific community now accepts that the specialized motor centers defined so painstakingly and accepted so enthusiastically in the latter years of the nineteenth century in animals and in the twentieth century in humans have a more limited role in the regulation of movement. Phillips and Porter, in a monograph published in 1977, remarked that, "... the 'motor' cortex [has an] ... intermediate position in relation to ... structures which 'command' it from upstream and to the structures which it excites and inhibits in the brainstem and spinal cord .... The locations and structure of the 'higher-level' programmes which provide the ... central inputs remain elusive."[53] It was the structural components of these functional command-programs that Brown-Séquard viewed as localized diffusely within the brain, beyond the confines of any single structure and varying, of necessity, with the function to be generated. It seemed a logical step to conclude on theoretical grounds that, if this were the case, a lesion within a discrete region of the brain could inhibit or excite nerve cells involved in specific functions, regardless of their location in the brain or spinal cord, in order to ensure that the system operated in a coordinated fashion. Thus, he argued against the localization or absolute lateralization of cerebral function.

Brown-Séquard believed that a similar arrangement existed for motor, sensory, or cognitive functions. Interestingly, at a meeting of neuroscientists held in Oxford one hundred years after the celebrated International Medical Congress of 1881, it was apparent that, although different parts of the cerebral cortex clearly perform distinct functions, specific cortical areas are more difficult to define than had been envisioned earlier, and agreement is lacking about the precise functions that are actually localized.[54] Cortical areas once defined by coarse electrical stimulation or microscopic anatomy can now be defined by more subtle features using advanced investigative techniques. Function within a cortical area, as depicted by maps, are not as orderly, constant, or consistent between subjects as once supposed. Instead, they are plastic, dynamic, and changed by preceding activity and other factors. Specific functions or types of function may involve multiple cortical areas. The subjective appreciation of color, for example, requires the activity of different areas. If different cortical areas are specialized to analyze different aspects or components of motor, sensory, or other functions, a redistribution of information, either within or between areas becomes necessary, so that all this information can be brought together into a cohesive whole. The cells that interact must be interconnected in functional networks.[54] Through such networks, the dynamic interaction of different cortical and subcortical areas with multiple interconnections must underlie the organization of specific functions. Most cognitive processing begins with sensory input (as also does motor activity), and "higher" cognitive functions may necessitate the integration of information from multiple modalities.[55]

Brown-Séquard would have been gratified to learn that, a century after he aired his views, advanced techniques—such as functional magnetic resonance imaging—have confirmed the functional connectivity of many areas of the brain, showing that spatially distinct cortical and subcortical regions are activated during performance of specific tasks.[56,57] Behavioral neurologists now accept that the consequences of a focal lesion are best interpreted by regarding the affected area as part of a neural network mediating a specific function,[58] and that disconnection of specific areas of the brain may lead to major behavioral disturbances.[59] It has even been suggested that neurodegenerative diseases, rather than involving random or confluent parts of the brain, target intrinsic neural networks related to specific functions.[60] Although Brown-Séquard may have erred in the details, he had intuitively conceived of an approach that few of his peers could even understand, let alone accept seriously, but which time has vindicated. The concepts that he had tried unsuccessfully to communicate to others without substantive experimental support—views that helped to relegate him to the fringe of the academic enterprise—may have been closer to the constructs of modern neuroscience than his contemporaries could have imagined.

The Duality of the Brain

The emerging doctrine of cerebral localization constituted a rejection of the prior belief of cerebral equipotentiality. By opposing aspects of the concept that certain functions were localized in the cerebral hemispheres, Brown-Séquard came ultimately to believe that in its potential "... each of the cerebral hemispheres is a complete brain, endowed with all the powers that we know belong to the whole cerebrum."[61] His views in this regard encompassed those of Arthur Wigan, an English general practitioner who—in *The Duality of Mind*, published in 1844—argued that the two cerebral hemispheres were essentially two independent brains that functioned either in concert or in place of each other, depending on the occasion. Variations of this theory concerning the duality of the brain were common in the nineteenth century and were used to explain the occurrence of split or multiple personalities. It is said that Robert Louis Stevenson was influenced by Brown-Séquard, when he wrote *The Strange Case of Dr Jekyll and Mr Hyde*.[62] In his provoking paper—"Have we two brains or one?"—Brown-Séquard himself maintained that each cerebral hemisphere is capable of generating voluntary activity and of receiving sensory information from both sides of the body. With regard to movement, he stated explicitly that "... each half of the brain can originate all the voluntary movements of the two sides of the body, and, therefore, we have two brains for all the muscular actions caused by our will in the four limbs. ..."[61] This conclusion seemed to follow from his previously discussed views concerning the diffuse nature of the cerebral mechanisms regulating motor activities, the remote effects of focal cerebral lesions, and the functional processes permitting the interaction of different parts of the nervous system.

He also pointed to the plasticity of the brain as further evidence against the concept that localized anatomical regions have fixed and specific functions, and that both cerebral hemispheres are required for normal function. In many animals, destruction of one hemisphere leads to no permanent gross behavioral abnormality, presumably because other areas of the brain assume the functions of the extirpated hemisphere. Similarly, certain patients seem to recover completely—or virtually so—from a lesion destroying one hemisphere, especially when such pathological involvement occurs at an early age, thus suggesting that the functions of the affected region are taken over by the other hemisphere. Such plasticity has major implications not only for the operation of the nervous system but for the rehabilitation of patients with neurological injuries.

Brown-Séquard regarded each half of the brain to be complete in itself and capable of regulating the activities of both sides of the body, as well as of other cerebral activities, but concluded that the left hemisphere was normally the "predominant" one in humans. More specifically, in normal circumstances, the left hemisphere was chiefly the

> organ serving the mental functions, either in speech, or in intelligence, or in gesture, or in writing. That organ, therefore, is the important organ in our system adapted to the life of communication between ourselves and our brethren in a mental way. But the other organ—the right side of the brain, in some individuals ... has the power of the left side, and in all, perhaps, it might have had if the proper development had taken place; but this right side has also additional functions. The right side of the brain serves chiefly the emotional manifestations ... [but] can be educated to become a leader in mental faculties as well as the left side of the brain.[34]

He attributed the importance of the left hemisphere for communication to its greater role in controlling the right-sided limbs, which are the preferred limbs for most people, rather than to innate differences between the two hemispheres. Greater use of the left hemisphere, he suggested, permitted it to assume a predominant role. He thus urged the educational authorities to endeavor, by developing motor skills of the left-sided limbs, to develop the capabilities of the right hemisphere (that is., of our second brain). A number of schools in America and Britain put this approach into practice, at least for a period, but it eventually fell into disfavor when no practical benefit was seen to emerge and evidence began to accumulate that training children to use their nondominant hand was sometimes detrimental to their development, leading, for example, to stammering.

Brown-Séquard's views, published in 1874,[34] concerning the predominance of the left hemisphere for certain functions are now generally accepted. At the time that he first wrote on this theme, however, the concept was still developing. His beliefs were not dissimilar to those of Hughlings Jackson who, also in 1874, wrote of the left hemisphere as the leading one.[31] But Brown-Séquard's views concerning the equipotentiality of the two hemispheres have been overtaken by advances in the neurosciences; the developments that occur during the first few years of life lead to changes in the hemispheres that seem to dissipate their equipotentiality. The brains of infants and young children have many more neurons and connections than those of adults. There is marked neuronal loss and alterations in neuronal connectivity (synaptic pruning and rearrangement of dendrites) during childhood. The pathways that are used often will survive, whereas those that are used rarely will disappear.

With regard to mental duality in the intact brain,[1] the fact are less clear. Most scientists believe that we have only a single mind, reflecting the operation of the duplicated brain. The two sides of the brain act in harmony together, collaboratively in an integrated manner, to make us what we are. Nevertheless, patients who have undergone the surgical procedure of hemispherectomy (removal of much of one cerebral hemisphere, for example, for intractable epilepsy) retain a mind of their own. In animals or patients who have undergone a surgical procedure ("split brain") to disrupt the corpus callosum (which connects much, but not all, of the two hemispheres), mental processes limited to each hemisphere can be demonstrated and behavioral changes may be relatively subtle. Such individuals can be said to have two minds, with separate discriminative and volitional capacities.[1] Thus, the *potential* remains for the operation of two minds in humans with an intact brain (with two cerebral hemispheres), particularly as the connections between the two intact hemispheres are insufficient to unify all the information contained within them so that there is some independence of hemispheric function.[1] At the same time, the two hemispheres also act in concert. Components of complex stimuli can be processed concurrently and independently by the two hemispheres, depending on which hemisphere is dominant for the factor under analysis.[63] At present, then, the existence and extent of mental duality in intact human subjects remains open to discussion and reflects, perhaps, a semantic issue that has yet to be resolved.

References and Source Notes

1. Bogen JE. Mental duality in the intact brain. *Bull Clin Neurosci*, 51:3–29, 1986.
2. Sherrington CS. Inhibition as a coordinating factor. Nobel Lecture, 12 December 1932. In: *Nobel lectures, including presentation speeches and laureates' biographies: Physiology or medicine, 1922–1941* (pp. 278–289). Amsterdam: Elsevier (for the Nobel Foundation), 1965.
3. Brown-Séquard CE. *Course of lectures on the physiology and pathology of the central nervous system* (pp. 187–192). Philadelphia: Collins, 1860.
4. Brown-Séquard CE. On the mechanism of production of symptoms of diseases of the brain. *Arch Sci Pract Med (NY)*, 1:251–266, 1873.
5. Brown-Séquard CE. Faits montrant que des lésions de diverses parties de l'encéphale peuvent déterminer l'inhibition des cellules nerveuses et d'autres éléments de la moelle épinière, servant aux mouvements réflexes. *C R Soc Biol (Paris)*, 31:129–131, 1879.

6. Brown-Séquard CE. Expériences montrant: 1, que l'excitation galvanique des parties considérées comme motrices à la base de l'encéphale produit plus souvent des mouvements du côté correspondant que du côté opposé; 2, qu'une lésion d'un côté de la moelle épinière ou d'un des nerfs sciatiques peut produire l'inhibition des cellules motrices et sensitives du bulbe et de la protubérances. *C R Soc Biol (Paris)*, 31:200–201, 1879.
7. Brown-Séquard CE. Faits nouveaux relatifs à la mise en jeu ou à l'arrêt (inhibition) des propriétés motrices ou sensitives de diverses parties du centre cérébro-rachidien. *Arch Physiol Norm Pathol (2nd Series)*, 6:494–499, 1879.
8. Brown-Séquard CE. Expériences montrant: 1, Que la même lésion d'un centre nerveux peut déterminer un état paralytique avec perte du ton musculaire ou une contracture; 2, Qu'une irritation mécanique violente de l'encéphale peut produire de l'inhibition dans certaines parties de la moelle épinière et de la dynamogénie dans d'autres. *C R Soc Biol (Paris)*, 31:296–297, 1879.
9. Brown-Séquard CE. Recherches montrant la puissance, la rapidité d'action et les variétés de certaines influences inhibitoires (influences d'arrêt) de l'encéphale sur lui-même ou sur la moelle épinière, et de ce dernier centre sur lui-même ou sur l'encéphale. *C R Acad Sci*, 89:657–659, 1879.
10. Brown-Séquard CE. The effects produced by various lesions of the base of the brain on the excitability of the so-called motor centres. *Br Med J*, 2:383, 1880.
11. Brown-Séquard CE. Phénomènes d'inhibition et de dynamogénie. *Gaz Hebd Med (2nd Series)*, 18:380–381, 1881.
12. Brown-Séquard CE. Recherches expérimentales et cliniques sur l'inhibition et la dynamogénie. Application des connaissances fournies par ces recherches aux phénomènes principaux de l'hypnotisme, de l'extase et du transfert. [In several parts.] *Gaz Hebd Med (2nd Series)*, 19:35–36, 53–55, 75–77, 105–107, and 136–138, 1882.
13. Brown-Séquard CE. Recherches expérimentales et cliniques sur le mode de production de l'anesthésie dans les affections organiques de l'encéphale. *C R Acad Sci*, 96:1766–1769, 1883.
14. Brown-Séquard CE. De l'importance du rôle de l'inhibition en thérapeutique. *C R Acad Sci*, 96:617–620, 1883.
15. Smith R. *Inhibition: History and meaning in the sciences of mind and brain.* Berkeley: University of California Press, 1992.
16. Bert P. Prix Lallemand. *C R Acad Sci*, 100:535–537, 1885.
17. Sherrington CS. Sur une action inhibitrice de l'écorce cérébrale. *Rev Neurol (Paris*, 1:318–319, 1893.
18. Tizard B. Theories of brain localization from Flourens to Lashley. *Med Hist*, 3:132–145, 1959.
19. Swazey JP. Action propre and action commune: The localization of cerebral function. *J Hist Biol*, 3:213–234, 1970.
20. Young RM. The functions of the brain: Gall to Ferrier (1808–1886). *Isis*, 59:251–266, 1968.
21. Walker AE. The development of the concept of cerebral localization in the nineteenth century. *Bull Hist Med*, 31:99–121, 1957.
22. Critchley M. Neurology's debt to F.J. Gall (1758–1828). *Br Med J*, 2:775–781, 1965.
23. Young RM. *Mind, brain and adaptation in the nineteenth century* (pp. 58–75). Oxford: Clarendon Press, 1970.
24. Clarke E, Jacyna LS. *Nineteenth-century origins of neuroscientific concepts.* Berkeley: University of California Press, 1987.
25. Broca P. Perte de la parole, ramollissement chronique et destruction partielle du lobe antérieur gauche du cerveau. *Bull Soc d'Anthropol (Paris)*, 2:235–238, 1861.

26. Broca P. Remarques sur le siège de la faculté du langage articulé, suivies d'une observation d'aphémie (perte de la parole). *Bull Soc Anat (Paris)*, 36:330–357, 1861.
27. Broca P. Nouvelle observation d'aphémie produite par une lésion de la moitié postérieure des deuxième et troisième circonvolutions frontales. *Bull Soc Anat (Paris)*, 36:398–407, 1861.
28. Broca P. Localisation des fonctions cérébrales. Siége du langage articulé. *Bull Soc d'Anthropol (Paris)*, 4:200–204, 1863.
29. Finger S, Roe D. Gustave Dax and the early history of cerebral dominance. *Arch Neurol*, 53:806–813, 1996.
30. Head H. Hughlings Jackson on aphasia and kindred affections of speech. *Brain*, 38:1–27, 1915.
31. Hughlings Jackson J. On the nature of the duality of the brain. *Brain*, 38:80–86, 1915. [Reprinted from *Medical Press & Circular*, January 14, 1874.]
32. Hughlings Jackson J. On affections of speech from disease of the brain. *Brain*, 2:203–222, 1879.
33. Brown-Séquard CE. Aphasia as an effect of brain-disease. *Dublin J Med Sci*, 63:209–225, 1877.
34. Brown-Séquard CE. Dual character of the brain. (The Toner Lectures: Lecture 2: Delivered 22 April 1874.) Article 3. *Smithsonian Miscellaneous Collections, Volume 15*. Washington: Smithsonian Institute, 1878.
35. Hughlings Jackson J. On the anatomical and physiological localisation of movements in the brain. [In several parts.] *Lancet*, 1:84–85, 162–164, and 232–234, 1873.
36. Taylor J, ed. *Selected writings of John Hughlings Jackson. Volume 1. On Epilepsy and Epileptiform Convulsions*. London: Hodder & Stoughton, 1931.
37. Fritsch G, Hitzig E. Über die elektrische Erregbarkeit des Grosshirns. *Arch Anat Physiol (Lpz)*, 37:300–332, 1870.
38. Ferrier D. *The functions of the brain*. London: Smith, Elder & Co., 1876.
39. Young RM. *Mind, brain and adaptation in the nineteenth century* (pp. 234–240). Oxford: Clarendon Press, 1970.
40. Bartholow R. Experimental investigations into the functions of the human brain. *Am J Med Sci*, 67:305–313, 1874.
41. Harris LJ, Almerigi JB. Probing the human brain with stimulating electrodes: the story of Roberts Bartholow's (1874) experiment on Mary Rafferty. *Brain Cogn*, 70:92–115, 2009.
42. Bennett H, Godlee RJ. A mirror of hospital practice: British and foreign. Hospital for Epilepsy and Paralysis, Regent's Park. Excision of a tumour from the brain. *Lancet*, 2:1090–1091, 1884.
43. Tyler KL, Malessa R. The Goltz–Ferrier debates and the triumph of cerebral localizationalist theory. *Neurology*, 55:1015–1024, 2000.
44. Klein E, Langley JN, Schäffer EA. On the cortical areas removed from the brain of a dog, and from the brain of a monkey. *J Physiol*, 4:231–326, 1884.
45. Brown-Séquard CE. On localization of functions in the brain. *Boston Med Surg J*, 93:119–124, 1875.
46. Brown-Séquard CE. Cerebral localization. *Forum*, 5:166–177, 1888.
47. Brown-Séquard CE. Lectures on the diagnosis and treatment of the various forms of paralytic, convulsive, and mental affections, considered as effects of morbid alterations of the blood, or of the brain or other organs. Lecture 1 – Part 2. On the mode of origin of symptoms of disease of the brain. *Lancet*, 2:29–30, 1861.
48. Brown-Séquard CE. Introduction à une série de mémoires sur la physiologie et la pathologie des diverses parties de l'encéphale. *Arch Physiol Norm Pathol (2nd Series)*, 4:409–423 and 655–694, 1877.

49. Brown-Séquard CE. Sur l'apparition d'une paralysie du coté d'une lésion encéphalique. *C R Soc Biol (Paris)*, 27:424, 1875; *C R Soc Biol (Paris)*, 28:2 and 13, 1876.
50. Brown-Séquard CE. A lecture on the appearances of paralysis on the side of a lesion of the brain. [In several parts.] *Lancet*, 1:2–4, 79–80, and 159–161, 1876.
51. Brown-Séquard CE. Introductory lecture to a course on the physiological pathology of the brain. *Lancet*, 2:75–78, 1876.
52. Brown-Séquard CE. Experimental facts showing that the admitted views relating to paralysis of cerebral origin and to the physiology of the so-called motor tract in the brain must be rejected. *Lancet*, 2:254–255, 1881.
53. Phillips CG, Porter R. *Corticospinal neurones: Their role in movement* (pp. 402–406). London: Academic Press, 1977.
54. Phillips CG, Zeki S, Barlow HB. Localization of function in the cerebral cortex. Past, present and future. *Brain*, 107:327–361, 1984.
55. Rosen HJ, Viskontas IV. Cortical neuroanatomy and cognition. *Handb Clin Neurol*, 88:41–60, 2008.
56. Fox MD, Raichle ME. Spontaneous fluctuations in brain activity observed with functional magnetic resonance imaging. *Nat Rev Neurosci*, 8:700–711, 2007.
57. Greicius M. Resting-state functional connectivity in neuropsychiatric disorders. *Curr Opin Neurol*, 21:424–430, 2008.
58. Damasio AR, Geschwind N. Anatomical localization in clinical neuropsychology. In: Frederiks JAM, ed., *Handbook of clinical neurology* (Vol. 45, pp. 7–22). Amsterdam: Elsevier, 1985.
59. Geschwind N. Disconnexion syndromes in animals and man. *Brain*, 88:237–294, and 585–644, 1965.
60. Seeley WW, Crawford RK, Zhou J, Miller BL, Greicius MD. Neurodegenerative diseases target large-scale human brain networks. *Neuron*, 62:42–52, 2009.
61. Brown-Séquard CE. Have we two brains or one? *Forum*, 9:627–643, 1890.
62. Stiles A. Robert Louis Stevenson's *Jekyll and Hyde* and the double brain. *Studies in English Literature*, 46:879–900, 2006.
63. Bradshaw JL, Nettleton NC. *Human cerebral asymmetry*. Englewood Cliffs, NJ: Prentice-Hall, 1983.

11

The Disease of Devils and Demons

THE TERM *epilepsy* refers to a group of disorders in which there is a tendency to recurrent, unprovoked seizures. Seizures are due to an abnormal, sudden, and excessive discharge of neurons. They may consist of an alteration in mental state that ranges from loss of consciousness to a dreamlike state or a brief blank period in which there is loss or limited awareness of external events; psychic symptoms such as fear, déjà vu (the feeling of having experienced a new situation previously), or jamais vu (the feeling of never having experienced a situation previously experienced) also occur. There may be involuntary stiffening or jerking movements—or abnormal sensations—in some or all of the limbs, and other behavioral changes. Seizures may also occur in nonepileptic individuals as, for example, when they are provoked by abnormal levels of certain chemicals, such as glucose, in the blood. Modern classifications divide seizures into generalized seizures, which involve the entire brain, and partial seizures, which involve a localized part of the brain.

Julius Caesar, Alexander the Great, Napoleon, Lenin, Charles Dickens, Dostoevsky, Byron, Molière, Flaubert, de Maupassant, Van Gogh, and Alfred Nobel were all said to have had epilepsy. Epilepsy has always engendered fear in those so afflicted and in the general public, and has been variously attributed to the anger of the gods, to devils and demons, and to possession by unclean spirits. Both Hippocrates and Galen are said to have recognized that epilepsy or epileptic seizures originate in the brain. Galen also pointed out that epilepsy may result either from a primary (idiopathic) or secondary disorder of the brain, and that the seizures may take a variety of forms. Seizures occurring as a secondary phenomenon were related to involvement of the brain "in sympathy" with disease in other parts of the body, especially the stomach. Such a division of epilepsy continued, with only minor modifications, into the twentieth century.

In the nineteenth century, the repertoire of epileptic phenomena increased and attempts were made to provide a physiological explanation for the occurrence of seizures. Seizures were for a time attributed to cerebral congestion. Marshall Hall, the physiologist who really established the concept of reflexes on a solid framework (discussed in Chapter 3), applied them to the genesis of epilepsy.[1] Specifically, he referred, in an 1833 communication to the Royal Society, to the possibility that a number of medical disorders, including epilepsy, relate to disturbances of reflexes.[1,2] He defined *centric epilepsy* as arising from the spinal cord and base of the brain (i.e., the central nervous system), and distinguished it from *eccentric (sympathetic) epilepsy*, in which the underlying cause was distant from these regions of the nervous system but involved them reflexly.[2] A reflex response is an involuntary or automatic reaction of the body to a specific stimulus, for example, the sudden withdrawal of a limb from a painful stimulus or the narrowing of the pupil of the eye exposed to a bright light. Reflexes involve sensory or afferent input, and motor or efferent output from the central nervous system; depending on the type of reflex, there may also be intermediate components between the afferent and efferent paths of the reflex. According to Hall, increased afferent activity led to eccentric epilepsy, with secondary involvement of the entire brain occurring from venous congestion, which was attributed to "forcible closure of the larynx and expiratory efforts." The loss of consciousness in both types of epilepsy was believed to result from involvement of the cerebral hemispheres.[3] However, this failed to explain the occurrence of seizures that began simply with a loss of consciousness. Others held and extended these views—the eminent pathologist Jakob Henle,[A] for example, attributed convulsions to the pressure of accumulated blood in the vessels at the base of the brain, with loss of consciousness resulting from altered (increased or diminished) blood flow to the hemispheres.[3,4]

[A] Friedrich Gustav Jakob Henle (1809-1885), Bavarian anatomist and pathologist, probably the foremost histologist of his time, after whom are named various anatomical structures but especially an important structure in the kidneys. He believed that microscopic living organisms caused many diseases, especially those occurring in epidemics, and the germ theory was subsequently established by his student Robert Koch. A talented musician and poet, he had many friends in the world of the arts including Felix Mendelssohn.

Others came up with equally fanciful explanations for seizures, but the common thread was that convulsive movements related to involvement of the spinal cord, medulla, or other brainstem structures (that were then thought to represent the "motor" parts of the brain), whereas loss of consciousness reflected a disturbance of the cerebral hemispheres. It is in this context that Brown-Séquard's work on epilepsy must be considered. Between 1850 and 1872, he published twenty-two scientific papers directly related to epilepsy, some in several parts and one of which was also published as a book.[5] His views were influenced by the experimental observations he made in the laboratory, and were not simply theoretical concepts. In brief, he believed that external stimuli led to activation of the medulla (a portion of the hindbrain concerned especially with regulation of the circulation), with resultant constriction of the cerebral blood vessels leading to loss of consciousness.

> Epilepsy seems to consist essentially in an increased reflex excitability of certain parts of the cerebro-spinal axis, and in a loss of the control that, in normal conditions, the will possesses over the reflex faculty. The base of the encephalon, and especially the medulla oblongata, is the most frequent seat of the increase in reflex excitability, so that this part of the nervous system is the ordinary seat of epilepsy.... I have tried to show that the same cause that produces the first convulsions in some muscles ... produces also a contraction of the blood vessels of the brain proper, which contraction is necessarily followed by loss of consciousness.[6]

Thus, he attributed the onset of seizures to increased reflex excitability,[B] and this—he believed—was related in many instances to afferent input from the skin. Within this substrate of epilepsy he found a role for the vasomotor nerves, whose existence he had demonstrated so recently. In particular, he suggested that excitation of the spinal cord or brainstem (medulla) led to excitation of sympathetic vasomotor fibers passing to the blood vessels of the head, and this, in turn, caused facial pallor and an impairment of the blood supply to the cerebral hemispheres; the blood accumulating about the brainstem and the spinal cord provoked convulsions, either in the manner proposed by Henle or, more probably, because of its reduced oxygen content and increased

---

[B] Seizures, usually convulsions or episodes of impaired external awareness, may indeed occur in some patients as a response to a specific external stimulus such as a flashing light (photogenic epilepsy), music or even a particular bar of music (musicogenic epilepsy), sounds, touch or pressure on the skin, and reading. Only a few patients with epilepsy, however, have seizures that can be evoked by specific sensory stimuli or the cognitive processing related to such stimuli. Patients with such seizures are said to have *reflex epilepsy*, which may have a genetic basis.

concentration of carbon dioxide as a result of impaired ventilation.[C] He later showed by experiment, however, that loss of consciousness could occur in guinea pigs without constriction of the cerebral blood vessels, and noted that treatment of epileptic patients by cutting the sympathetic nerves on both sides in the neck (i.e., bilateral cervical sympathectomy) was unsuccessful.[7] He eventually concluded, therefore, that the loss of consciousness during seizures was related to cerebral inhibitory phenomena, but was not more specific in this regard.[7]

Even today, the pathophysiological mechanisms responsible for the occurrence of epileptic seizures remain opaque. No single mechanism provides a fully adequate explanation, and evidence has accumulated of a complicated series of changes affecting the structure and function of the nervous system at many levels. An epileptic seizure seems to result from an imbalance between excitatory and inhibitory inputs in the brain, but the precise details and their application to different seizure types remain to be elucidated. Brown-Séquard was beginning to grope vaguely toward such a belief at the end of his long career, well ahead of many of his contemporaries, although his beliefs were based more on intuition that scientific evidence and were too ill-defined to be of any utility.

In any event, Brown-Séquard recommended cauterization of the skin with a hot iron to cure the irritative skin lesion that—he felt—was causing the seizures by exciting the afferent part of the involved reflexes. He used ligatures to localize the likely site of involvement, presumably by interfering with afferent nerve function, although this was never stated explicitly[8]:

> [Localization involves the] application of ligatures in each limb alternately. Suppose a case of epilepsy in which the fits are frequent ... a very tight ligature is put on one limb; and if the fit does not come, it is extremely probably that it depends on the irritation ...; if it comes, the ligature is applied on the other limbs at other times.[9]

In keeping with the seeming importance of forcible closure of the larynx in the genesis of eccentric epilepsy, Brown-Séquard proposed that the larynx

---

[C] Brown-Séquard's early studies were used by others in the 1880s to support the belief that epileptic seizures relate to disturbances in the flow of blood to the brain (the so-called vasomotor theory of epilepsy). The "seizures" occurring in this context, however, are probably examples of convulsive syncope (faints accompanied by muscle twitching and stiffening) rather than true epileptic seizures. Further details are provided elsewhere. See, for example, Bladin PF. The great deceiver: the role of convulsive syncope in the history of epilepsy. *J Clin Neurosci*, 3:354–357, 1996.

also be cauterized—with silver nitrate as an alternative to the tracheotomy (i.e., direct incision into the trachea or windpipe to bypass any obstruction at the larynx) proposed by Marshall Hall. In reviewing his researches in 1853, he wrote,

> As I have had the opportunity during the last three or four years of observing every day a great many animals (more than a hundred) which had a convulsive affection resembling epilepsy very much, I have been able to discover some very interesting facts, among which are the following ... cauterization of the mucous membrane of the larynx is able either to cure or to relieve these epileptic animals ... I knew that an animal was cured, not only by the absence of spontaneous fits, but when I could not produce a fit ... some physicians in this country have already tried on man the mode of treatment that I have found so successful on animals ....[10]

Within a short time, such approaches fell out of favor as bromides became increasingly popular for treating epilepsy, after their introduction for this purpose by Sir Charles Locock, as noted in Chapter 7. Brown-Séquard was one of the first to use them and helped to popularize their use, advising his students to prescribe treatment for at least twelve to fifteen months after the last seizure, and to continue it through any concurrent illnesses,[11] an approach that is still followed today. Bromides continued to be used to prevent seizures until the twentieth century.

Although the concept of altering sensory input to abort or prevent seizures has now been largely forgotten, it has been known for centuries that a specific sensory stimulus can sometimes arrest a seizure, by uncertain mechanisms. Various modern accounts suggest that such an intervention may sometimes be worthwhile. Efron, for example, reported a patient who was able to arrest his focal (partial) seizures by exposure to an unpleasant odor and learned to arrest them also by visual stimuli.[12] Forster found that conditioning could affect which stimuli elicit or suppress seizures, and that increased exposure to seizure-eliciting stimuli could lead to desensitization, so that seizure frequency is eventually reduced.[13] In other words, he showed that behavioral techniques could modify the course of patients with reflex epilepsies, reducing the seizure frequency. Despite the therapeutic implications of such studies,[14,15] the primary approach to seizure control in epileptic patients remains pharmacological. More recently, electrical stimulation of the vagus nerve (a nerve that arises from the brain itself and innervates the heart, lungs, larynx, and various abdominal organs) has been shown to reduce experimentally induced seizures in various animals and to diminish the frequency of seizures in selected patients with so-called complex partial seizures[D] refractory to antiepileptic medication. Curiously, vagal nerve stimulation had originally been used in the 1880s by the American neurologist James Corning, but then fell into disrepute until recently.[16] The mechanisms involved in affecting seizures are unclear but—interestingly in view of Brown-Séquard's early views on the involvement of the blood supply of the brain in the genesis of some aspects of seizures—such stimulation has been shown to increase blood flow to certain parts of the brain and also to alter various neurotransmitters in the brain.[17]

Brown-Séquard's localization of epilepsy to the brainstem was superseded within a few years by the work of Hughlings Jackson, who considered that seizures arose in the cerebral cortex, a view that gained overwhelming support once it was shown experimentally, in the 1870s, that certain regions of the cortex have motor functions. Jackson came to the conclusion from a study of unilateral or focal seizures (i.e., seizures involving one side or a localized region of the body) that these originated from discrete parts of the cortex. His views received substantial support from the experimental work of Fritsch and Hitzig (see Chapter 10), who showed that weak electrical stimuli of discrete cortical regions led to contractions of certain muscles, whereas stronger stimuli led to more widespread motor activity or to convulsions, sometimes preceded by localized muscle activity.[18] This work, and that of Ferrier in monkeys,[19] supported the belief that certain seizures begin locally in the cortex and then spread to other regions or become generalized. It also led to Jackson's eventual definition of epilepsy as a disorder marked by "occasional, sudden, excessive, rapid and local discharges of grey matter."[20,21] In the early part of the twentieth century, Hans Berger[E] demonstrated the possibility of recording the electrical activity of the brain (that is, of recording the electroencephalogram or EEG) from the scalp, and he described the cyclical fluctuations in voltage (brain waves) that occur. The presence of abnormalities in this activity during seizures indicated that the abnormal discharges of gray matter postulated by Hughlings Jackson were electrical in nature. The EEG is now widely used as an aid to the detection, diagnosis, and classification[D] of seizures. The EEG has also revealed that the "seizures" related by Brown-Séquard and others to disturbances in the flow of blood to the brain are often probably examples of

---

[D] Complex partial seizures are seizures that lead to an impairment of consciousness (hence, *complex*) but involve only a limited part of the brain (thus, *partial*), typically the temporal or frontal lobe. They occur in about one-third of patients with epilepsy.

[E] Hans Berger (1873–1941), German neuropsychiatrist and the first to record the electroencephalogram of human subjects in health and disease. He was humiliated and forced into retirement by the Nazis and eventually hanged himself in a fit of depression during World War II.

convulsive syncope (faints accompanied by muscle stiffness, twitching, and jerking) rather than true epileptic seizures, a distinction that may be difficult to make on clinical grounds alone.

An Experimental Model of Epilepsy

While Brown-Séquard was studying the sensory pathways, he cut various nerves in the extremities and made lesions in the spinal cord. In 1850, he described "a convulsive affection, very much resembling epilepsy"[22] that he could induce in guinea pigs with lesions in a variety of locations involving the spinal cord, especially in the thoracic or lumbar region.[23,24] Lateral hemisection or more discrete lesions of the cord led, usually after about three or four weeks, to convulsive movements resembling seizures that occurred spontaneously or following stimulation of certain regions of the skin. At first, the seizure involved only the muscles of the face and neck on one or both sides, depending on the extent of the injury, but after a few days all nonparalyzed parts of the body exhibited violent repetitive muscle contractions lasting for up to about five minutes. At the onset of such attacks, animals often uttered hoarse cries, as if the vocal cords were partially closed. With complete transection of the spinal cord, the attacks differed in that the paralyzed lower part of the body did not become involved.[25]

> When the attack begins, the head is drawn first, and sometimes violently, towards the shoulder, by the contraction of the muscles of the neck, on the side of the irritation; the mouth is drawn open ... and the muscles of the face and eye (particularly the orbicularis) contract violently .... Frequently at the same time, or very nearly so, the animal suddenly cries with a particularly hoarse voice, as if the passage of air were not free through the vocal cords, spasmodically contracted. Then the animal falls ... and then all the muscles of the trunk and limbs that are not paralyzed become the seat of convulsions, alternate clonic and tonic .... Respiration takes place irregularly, on account of the convulsions of the respiratory muscles. Almost always there is an expulsion of faecal matter, and often urine.[5]

In the following years, Brown-Séquard provided more details of the disorder,[24,26] which could also be provoked by amputation of the leg or cutting the great sciatic nerve (the main nerve to the leg) or the posterior spinal roots with which it is connects. The convulsive movements were induced particularly by light pressure on the skin over the face or neck on the same (but not the opposite) side as the lesion (the "epileptogenous zone"). Trophic changes occurred with time in the epileptogenous zone, with loss of hair, changes in cutaneous sensation, and the accumulation there of lice.[26] There was sometimes an apparent loss of consciousness followed by a period of drowsiness.[27,28] Urinary and fecal incontinence were common during the attacks.[24] The convulsive movements were sometimes restricted to the limbs of one side, but they frequently then alternated from one side to the other. He concluded that "the spinal cord in animals may be the *cause* (I do not say the *seat*) of an epileptic affection" (emphasis in original), that epileptiform convulsions may be a "constant consequence of slight irritations" on certain nerves, and that there was a relation between the skin of the face and neck and certain parts of the spinal cord.[29] Although Brown-Séquard pointed out the obvious similarities between epileptic seizures in humans and the behavioral disturbance in his guinea pigs, he was cautious enough to indicate "that if the convulsions of these animals are not truly epileptic, they are at least epileptiform,"[30] even if the distinction sometimes seems blurred in his writings. He initially attributed the loss of consciousness to a constriction of the cerebral blood vessels during attacks,[27,28] but subsequently showed that loss of consciousness could be induced in guinea pigs even when such a constriction was prevented experimentally (by destroying the superior cervical ganglion on both sides).[7]

Others confirmed Brown-Séquard's findings about the occurrence of "epileptiform convulsions" with spinal lesions, including Vulpian,[31] Victor Horsley[32,33] (the noted British neurosurgeon, who also confirmed that consciousness was indeed lost during the attacks[32]), and Graham Brown,[F] a young physiologist who studied and worked with Sir Charles Sherrington.[34] It seemed that "spinal epilepsy" or "Brown-Séquard's epilepsy" might serve as an experimental model of epilepsy in humans and provide some clue as to its basis.

Over the following years, spinal epilepsy aroused considerable interest among clinicians. Wilhelm Heinrich Erb,[G] for example, sought a relation between spinal epilepsy and ankle clonus, as did the French master clinician, Jean-Martin Charcot.[35] The term *clonus* refers to the repetitive involuntary

---

[F] Graham Brown (1882–1965), British neurophysiologist who studied reflex movements, gait, and the control of posture. He seemed in his later years to be more interested in mountain climbing than physiology, became editor of the *Alpine Journal*, and found several new routes to the summit of Mount Blanc in the Alps.

[G] Wilhelm Heinrich Erb (1840–1921), German neurologist, has named after him an anatomical point and a neuromuscular disorder of the arm that follows injury at birth (Erb's palsy). He also described many of the features of the disease now known as myasthenia gravis, which is characterized by fluctuating weakness of muscles that increases with activity and improves with rest. The weakness results from abnormal transmission of nerve impulses to muscles.

contractions and relaxations of a muscle that follow its sudden stretch in patients with abnormally brisk stretch reflexes (such as may occur after a stroke or in spinal cord disease); clonus is not an epileptic phenomenon but simply a manifestation of the brisk stretch reflexes.

The nature and basis of spinal epilepsy came into question in the latter part of the nineteenth century. The initial repetitive limb movements of the attacks were shown by Graham Brown to be similar to the scratch reflexes that Sherrington described in dogs whose spinal cord had been severed.[34,36] Scratch reflexes are components of normal grooming behavior but are elicited by a variety of innocuous or inappropriate mechanical stimuli, such as rubbing the skin. Sherrington attributed their appearance after spinal cord transection to the loss of an inhibitory cerebral influence on the cord,[37] and believed that they are generated within the cord by the increased excitability of a neuronal arrangement that permits an integrated, coordinated response to the stimulus. Graham Brown found that the epileptogenous zone of Brown-Séquard resembled the receptive field that Sherrington subsequently noted as the area within which stimulation elicited scratch reflexes, suggesting an analogy between the two phenomena. There were, however, differences between various aspects of the Brown-Séquard phenomenon and the scratch reflex; in particular, the tonic phase of muscle stiffening was much more pronounced in the former, and in the complete Brown-Séquard reaction there was marked overflow of the movements from one side of the body to the other.[34]

In interpreting his findings, Graham Brown concluded that the entire Brown-Séquard phenomenon was simply a specific instance of the scratch reflex,[36] and most authorities subsequently accepted this view, even though it did not account for the complete behavioral disturbance[38] or the loss of consciousness that sometimes occurred. However, the phenomenon seems more than a simple scratch reflex and has several obvious similarities to the convulsions occurring in humans with epilepsy. Its precise basis remains unclear. It has been suggested by certain recent writers that the disorder in guinea pigs relates specifically to the accumulation of a particular species of louse on affected animals and that "seizures" are abolished by delousing infested animals.[39] Brown-Séquard himself noted that lice infestations followed placement of the lesions that led to "epileptiform seizures" in his animals; limb disabilities (or amputations) certainly lead to localized infestations or population-expansion of lice as a result of impaired grooming behavior. Even so, the nature of the reaction remains uncertain. Whether it is truly epileptic, and thus whether Brown-Séquard had developed an acceptable animal model of epilepsy is unclear, but modern definitions of an epileptic seizure require that the episodic behavioral disturbance results from an abnormal discharge of *cerebral* neurons with certain specific physiological characteristics.

Despite this ambiguity, Brown-Séquard's work suggested that experimental models of epilepsy can be developed in animals to permit detailed analysis of the pathophysiological basis of the naturally occurring disease, a viewpoint that is now widely accepted. It also implied that proposed therapies for epilepsy could be tested experimentally. The treatment for epilepsy when he first began to practice medicine included the traditional approach of blood-letting, as well as a variety of other more enthusiastic and extravagant therapies, depending on the whim or enterprise of individual physicians.[40] For patients with sympathetic (reflex) epilepsy, surgical procedures involved isolation or removal of the supposed site of the peripheral stimulus, and there are published accounts of division of nerves, ligature of arteries, and amputation of various body parts with this aim in mind. Within five years of his graduation in 1846, Brown-Séquard was challenging such therapeutic adventurism based on his experimental studies. Although his own therapeutic approach is now largely forgotten, there is no doubt that close ties between experimental studies in the laboratory and clinical care have improved the management of epileptic patients.

A more controversial aspect of Brown-Séquard's work was to do with the inheritance of acquired epilepsy. Brown-Séquard believed that the "epileptiform" abnormalities[41] that he induced in guinea pigs could be passed on to their offspring, and other contemporary investigators confirmed his observations. He returned to the inheritance of such acquired characteristics several times over the years, noting, for example, that his guinea pigs with sectioned sciatic nerves developed trophic changes (such as the tendency to nibble off their anesthetic toes) that appeared to be passed on to their offspring, who were sometimes born with missing toes as well as a tendency to epileptiform convulsions.[42] The evidence impressed Charles Darwin, who referred directly to Brown-Séquard's work in one of his books as "the evidence which admits of no doubt" with regard to the inheritance of certain acquired characteristics.[43] Nevertheless, others had doubts. Some years later, the suggestion was made that—if heredity was involved at all in the development of epileptiform convulsions in his guinea pigs—it involved the inheritance of a state of increased excitability of an existing spinal reflex mechanism, rather than of a novel acquired mechanism.[36] Moreover, an explanation other than heredity was also put forward for his findings, namely that animals with a severed sciatic nerve tend to nibble off the toes of their newborn offspring (as well as their own anesthetic toes), and this leads to a behavioral disturbance resembling seizures in the offspring[36] as their grooming ability is impaired and lice accumulate on them.

Brown-Séquard's results are now regarded as anomalous, even though similar effects were observed by others. It seems presumptuous, however, to be dogmatic about the heritability of the behavioral disturbance—be it epileptic or otherwise—described by Brown-Séquard when the very nature of the disturbance remains uncertain. The tendency to dismiss the possibility simply because it is at odds with accepted views on heredity is unfortunate, if only because evidence is accumulating that the way genes are expressed can be modified by various experiences, and the change in gene function (but not structure) can then be passed on to future generations. The new science of epigenetics is exploring the way in which genes can be switched on and off in this manner.

References and Source Notes

1. Eadie MJ. Marshall Hall, the reflex arc and epilepsy. *J R Coll Physicians Edinb*, 38:167–171, 2008.
2. Hall M. On the reflex functions of the medulla oblongata and medulla spinalis. *Philos Transact R Soc Lond*, 123: 635–665, 1833.
3. Temkin O. *The falling sickness*, 2nd edition (pp. 278–299). Baltimore: Johns Hopkins Press, 1971.
4. Brown-Séquard E. Experimental and clinical researches applied to physiology and pathology. *Boston Med Surg J*, 56: 220, 1857.
5. Brown-Séquard CE. *Researches on epilepsy. Its artificial production in animals and its etiology, nature and treatment in man.* Boston: Clapp, 1857.
6. Brown-Séquard CE. *Course of lectures on the physiology and pathology of the central nervous system* (p. 183). Philadelphia: Collins, 1860.
7. Brown-Séquard CE. De la perte de connaissance dans l'épilepsie après l'ablation du gangion cervical supérieur du nerf grand sympathique, des deux côtés, chez l'homme et chez le cobaye. *Arch Physiol Norm Pathol (5th Series)*, 3:216–218, 1891.
8. Eadie MJ. The ligature in the management of epilepsy. *J Clin Neurosci*, 3:75–78, 1996.
9. Brown-Séquard CE. *Course of lectures on the physiology and pathology of the central nervous system* (p. 182). Philadelphia: Collins, 1860.
10. Brown-Séquard E. On the treatment of epilepsy. *Med Exam (Philadelphia)*, 9:205–209, 1853. [*Experimental researches applied to physiology and pathology* (pp. 80–84). New York: Bailliere 1853.]
11. Bowditch HP. Lecture notes taken at Harvard Medical School 1866–1867: Dr. Brown-Séquard. Harvard Medical Archives, CB 1869.9. Countway Library of Medicine, Boston.
12. Efron R. The conditioned inhibition of uncinate fits. *Brain*, 80:251–262, 1957.
13. Forster FM. *Reflex epilepsy, behavioral therapy and conditional reflexes*. Springfield, IL: Charles C. Thomas, 1977.
14. Fenwick P. The behavioral treatment of epilepsy generation and inhibition of seizures. *Neurol Clin*, 12:175–202, 1994.
15. Fenwick P. Precipitation and inhibition of seizures. In: Reynolds EH, Trimble M, eds., *Epilepsy and psychiatry* (pp. 306–321). London: Churchill Livingstone, 1981.

16. Lanska DJ. J.L. Corning and vagal nerve stimulation for seizures in the 1880s. *Neurology*, 58:452–459, 2002.
17. Ben-Menachem E. Vagus-nerve stimulation for the treatment of epilepsy. *Lancet Neurol*, 1:477–482, 2002.
18. Fritsch G, Hitzig E. Über die elektrische Erregbarkeit des Grosshirns. *Arch Anat Physiol (Lpz)*, 37:300–332, 1870.
19. Ferrier D. *The functions of the brain*. London: Smith, Elder & Co., 1876.
20. Temkin O. *The falling sickness*, 2nd edition (pp. 329–346). Baltimore: Johns Hopkins Press, 1971.
21. Eadie MJ. The understanding of epilepsy across three millennia. *Clin Exp Neurol*, 31:1–12, 1994.
22. Brown-Séquard CE. *Course of lectures on the physiology and pathology of the central nervous system* (p. 178). Philadelphia: Collins, 1860.
23. Brown-Séquard E. D'une affection convulsive qui survient chez les animaux ayant eu une moitié latérale de la moelle épinière coupée. *C R Soc Biol (Paris)*, 2: 105, 1850.
24. Brown-Séquard E. Experimental and clinical researches applied to physiology and pathology. *Boston Med Surg J*, 55:337–342, 377–380, 421–427, and 457–461, 1856/1857; 56:54–58, 112–115, 155–158, 174–176, 216–220, 271–278, 338–340, 433–437, and 473–478, 1857. [This series of papers summarizes Brown-Séquard's researches and opinions on epilepsy.]
25. Brown-Séquard E. D'une affection convulsive consécutive à la section transversale de la moelle épinière. *C R Soc Biol (Paris)*, 2:169, 1850.
26. Brown-Séquard CE. Nouvelle recherches sur l'épilepsie due a certaines lésions de la moelle épinière et des nerfs rachidiens. *Arch Physiol Norm Pathol*, 2:211–220, 422–438, and 496–503, 1869.
27. Brown-Séquard E. Note sur des faits nouveaux concernant l'épilepsie consécutive aux lésions de la moelle épinière. *J Physiol (Paris)*, 1:472–478, 1858.
28. Brown-Séquard E. Sur une modification spéciale de la nutrition dans une partie limitée du corps sous l'influence d'irritations de l'encéphale ou de la moelle épinière dans certains cas d'epilepsie. *J Physiol (Paris)*, 3:167–173, 1860.
29. Brown-Séquard CE. *Course of lectures on the physiology and pathology of the central nervous system* (p. 179). Philadelphia: Collins, 1860.
30. Brown-Séquard E. Experimental and clinical researches applied to physiology and pathology. *Boston Med Surg J*, 55:341–342, 1856.
31. Vulpian A. Epilepsie observée chez un cochon d'inde qui avait subi la section d'un des nerfs sciatiques. *Arch Physiol Norm Pathol*, 2:297–299, 1869.
32. Horsley V. Epileptic guinea-pigs. *Lancet*, 2:975, 1886.
33. Horsley V. Abstract of the Brown Lectures delivered at the University of London: Epilepsy. *Lancet*, 2:211–213, 1886.
34. Brown TG. Studies in the reflexes of the guinea-pig. I. The scratch-reflex in relation to "Brown-Séquard's epilepsy." *Q J Exp Physiol*, 2:243–275, 1909.
35. Koehler PJ. Brown-Séquard's spinal epilepsy. *Med Hist*, 38:189–203, 1994.
36. Brown TG. An alleged specific instance of the transmission of acquired characters—Investigation and criticism. *Proc R Soc Lond (Ser B)*, 84:555–579, 1912.
37. Sherrington CS. The spinal cord. In: Schafer EA, ed., *Textbook of physiology* (Vol. 2, pp. 837–844). New York: Macmillan, 1900.
38. Randall W. Grooming reflexes in the cat: endocrine and pharmacological studies. *Ann N Y Acad Sci*, 525:301–320, 1988.
39. Plichet A. Brown-Sequard epilepsy induced by cutaneous parasites. *J Int Coll Surgeons*, 13:637–639, 1950.

40. Temkin O. *The falling sickness*, 2nd edition (pp. 291–299). Baltimore: Johns Hopkins Press, 1971.
41. Brown-Séquard E. Hereditary transmission of an epileptiform affection accidentally produced. *Proc R Soc Lond,* 10:297–298, 1860.
42. Brown-Séquard CE. On the hereditary transmission of effects of certain injuries to the nervous system. *Lancet,* 1:7–8, 1875.
43. Darwin C. *The variation of animals and plants under domestication.* London: Murray, 1868.

⌒ 12 ⌒

The Magnificent Maverick

THE MAN WHO returned to Paris as professor at the Collège de France was very different from the medical scientist who had made his name there in the 1840s and 1850s. The quick young man with dark hair, expressive eyes, and restless energy had certainly not become a tired old man, but his face was now framed by long white hair and a well-trimmed white beard and was dominated by intense dark eyes that shone beneath two black eyebrows. Even though there was a more gentle air about him, the inner sense of relentless purpose remained, coupled with bounding enthusiasm for whatever captured his interest. He would jump from one topic to another without seeming connection when speaking, as if he could not control the flow of his ideas. It is remarkable—and telling—how the calm and deliberate atmosphere in the laboratories that Brown-Séquard took over from Claude Bernard soon changed to one of restless excitement as he came up with new hypotheses on a variety of often unrelated topics and devised new experiments to test them before those already under way had even been completed. If, indeed, he suffered with bipolar disease, as suggested in Chapter 8, he was clearly on the upswing as he turned the obscurity to which he had seemed destined into a stunning professional acceptance. He focused initially on studying how one region of the brain influences the function of another, using electrical stimulation to activate various brain regions in an attempt to discredit the emerging concepts of cerebral localization, as discussed in Chapter 10. His work on this and on epilepsy and the inheritance of acquired characteristics (Chapter 11), the toxicity of expired air (Chapter 14), and the role of tissue extracts as therapeutic agents

(Chapter 13), was published in his *Archives de Physiologie,* as well as in other prominent scientific journals of the day.

His assistant was the talented Jacques Arsène d'Arsonval (1851–1940), who came from an ancient and aristocratic family of country doctors and had himself intended to follow a career in clinical medicine. In 1873, as a 22-year-old medical student with a particular interest in the physical sciences, he had gone on a whim to one of Bernard's lecture-demonstrations, during which a galvanometer broke down, bringing to a halt the experiment in progress. At the end of the lecture, d'Arsonval took a look at the faulty instrument and quickly put it right. Bernard invited the young man to lunch, a meal over which both men lingered in conversation, and invited the student to return to the Collège as often as he liked. Within a few months, d'Arsonval had become Bernard's part-time assistant, while continuing his own medical studies. In 1876, when Bernard's full-time assistant left the laboratory for a position at the University of Paris, d'Arsonval agreed to take his place despite the wishes of his father, and thereby finally abandoned any intention of following a clinical career. Nevertheless, he submitted his thesis—on the role of the elasticity of the lungs in circulatory phenomena—and, in August 1877, gained his doctorate in medicine. The thesis was dedicated to Claude Bernard. Meanwhile, Bernard wrote to his father that he understood and respected the conflict between the heart of a good father and that of his son, adding that

> since I took your son to join me, I have come to appreciate him more and more. I have seen few young men as gifted as him for the culture of science. He has extensive training, an inventive mind, a taste and passion for theoretical questions and their application accompanied by a kind and helpful character that make him beloved by all his friends and those who know him .... It is difficult for me in these circumstances to not encourage him and to not believe my duty [is] to give him my love and my support along a path where I believe he is destined to succeed.[1]

Relations between Brown-Séquard and d'Arsonval initially became strained when the young man used Claude Bernard's name somewhat unwisely to support his case during a disagreement with his new master. The angry exchange that followed culminated in d'Arsonval and *père* Lesage, the laboratory technician (who had been there since the days of Magendie), storming out to join the laboratory staff of Etienne-Jules Marey (1830–1904), another of the professors and the inventor of many of the devices used for recording physiological phenomena (including the sphygmograph).[2] Happily, the two became reconciled—d'Arsonval suggested that Brown-Séquard sought him out,[2] whereas Brown-Séquard wrote to Emma that d'Arsonval had asked through colleagues to be taken back, indicating that he was not well off and that if he lost the position he would have to give up science and return to the country to practice medicine.[3] Regardless of how it happened, d'Arsonval returned to work as Brown-Séquard's deputy, became his friend and indispensable collaborator, and eventually succeeded him in the chair.

Honors and Awards

The next ten years were as exciting as the previous decade had been drab and difficult. As is common in life, success brought further rewards to Brown-Séquard. Indeed, they came so thick and fast that it is legitimate to wonder whether they came to honor the man or the office that he held. He became a chevalier of the Legion of Honor in 1880 and, shortly thereafter, received the Prix Lacaze of the Académie des Sciences. This prize, awarded every second year to the person whose works had contributed most to the advancement of physiology, was worth ten thousand francs. The award committee of nine included Robin and Marey, and was chaired by Vulpian, who critically appraised Brown-Séquard's published contributions[4] and—in his report to the Académie—emphasized some of Brown-Séquard's most important work, especially his studies on the route taken by sensory fibers in the spinal cord, on experimentally induced epilepsy and its transmission by heredity, on the contractility of blood vessels and their regulation by the vasomotor nerves, and on the irrigation of dying tissues with blood (which suggested that severed limbs might be reconnected), and his demonstration that portions of the brain can exert an inhibitory influence on other distant regions.[5]

A short time later, he was named recipient of the 1884 Prix Lallemand of the Académie, as mentioned in Chapter 10. This time, Paul Bert (p. 163) reported on the committee's deliberations,[6] emphasizing his work on the excitatory and inhibitory effects of one part of the nervous system on more distant parts and his demonstration that a single lesion could exert both inhibitory and excitatory effects on different regions. The committee also indicated that the manner in which Brown-Séquard had interpreted his experimental observations had led him to combat the newly accepted concept of motor centers on the surface of the cerebral hemispheres, even as he revealed new properties and functions of the nervous system.

There was more to come, even bigger prizes. The Institut de France awarded a prize (the Prix Biennal) of twenty thousand francs every two years for the most significant work or discovery made in the preceding ten years. Its five constituent Académies took turns in nominating a candidate, who then had to be approved by the whole institute. In 1885, it was the turn of the Académie des Sciences to select the candidate, and several of its sections put forward nominees for consideration.[7] Brown-Séquard was chosen by the Section of Medicine and Surgery,[8] whereas Pierre Paul François Camille Savorgnan de Brazza—the well-born, Franco-Italian explorer to whom France was indebted for much of the territory she possessed on the Congo and after whom is named the city of Brazzaville—was the choice of the Section of Geography and Navigation. Five other sections also proposed persons for consideration. At the first ballot, Brown-Séquard received twenty votes and de Brazza gained fifteen, the remaining twenty votes being distributed among the other five competitors.[7,9,10] On the second ballot, Brown-Séquard—sponsored by Paul Bert[9]—won forty votes, whereas de Brazza merely retained his previous supporters. Brown-Séquard was therefore chosen by the Académie to receive the prize,[11] which was then worth four thousand American dollars, his selection being approved by the entire institute with an overwhelming majority of seventy-four votes to seven.[7,9,10,12,13] Soon thereafter, in 1886, Brown-Séquard was himself elected to the Académie des Sciences in place of Vulpian, who was made permanent secretary.

The Institut de France, created in 1795 after the Revolution, was reorganized in the early nineteenth century as a body charged with bringing together human endeavor in the arts and sciences. It is made up of five Académies, of which the most illustrious are the venerable Académie française (which is responsible for the safekeeping of the French language and consists of forty members who are elected for life and occupy numbered seats) and the Académie des Sciences.[A] Each academy has its own organization and focus, but there is a common library, archives, and funds. Election is by ballot, and membership is strictly limited in number. Brown-Séquard's election provided him with national recognition and the highest honor that a scientist could attain. In his day, the Académie met on Mondays, and the public proceedings were awaited with excitement by Parisians, who believed that men of distinction came to learn of important advances in the field and not simply to gossip or be seen in exalted circles. A description of the working of the Académie during the nineteenth century provides some insight to the respect accorded Brown-Séquard:

> On great occasions, of course, the aspect of the *seance* is different and practical demonstrations, such, for instance, as Dr. Brown-Séquard's explanation of his

---

[A] The other three academies are the Académie des Inscriptions and Belles-Lettres (devoted to the humanities), the Académie des Beaux-Arts (Academy of Fine Arts), and the Académie des Sciences Morales and Politiques (Academy of Moral and Political Science).

apparatus for analyzing the air breathed by consumptive patients, rivet the attention ....[14]

The honor that Brown-Séquard most prized came on 26 March 1887, when he was elected to a five-year term as president of the Société de Biologie (receiving forty-two votes against fifteen for his leading opponent) on the death from dysentery of Paul Bert, the physiologist who had become his friend and patron, and the politician who, as minister of education, had provided additional laboratory facilities for d'Arsonval to pursue his interest in electrophysiology.[B] This was the society that he had helped to found as a young man, that had vindicated his work on the sensory pathways in the spinal cord, and that he most enjoyed attending. He was its fourth president, succeeding Rayer (its founding president), Claude Bernard, and the unfortunate Paul Bert. His pleasure was absolute.

International honor also came to Brown-Séquard. In August 1880, he was awarded an honorary doctorate in law by the University of Cambridge, this being its highest honorary degree. Among the other eleven recipients were Franciscus Donders, the Dutch ophthalmologist[C]; Samuel Gross, professor of surgery at Jefferson Medical College of Philadelphia; William Jenner, physician to Queen Victoria and the Prince of Wales[D]; William Gull, another outstanding clinician (p. 91); William Bowman, the anatomist (p. 98); and Joseph Lister, the surgeon who introduced antisepsis and asepsis into the operating room before the germ theory of disease was widely accepted. "Brown-Séquard, Gross, and Donders could not [have been] more gratified with the rare honour of receiving the honorary degree of LL.D. Cantabriensis, than the profession of Britain will be gratified to know that they have received it."[15] Shortly after, in 1883, he was named the recipient of the prestigious Baly Medal, a gold medal awarded by the Royal College of Physicians of London every two years for accomplishments in physiology. In Brazil, the emperor Pedro d'Alcantara,[E]

[B] Paul Bert's seat in the Academie des Sciences went to Charles Bouchard.
[C] Donders (1818–1889), one of the fathers of modern ophthalmology, introduced various lenses for the treatment of astigmatism. He also studied human reaction time to understand stages in cognitive processing.
[D] Sir William Jenner (1815–1898) distinguished typhus from typhoid fever; others had done so earlier, but Jenner's study was the most persuasive. He had enormous court connections and a huge private practice. He allowed fifteen minutes for each consultation, believing that if he could not sort out a case in ten minutes, he never would.
[E] Dom Pedro d'Alcantara was friends with many European physicians and scientists, including Brown-Séquard, whose experimental studies in animals must have been somewhat abhorrent to this lover of animals. Because of ill health from diabetes, overwork, and, possibly malaria, he consulted—accompanied by his personal physician, the Brazilian Cláudio Velho de Motta Maia (1843–1897)—a number of eminent Parisian physicians, including Bouchard,

who had earlier (1872) made him a commander of the Imperial Order of the Rose, awarded him in 1889 the Grand Cross of the Order, its highest rank.

Brown-Séquard served as an honorary vice-president of the splendid seventh International Medical Congress held in London in August 1881.[16] This brought together physicians and scientists from many different countries to discuss the field in an age that had "... produced the ophthalmoscope, otoscope and laryngoscope, the sphygmograph and haemodynamometer; which has created the cell-theory, and placed pathology on a new basis by its application; which has revolutionised surgery by the enunciation and application of antisepticism; in which physiology has been completely reconstituted, both by the suggestion and perfecting of new instruments of research, and by the comparison of human processes with those which obtain in other organised beings ...."[17] Presided over by Sir James Paget, the Congress was attended by more than three thousand persons,[18,19] among whom were such illustrious figures as Jenner, Gull, Bowman, Lister, Pasteur, Charcot, Pancoast, Esmarch, Volkmann, and Virchow. The festivities were magnificent, beginning with a *conversazione* at the South Kensington Museum attended by the Prince of Wales (later King Edward VII) and Crown Prince Friedrich of Germany.[20,F] On the next evening, the Lord Mayor of London held a banquet at the Mansion House for some of the eminent persons attending the Congress, with music provided by two military bands and a company of glee-singers. Brown-Séquard was seated opposite Pasteur and Dr. Acland (President of the British Medical Council) at the head table, with Sir James Paget and such other celebrities as Goltz, Burdon Sanderson, Charcot, Huxley, Virchow, and Bowman.[21] Other social events during the week of the Congress included garden parties, fetes, and soirées, a reception by the Lord Mayor at the Guildhall and another by the foreign secretary for foreigners attending the Congress, trips on the River Thames, and visits to the Croydon sewage farm (a "thriving sewage-fed 460-acre piece of land"), a Female Orphan Asylum, Hanwell Lunatic Asylum, the Bethlem Convalescent Home, the Royal Sea-Bathing Infirmary (a hospital for the diseased poor), Apsley House (home of the Duke of Wellington), and various medical and nonmedical museums, galleries, and gardens in and about the capital. There was even a visit to the home of the anatomist, John Hunter,

---

Brown-Séquard, and Charcot. The deposed emperor was especially close to Charcot, who signed his death certificate when he died in Paris from pneumonitis. He was afforded a state funeral by the French, and some years later his remains were returned to Brazil. (See also footnote I, Chapter 9, p. 146.)

[F] The unfortunate Friedrich, a liberal, served as Kaiser for just a few months in 1888 before dying from throat cancer. He was succeeded by his militaristic son Wilhelm, who was emperor during World War I.

where a variety of human bones recently found in the grounds were displayed. Finally, an informal dinner at the huge glass-and-steel Crystal Palace was followed by a fireworks display featuring the fire-portraits of Sir James Paget, Charcot, and von Langenbeck.[20,G] Brown-Séquard also had occasion to lunch with Paget in the company of the Prince of Wales during the course of the Congress.

Despite such distractions, much was accomplished at the Congress. Brown-Séquard attended especially the gatherings of the section of physiology.[22] This was where the famous debate on cerebral localization took place between Ferrier and Goltz, as discussed in Chapter 10. The subject was one on which Brown-Séquard held strong views, and he refused to be seduced by the new concept of cerebral localization of function that was gaining wide acceptance, and thereby seemed to have been left behind by the advance of medical science. There were many other discussions on important topics, and Brown-Séquard was actively involved in debates concerning mechanisms for regulating the heart beat and on the innervation of blood vessels[22]; in these areas also, however, he was seen more as a has-been, an illustrious pioneer from the past, rather than an investigator in the vanguard of scientific progress.

Experimental Work: The Start of Hormone Replacement Therapy

Although Brown-Séquard was gratified by the various honors that he received, he seemed unaffected by them except insofar as they facilitated the pursuit of his intellectual interests. They did, however, embolden him to abandon the consulting room in favor of the laboratory, although he remained available to special patients. He is even said to have consulted by telegraph with those caring for the stricken President James Garfield, twentieth president of the United States, who was shot twice by a would-be assassin in 1881, one bullet grazing his arm and the other hitting him in the back, piercing a lumbar vertebra, and lodging within his body. If Brown-Séquard was indeed consulted, his advice went unheeded, and Garfield died several weeks later, at least partly from infection induced by the repeated and injudicious probing of his wound by the dirty fingers and instruments of his doctors in their search for the bullet. The importance of the antiseptic technique developed some years earlier by

---

[G] Bernard Von Langenbeck (1810–1887), German surgeon who devised many new operative procedures, was an authority on gunshot wounds (having served in wars in which Prussia was engaged against Denmark in 1864, Austria in 1866, and France in 1870), and he was director of the Clinical Institute for Surgery and Ophthalmology in Berlin.

Joseph Lister[H] was generally accepted in England and France, but not yet in the United States.[I] Curiously, Alexander Graham Bell—inventor of the telephone—helped to devise a metal detector that was also used in an attempt to locate the bullet in Garfield's body. The results were unrevealing, perhaps because Garfield was lying on the newly invented metal coil-spring mattress, an invention of which most people were unaware, and the detector thus indicated the presence of metal no matter where it was placed over the president. If Garfield had been moved off the bed, the bullet may well have been detected and Garfield's life saved thereby. Indeed, at his trial, the gunman admitted to shooting the president but not to killing him, alleging that his doctors bore that responsibility.

The peripatetic Brown-Séquard felt at home in Paris, the city of his student days, the center of French culture, and a city at the center of world events. French scholarship in medicine and science was highly regarded, and educated Parisians shared in each new triumph and advance, making known their views on important issues, regardless of their qualifications to do so. It was in Paris that the remarkable clinical advances of the previous quarter-century had led to the characterization of many previously unrecognized disorders of the nervous system, and public demonstrations of these neurological derangements were held every Tuesday in the famous amphitheater of the Salpêtrière Hospital by the imperious Charcot, who was not one to avoid the limelight, before an audience consisting not only of physicians but also of writers, actors, and the well-to-do.

Not surprisingly, the powerful example and responsibilities of French academic leaders engendered professional hostilities and jealousies. Brown-Séquard had his detractors, both among the general public and within the realm of medical science. His advocacy of the experimental method as an essential means of gaining fresh knowledge about the functioning of the body and the changes that lead to or result from disease states,[23] and his use of animals as subjects in his own studies had for years brought on him the enmity of the antivivisectionists. They felt that such an approach was unnecessary, unjustifiable, and immoral, and were becoming increasingly visible as they made their beliefs known to the world. Their hostility and reactions to him were discussed in earlier chapters. The nature of his experimental work in the late

---

[H] See footnote G, Chapter 7.
[I] G. G. Moore, in his book *Society Recollections in Paris and Vienna* (London: John Long, 1907, pp. 73–75), claims to have been with Brown-Séquard when the professor was consulted at the recommendation of the American Government, but I have been unable to verify this account.

1880s brought him into conflict with another segment of the general public and with many of his professional colleagues.

On 1 June 1889, he read a paper to the Société de Biologie that startled some, shocked others, and made him a figure of fun to many people.[24] After preliminary studies in animals, he had begun in May to inject himself subcutaneously with the liquid obtained by grinding the testicles of dogs and guinea pigs in a little water. After injecting about 1 cc of this mixture into himself on several occasions over a two-week period, he reported a marked increase in his strength and stamina, improved mental energy and concentration, an increase in force of his urinary stream, and greater regularity in his bowel movements. These changes persisted for about a month after the last injection before waning. Why had he injected himself in this way? The work was based on an idea that he had first expressed in one of his lectures at the Paris Faculty of Medicine in 1869, and to which he had returned in 1875 while working in the private laboratory that Agassiz had established near Boston. He had come to believe that the testicles manufacture a substance that enters the blood stream and in some manner energizes the nervous system and probably also the muscles. Castration during childhood or adolescence was known to affect the physical and behavioral development of men, and he had concluded that the weakness that develops in the elderly may relate at least in part to a decline in function of the genital glands.

This dramatic account attracted considerable attention not only among the medical establishment—who received it with amazement and incredulity—but also among the general public and in the popular press. The public attention that it received was hardly surprising, as the approach involved sex, the testicles, aging, rejuvenation, and the use of animal extracts.[25] It was to be the first of a number of reports from Brown-Séquard on the use of testicular extracts to reverse certain of the changes that occur with age. His observations led to their use not simply in the elderly whose powers were declining but also—at least by other physicians—in patients with a variety of neurological and other medical disorders. Remarkable cures were claimed, but not by Brown-Séquard, who denied that the administration of testicular extracts could cure infections or cancers, or provide any benefit other than as a nonspecific tonic that improved the appetite and sleep, and reduced malaise and lassitude. His reports were picked up by the popular press, taken out of context, exaggerated and distorted, and led to increasing public scorn and derision. Cartoons of him were published in both Europe and America, his work was caricatured, and music-hall comedians had a field-day at his expense. His concepts came to be coupled by the press with the rash statements and extravagant claims made by the opportunist fringe of medical society, which began marketing testicular extracts as "The Elixir of Life" or "The Universal Panacea" after Brown-Séquard, without thought of monetary gain, had published a full account of the technique he used to prepare his extracts and the manufacturing process, so that others might explore their uses and limitations.[26] Indeed, the term "Elixir of Life" was coupled with Brown-Séquard's name in full-color double-page centerfold political cartoons in magazines favored by both the Democrats and the Republicans in the United States within three months of his original presentation,[25] and a song—"Brown-Séquard's Elixir"—by Winchell Forbes soon became popular.[J] Its words did not spare him:

> The world has gone daft on the latest new fad
> For the fountain of youth has been found
> And nobody dies in the old-fashioned way
> To be tucked away under ground.
> It's a peripatetical fountain of course
> For every cheap medicine mixer
> Is posing as chief engineer of the spring
> That pumps out the genuine elixir.
> The latest sensation's the Sequard Elixir
> That's making young kids of the withered and gray
> There'll be no more pills or big doctor bills
> Or planting of people in churchyard clay
> And even the doctors are rattled at last
> For when their best patients are sick, sir
> They just step around to the corner drug store
> And "shake" for a dose of Elixir
> It's awful to think that some folks I know
> Forever among us may stay.
> By chinning some druggist when pay day comes
> For a dose of this cussed Elixir.

In fact, the aging professor refused to endorse any commercial products based on his preparations and did not allow the use of his name by any of the medical profiteers who sought to capitalize on his work. Nevertheless, he was

---

[J] Max Morath, the contemporary general entertainer and authority on ragtime, made a recording entitled "Drugstore Cabaret" for the 1991 annual meeting of the American Pharmaceutical Association, and this contained a number of songs on the history of the drugstore. It was prepared on analog cassette in a boxed set, with notes by Allen Debus, but later released commercially on a compact disk. Featured among the songs is "Brown-Séquard's Elixir." He generously provided me with a copy of his production notes and the recording, for which I am grateful.

blamed because others used his name. As one American medical correspondent wrote

> Quackery is rampant in Paris ... regularly educated practitioners who, weary of the restraints imposed by the regular profession, boldly announce their wares through every sort of advertising medium. And why should they not, when the venerable scientist, Brown-Séquard, is the greatest sinner of them all? Everywhere, on lamp-posts, in urinals, in railway stations, and in the most out-of-the-way places ... one will see large banner posters advertising the *"Suc de Brown-Sequard, très précieux"* etc., *for nervousness, diminished sexual power in men or women, old or young*.[27] [emphasis in original]

It was apparently not public knowledge that Brown-Séquard had gone so far as to obtain legal advice to prevent the unauthorized use of his name, particularly when it became apparent that one enterprising but unprincipled speculator was planning a book promoting the use of testicular extracts.[28]

It soon became evident, of course, that treatment by the *methode séquardienne* did not prolong life. The fact that Brown-Séquard had never claimed otherwise was conveniently forgotten by his detractors, who did not hesitate to call him a charlatan because his extracts had not fulfilled their supposed promise. Regardless of the uproar that followed his studies, work which some ascribed to the ill-considered attempts by a failing old man to recapture his youth, Brown-Séquard carried on as before. He simply ignored the swipes of an ill-informed public, but he was hurt by the skeptical response of some of his friends and colleagues. He did not think that Alphonse Dumontpallier (see footnote B, p. 4, Chapter 1), who was later to be one of his pall-bearers, would follow through on experiments with the testicular extracts "because he is the most timorous man in the world. He is frightened that people will laugh at him."[29]

Many physicians or scientists, such as Dejerine[K] and countless lesser-known practitioners in France, Germany, and Russia; George John Romanes,[L] Victor Horsley, and Hughlings Jackson (see Chapter 7), David Ferrier (Chapter 10),

---

[K] Joseph Jules Dejerine (1849–1917), French neurologist who was eventually appointed to Charcot's chair at the Salpêtrière Hospital and who has named after him numerous neurological disorders and syndromes affecting different parts of the nervous system.

[L] George John Romanes (1848–1894), British physiologist who focused on evolution and was a friend of Charles Darwin and Thomas Huxley. He was interested particularly in Brown-Séquard's experiments on epilepsy, and Brown-Séquard gave him access to his laboratory at the Collège de France. The Romanes lecture, given annually at Oxford University, is named after him.

Brudenell Carter,[M] Fanton-Cameron,[N] and his wife's cousin, Dr. Waterhouse, in England; and Weir Mitchell and William Hammond (Chapter 8) in the United States, did give it a try—with varying success—and some became advocates. Samples of the extracts were also sent to Armand de Watteville, the editor of the journal *Brain*,[O] and, at their request, to physicians at the Hospital for the Paralysed and Epileptic in London. "My old hospital, which has become one of the most beautiful hospitals in the world and which has, among its physicians, the most celebrated practitioners in England, offers us the best field experience—the most decisive."[30]

The response of Charcot, who is said to have claimed acidly that injections of distilled water were as effective as injections of testicular extracts[31] and eventually abandoned Brown-Séquard's liquid altogether,[32] was particularly distressing. For some time, it seems that the relationship between the two giants—one a widely respected neuroscientist, the other a master clinician—had been strained. In his lectures of 1879–1880 on diseases of the spinal cord, for example, Charcot casually dismissed the importance of Brown-Séquard's work on sensory function: "[I]t is in regard to sensibility a matter of indifference by what elements of the cord the conduction is effected ...."[33] He apparently believed that "... in the case of the spinal cord the experimenter will be confounded with difficulties nearly insurmountable ...,"[34] an unfortunate viewpoint, as Brown-Séquard had made his name on experimental work on the spinal cord. And in discussing the results of spinal hemisections, he referred only to "the experiments of Schiff, repeated by Vulpian and others,"[35] as if Brown-Séquard's work was not worthy of consideration. It seems, as mentioned in an earlier chapter, that Charcot now viewed Brown-Séquard as a rival to be downplayed or marginalized.

Charcot had originally sent patients to Brown-Séquard for treatment with testicular extracts but then decided to examine for himself the effects of the orchitic fluid.[36] He began buying supplies of testicles from local slaughter houses to make his own preparations.[37] Brown-Séquard immediately worried

---

[M] Robert Brudenell Carter (1828–1918), accomplished British ophthalmic surgeon who was on the staff of several major London hospitals, including the National Hospital for the Paralysed and Epileptic. He served on the staff of *The Lancet* and wrote with facility on diverse topics, authoring books on hysteria and on education in preventing diseases of the nervous system, as well as on various ophthalmological topics.

[N] I have been unable to find any information about Dr. Fanton-Cameron.

[O] *Brain*, an influential British clinical and scientific journal devoted to neurology, was founded by J. Crichton Browne, J.C. Bucknill, David Ferrier, and J. Hughlings Jackson in 1878. In 1889, the journal became the official organ of the new London Neurological Society under the editorship of Armand de Watteville.

that use of a weak or poorly prepared liquid would lead to lack of a response[38] or that failure of the liquid to work when tested in England would have an instant impact on Charcot and others who were jealous of his success.[39] Indeed, Brown-Séquard concluded that Charcot wanted to "kiss us the better to throttle us" but that—if the extracts worked—he would claim to have altered the preparation and take credit for curing the patients.[38]

Brown-Séquard's growing distrust of Charcot and increasing friendship with the ambitious Charles Bouchard (1837–1915)—a former student and protégé of Charcot who had come to see his old mentor as a rival rather than friend, and whose work on hysteria he ridiculed—had professional consequences. The competitive national examinations for associate professorships (*professeur agrégé*) in 1892 had a particularly bitter note. Bouchard had been chosen by the minister of education to preside over the proceedings for the professorships in internal medicine. Bouchard did not include Charcot on the jury for the examinations, but instead included allies of his own or non-Parisians without especial loyalty to Charcot. It was not uncommon for established professors to advance their own candidates, and among the candidates on this occasion were two outstanding students of Charcot, namely, Joseph Babinski[P] and Georges Gilles de la Tourette,[Q] and several candidates of Bouchard. The results of the examinations created a storm when none of Charcot's students but four of Bouchard's former students or assistants were among the five successful candidates out of a total of sixteen. The controversy became public, with articles published in the daily and weekly newspapers,[40,41] as well as in the medical journals.[42–44] Brown-Séquard and d'Arsonval sided with Bouchard both in private and public,[45,46] to the extent that, at its conclusion, d'Arsonval was able to write to his master that "the reign of Charcot is finished ...."[46] Public opinion was divided as to whether an appeal was

---

[P] Joseph Babinski (1857–1932), born in Paris of Polish parents, became one of the most prominent clinical neurologists of his day, although he never competed again for the *agrégation* and thus never held a formal professorial appointment. Unmarried, he lived with his brother, a famed chef. He had a major role in the development of neurosurgery in France and published many original clinical observations, the most well-known being the so-called Babinski sign, a reflex response elicited by scratching or scraping the outer border of the sole of the foot: an upward movement (i.e., toward the head) of the big toe indicates an abnormality of the central nervous system (specifically, a disorder of the upper motor neurons or the corticospinal tract connecting these neurons with the spinal cord, such as may occur with spinal cord compression or after a stroke).

[Q] Georges Gilles de la Tourette (1857–1904), French neurologist after whom Tourette syndrome (of chronic multiple tics) is named. A moody and difficult man, he was shot by a delusional former patient but survived, dying several years later of what may well have been syphilis.

justified, but the minister turned it down. An appeal was taken to the Conseil d'État, a higher authority, which eventually ruled (in late 1894) that there were no legal or procedural grounds to invalidate the examination.[47] The entire episode left an unfortunate impression of academia for years, embittered Babinski and many others among the new generation of French neurologists, and raised disturbing questions about the French examination system. "It becomes more and more evident that these examinations furnish opportunities for intrigue and injustice. Bargains are made savouring more of the Bourse than of scientific impartiality. Professor So-and-So promises to vote for A, if Professor So-and-So votes for B .... Sometimes a distinguished candidate bears the brunt of the animosity felt for the professor whose pupil and *protégé* he is."[48]

Brown-Séquard had to face not just the scorn of the general public, but the incredulity of certain members of the medical and scientific community for the claims that were being made for the testicular extracts. He also met with the antagonism and outrage of clerics and religious bodies because he had suggested to some of his patients that, by analogous means as the injection of testicular fluids, sexual excitement (as by masturbation) without ejaculation might increase their general vigor.[49,50] Masturbation was frowned on by society in general and by the church in particular, and his suggestion aroused their fury and led to a debate about his motives. The antivivisectionists—already hostile to him—were upset even further by the idea that the testicles of innocent animals were being removed for such seemingly perverse reasons. Thus, the antivivisectionist Dr. Edward Berdoe, for example, circulated in July 1889 an extraordinary letter—that he earnestly warned should not be left where it could be read by innocent young persons—suggesting that the object of

> these abominable proceedings is to enable broken down libertines to pursue with renewed vigour the excesses of their youth, to rekindle the dying embers of lust in the debilitated and aged, and to profane the bodies of men which are the temples of God by an elixir drawn from the testicles of dogs and rabbits by a process involving the excruciating torture of the innocent animals, which elixir is then injected by a physician into the veins of his patient whom he has caused to practice a degrading and loathing vice ... we may also have a new race of beings intermediate between man and the lower animals as a remoter consequence of the boon to humanity conferred by French physiology.[51]

To others the issue was simpler: "Vivisection may be an open question, but self-abuse is not" wrote an outraged member of the medical profession.[52] Brown-Séquard's reaction was simply to ignore the vitriolic attacks made upon himself and his new approach.

In the following years, Brown-Séquard and d'Arsonval experimented with the administration of extracts of other animal organs in different diseases of humans, trying, for example, pancreatic extract for diabetes, extracts of the adrenal glands for Addison's disease, and muscle tissue in certain diseases of muscle. Tissue was dissolved in glycerine for subcutaneous injection or saline for intravenous administration. They gained no profit from this work. In fact, Brown-Séquard spent some ten thousand francs of his own money, just in the last one or two years of his life, to give out his preparations to physicians free of charge,[53] provided only that they would let him know of the indications for and outcome of their use. A letter from Sir Henry Thompson[R] to Ernest Hart, editor of the *British Medical Journal*, dated April 17, 1890, includes the telling comment

> I have had ever since the first appearance of Brown-Séquard's remarkable paper on the injection of fresh juices from the testicles for the human subject some correspondence with him and a long talk last summer .... He won't make a single experiment himself on any patient, lest he should be accused of desiring to obtain fees by the very tempting prospects held forth of his power to rejuvenate the old fellows on the border of the grave who would give half they possess for a reprieve![54]

Chapter 13 provides a detailed account of this work and its aftermath, which is now largely forgotten. It led directly to a new therapeutic method—hormone replacement therapy—that initially involved the administration of extracts of organs, selected on the basis of the disease to be treated, to restore to the blood substances normally secreted into it but which were lacking because of the underlying disease.

Experimental Work: More on Sensation

Brown-Séquard's concept of the sensory pathways within the spinal cord and on the effects of cord hemisection gained wide acceptance in the latter half of the nineteenth century. The loss of pain and temperature appreciation on the side opposite to the hemisection was attributed to an interruption of the crossed fibers that mediate these modalities and ascend in the spinothalamic

---

[R] An eminent genito-urinary surgeon who numbered Napoleon III and the King of the Belgians among his patients, Thompson was also a painter, novelist, amateur astronomer, and a well-known collector of Chinese porcelain, as well as a gourmet famous for the splendor of his dinner parties.

212 *Brown-Séquard: An Improbable Genius*

Uncrossed fibers passing to brain in posterior column (fibers cross in lower brainstem)

Crossed fibers passing to brain in the anterior and lateral spinothalamic tracts

touch, pressure, joint position, vibration

touch, pressure, pain, temperature

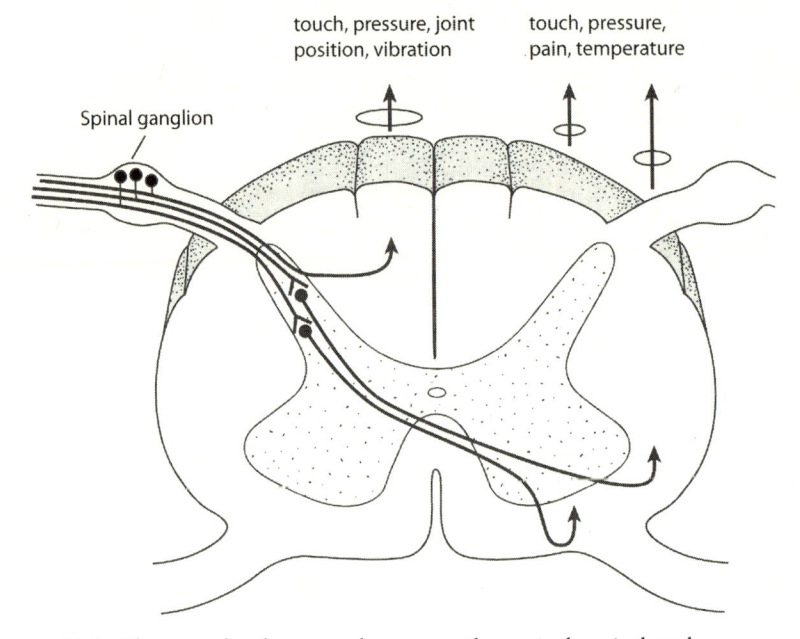

Spinal ganglion

FIGURE 12.1 The crossed and uncrossed sensory pathways in the spinal cord.

tracts to the brain (Figure 12.1). Nevertheless, certain of his findings remained difficult to explain, such as the ipsilateral hyperesthesia (increased sensitivity) below lateral hemisections of the cord, which most clinicians simply chose to ignore. Similarly, the contralateral sensory loss that Brown-Séquard found was more complete than is generally accepted, and the discrepancy was quietly forgotten. Nevertheless, his findings have been confirmed by other clinicians and scientists,[55] and cannot simply be dismissed.

In 1892, Frederick Mott,[s] a young and relatively unknown British neurologist, reported to the Royal Society of London his findings following hemisection of the spinal cord in monkeys.[56] Animals could usually localize a painful

---

[s] Frederick Mott (1853–1926), British physician, physiologist, and pathologist who made important contributions to neurology and psychiatry. He showed the relationship between syphilis and general paralysis of the insane (a form of neurosyphilis), made contributions to the physiology of speech and song, investigated the causes of insanity, worked on the inheritance of mental illness, and was a supporter of eugenics. He had a major role in the founding of the Maudsley Hospital (London, UK) for the study and treatment of mental disorders.

stimulus accurately only on the side that was not paralyzed (that is, the contralateral side), the exact opposite of the findings reported by Brown-Séquard. Moreover, rather than hyperesthesia occurring ipsilaterally below the cord hemisection, sensation was sometimes diminished or lost on that side and preserved contralaterally. These findings, which seemed the opposite of those reported by Brown-Séquard, questioned the very existence of the Brown-Séquard syndrome, which most clinicians now accepted as an established entity (and still do to this day). Two years later, Brown-Séquard published an extraordinary, four-page response to Mott's paper.[57] He began by praising the work but pointed out the difficulties of inferring the function of different parts of the nervous system from lesion experiments. Any loss of function that followed selective lesions could—he indicated—simply reflect an influence exerted on some distant part more directly involved in the lost function. He then indicated that he had revised—fifteen years earlier—his original views concerning the transmission of sensory information in the spinal cord based on additional experimental evidence that he himself had accumulated over the years. He had found, for example, that the analgesia produced on the side opposite a hemisection of the cervical cord is replaced by hyperesthesia when the cord is hemisected again on the same side as, but below, the original lesion, for example, in the thoracic region; the ipsilateral side (which was originally hyperesthetic) then becomes insensitive to pain.[58] This remarkable reversal of the sensory abnormalities suggested that the original analgesia had not occurred simply because the first (upper) lesion had cut ascending sensory fibers.

Various other experimental observations seemed to add to the confusion and suggested that to regard the sensory system simply as a hard-wired system was to fail to recognize its complexity and the manner of its operation. For example, he had found (as also had Vulpian) that a small lesion in the posterior column of the cord could produce contralateral analgesia, as if the cord had been hemisected.[59] Moreover, section of the posterior roots in the upper thoracic region on one side sometimes produced sensory changes on the opposite side, similar to those following cord hemisection.[59] Again, the analgesia of the hind limb that occurs below a hemisection of the thoracic cord was sometimes abolished by slight stretch of the sciatic nerve on the contralateral (anesthetic) side, suggesting that the sensory pathways could not have been transected by the cord lesion.[60] Such findings had led him to believe that the analgesia occurring in these experimental circumstances could result from an inhibitory effect, and the hyperesthesia from an excitatory effect, exerted on central sensory mechanisms as a consequence of the various lesions, rather than simply resulting from the interruption of hard-wired pathways.

Brown-Séquard's remarkable paper attests to the integrity of its author who, in his seventies, was prepared to retract or modify the work on which his reputation had first been established more than forty years earlier. He refused to adhere to a particular viewpoint simply because he had previously proposed it. His interest was in the correctness of the concepts that he advocated, and not in his image or reputation. His paper is noteworthy also for the respect and courtesy that he afforded a junior whose work seemed to challenge his own, and whom others in a similar position might have resented. The paper represents an extraordinary contribution, encapsulating an important concept of the spinal cord as an integrator of various excitatory and inhibitory inputs that determine the outcome to a particular event, such as a sensory stimulus, rather than acting simply as a conduit between the periphery and the brain.

Nevertheless, his experimental observations were quietly forgotten over the years, although pain specialists and neurologists have long been aware that ipsilateral hyperesthesia and spontaneous pain is encountered occasionally in humans with traumatic Brown-Séquard syndrome. Then, in 1979, Derek Denny-Brown (professor of neurology at Harvard Medical School) reverted to the topic.[55] He studied monkeys in which the spinal cord had been sectioned in the thoracic region, and confirmed that spinal cord hemisection that was not quite complete led to contralateral analgesia with ipsilateral hyperesthesia (that is, the Brown-Séquard syndrome), whereas complete hemisection caused the reverse (ipsilateral analgesia but contralateral hyperesthesia). When an animal with a Brown-Séquard syndrome underwent a second hemisection above the level of the original lesion, but one that extended just over the midline to the other side of the spinal cord to ensure that it completely interrupted the ipsilateral anterior column, the initial contralateral sensory loss disappeared and sensation was restored on that side, but sensory loss then occurred on the side of the lesion (Figure 12.2). When the new lesion interrupted the anterior columns bilaterally, touch and pain sensation returned to both sides. The sensory loss that occurred on the side opposite the hemisection could be replaced transiently by marked hyperesthesia if a subconvulsive dose of strychnine was administered, and by more permanent hyperesthesia if a second lesion was made above the level of the first lesion that hemisected the cord and destroyed also the contralateral anterior and posterior columns—after four weeks there was no cutaneous area in which stimulation failed to elicit a reaction.

Denny-Brown concluded from this work that incomplete cord hemisection leads to contralateral sensory loss that is due to an inhibitory influence and is reversible by strychnine. The sensory loss (and the inhibitory effect to which it relates) is abolished by complete section of the anterior column on the

Spinal Cord Lesion (shaded) Clinical Result

A: First lesion

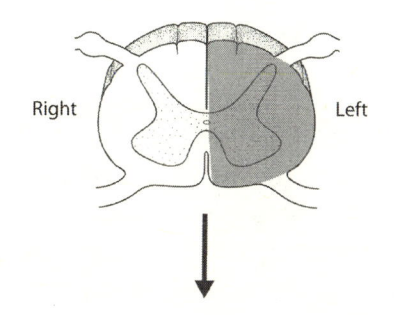

Right — Left

Contralateral (right) analgesia

Ipsilateral (left) hyperesthesia

B: Second lesion (rostral to first lesion)

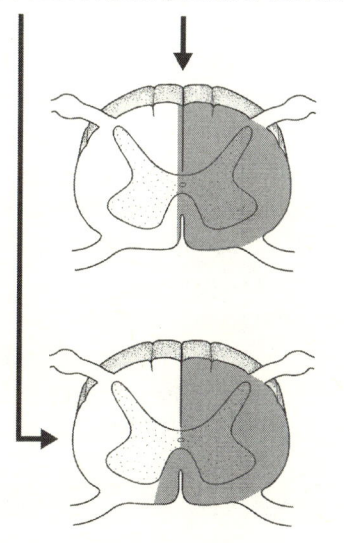

Contralateral hyperesthesia replaces analgesia

Ipsilateral analgesia develops

Sensory responses return bilaterally

FIGURE 12.2 An incomplete hemisection causes the Brown-Séquard syndrome (A). When a second lesion is made at a higher level than the first one, the sensory disturbance is either reversed or eliminated (B), depending on the extent of the lesion.

hemisected side, but the activity of the opposite anterior column then produces sensory loss ipsilateral to the lesion. He thus considered the descending pathways in the anterior columns on each side of the spinal cord to have a tonic suppressive effect on spinal mechanisms, an effect that is balanced against the function of the lateral spinothalamic tract in the lateral funiculus. There seemed also to be a large and direct crossing of sensory traffic in the posterior spinal commissure connecting certain parts of the spinal cord on the two sides, allowing for the bilateral transmission of touch, pain, and temperature sensation, with good localization from any point.

But things are not quite as simple as they appear. The lesion method used by Brown-Séquard, Mott, and Denny-Brown, while useful in its day, has certain limitations, especially when applied to the study of pain and sensory pathways in animals. Experimental studies of the sort that they undertook are often confounded by stimulus control and variables, variability in responses, and difficulties in interpreting the responses that are elicited, and by the fact that interpretation requires evaluation of both the short- and long-term consequences of such lesions.[61] They may lead to ambiguous results when behavioral responses are studied, particularly if the reflex responses to pain or other sensory stimuli are equated with perception of the sensory stimulus. Experiments in nonhuman primates have shown, for example, that reflex responses are modulated differently than are purposive responses to pain.[62] Nevertheless, modern neuroscientists still commonly use reflex measures of pain sensitivity in studies on animals, and thus the problem remains.

Patrick Wall, a contemporary expert on the pathophysiology of pain, has stressed the importance of the concepts proposed by Brown-Séquard in his 1894 paper,[T] emphasizing that dynamic mechanisms within the spinal cord may well account at least in part for the alteration in sensation that results from cord lesions.[63] It is likely, however, that the experimental work of Brown-Séquard and other investigators may well have been focused unwittingly more on the innate (reflex) behavioral responses to sensory stimuli in the animals that they studied than on sensory function itself. With regard to the dynamic cord mechanisms involved, these may involve the interaction of tonic excitatory and inhibitory mechanisms that relate to peripheral and descending inputs to segmental cells or may involve more prolonged alterations of excitability that are initiated by the segmental input and then sustained by local mechanisms. Other mechanisms may also be involved. The importance of these concepts is in their implication that it may be possible to restore certain functions, at least to some extent, after damage to the spinal cord, by altering the balance of interacting influences on the spinal mechanisms subserving sensation or behavior.

In the last quarter-century, more has been learned about the pain-modulating circuits in the central nervous system, and this work supports Brown-Séquard's concept of excitatory and inhibitory inputs acting both in the spinal cord and brain to influence the perception of pain or the innate (reflex) behavioral reactions to pain that he observed and attributed to pain perception.

[T] Wall, who died in 2001, wrote to this author concerning Brown-Séquard's paper. He rated it as one of the most important in neurology but felt that most neurologists had never heard of it and would be incapable of understanding it.

Central regions involved in the pathways subserving pain in animals seem to be involved similarly in humans, and pain perception in humans is blocked by selective lesions of these regions in the spinal cord and brain. Brief commentary on such sensory processing is provided here for the interested reader and to put Brown-Séquard's findings into a modern perspective. Excellent reviews of the topic are provided elsewhere by others.[64,65]

Neurons involved in pain-modulating circuits are tuned to detect tissue-damaging stimuli.[64] Sensory input from nociceptive stimuli (i.e., stimuli causing pain or injury) is transmitted by primary afferent fibers from the periphery to the posterior horns of the spinal cord. The posterior horns can be divided into various layers or *laminae*, each of which has distinctive physiological properties and some of which have an important role in relaying nociceptive stimuli. Stimulation of certain regions of the brain inhibits or relieves pain and inhibits neurons responding to nociceptive stimuli in the posterior horns. These regions project through pathways from the brainstem (in particular, from the pons and medulla) that traverse the posterolateral funiculus of the spinal cord and pass to the laminae of the posterior horns containing nociceptive relay neurons (Figure 12.3). In other words, this circuit controls pain by targeting neurons (and the input to them) in the posterior horns that respond to nociceptive stimuli. Thus, the posterolateral funiculus controls nociceptive transmission. Cutting this region of the spinal cord can lead to pain, hyperalgesia, or hyperesthesia, whereas stimulating these pathways may inhibit pain. The pain-modulating circuitry, however, can enhance as well as inhibit nociceptive transmission and the neuronal responses to noxious stimuli,[66-68] and prolonged nociceptor input can lead to hyperalgesia and hyperesthesia. These seemingly contradictory effects relate to the existence and activity of two distinct subpopulations of neurons within this circuit; their effects are mediated by opioid neurotransmitters.[64] Other pathways from brainstem structures that descend in the posterolateral funiculus to control nociceptive transmission in the spinal cord also exist and are distinct from those just described in that they involve different neurotransmitters; specifically, *serotonin* (which may have either facilitatory or inhibitory effect on spinal transmission), *norepinephrine* (primarily inhibitory), and *dopamine* (facilitatory or inhibitory) act on different subtypes of receptors to facilitate or inhibit spinal nociceptive transmission, affecting nociceptor afferent fibers, dorsal (posterior) horn neurons, and excitatory and inhibitory interneurons, and even glial (non-neuronal) cells.[69,70] Fibers from the brainstem (pons) may also travel in the anterior funiculus of the spinal cord and have pain-inhibitory effects,[69,71] although this is less clear. It appears, then, that neurons in the brainstem can turn the neural pain mechanisms on or off in the spinal cord (Figure 12.3). It is probably the target

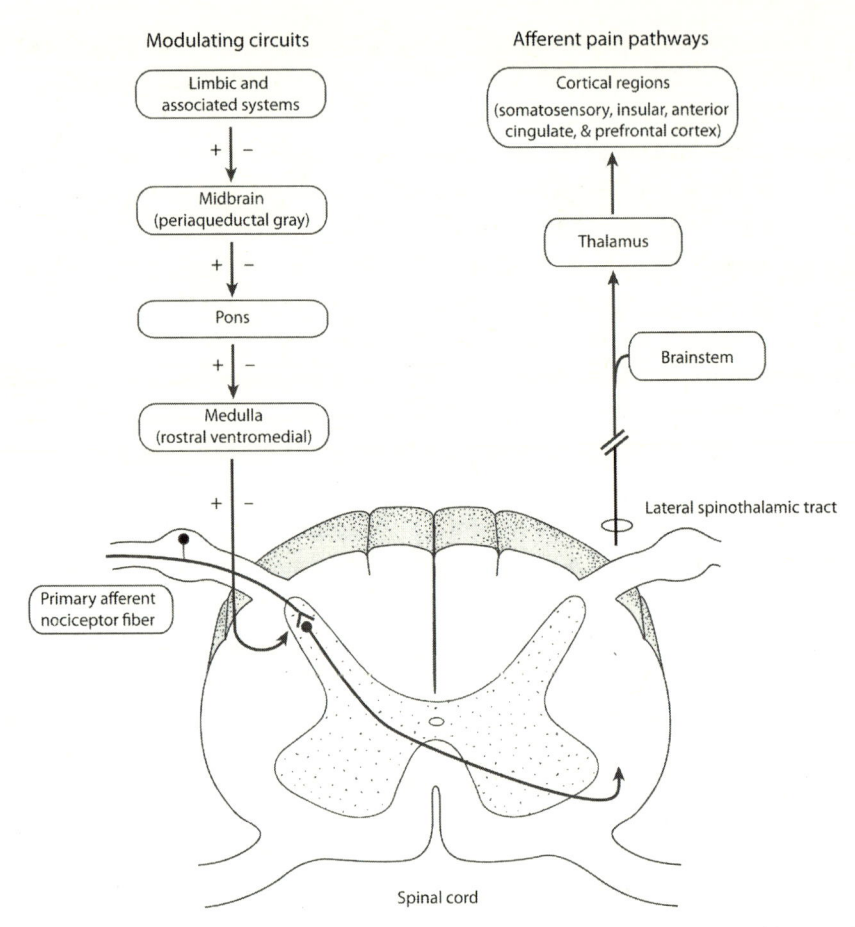

FIGURE 12.3 The right side of the illustration shows the pathway of the sensory fibers mediating pain. Having crossed in the spinal cord, the fibers ascend to the thalamus of the brain in the spinothalamic tract, and from there pass to various cortical regions. The left side of the figure shows some of the pain-modulating influences on the spinal pathways and processes mediating pain sensation. These descending fibers travel in the posterolateral funiculus of the spinal cord and may be excitatory (+) or inhibitory (−) in nature. Pain-modulating pathways may also descend in the anterior funiculus, but these are less clearly characterized and are not shown here.

receptors and their location in the spinal cord that define whether excitation or inhibition occurs in response to a particular neurotransmitter system. However, knowledge about the precise circuitry is still limited and the literature is confused, as it often fails to distinguish clearly between the types of response elicited by sensory stimuli and between nociceptive and non-nociceptive sensory stimuli.

In any event, it appears that Brown-Séquard's final concept of sensory function and, specifically, of pain physiology, in the spinal cord is not far removed in principle from the views that have evolved among modern neuroscientists, even though—like many modern neuroscientists—he may have confused sensory perception with reflex behavioral responses to pain. If his views seemed forbidding in their complexity to clinicians, they are in fact less daunting than the mechanisms now envisioned by neuroscientists, which remain to be elucidated more fully and which clinicians have yet to grasp.

So, what are the clinical consequences of an isolated lateral hemisection of the spinal cord? These are broadly as described by Brown-Séquard more than one hundred and fifty years ago, although more detail has since been added, and can be summarized as follows. There is ipsilateral impairment of tactile direction sensitivity and of repetitive stimulation (interruption of posterior columns),[71-73] two-point discrimination (posterior columns and spinocervical tracts),[72,73] and joint-position sense (posterior and posterolateral columns); ipsilateral hyperalgesia (interruption of the posterolateral column leading to loss of descending inhibitory influences)[74]; and ipsilateral weakness (corticospinal tract and posterior columns—it is difficult to move a limb if you do not know where it is in space). Contralaterally, pain and temperature appreciation are lost (spinothalamic and spinoreticulothalamic pathways).[75]

It should be noted parenthetically that contralateral pain and temperature sensation is reduced but not lost with lesions restricted to the spinothalamic tract in the lateral and anterior funiculi[62,76]; superficial lesions lead to little or no recovery, whereas medially extensive lesions involving gray matter are followed by some degree of recovery and some ipsilateral hyperalgesia. This is the reason that the surgical procedure of *cordotomy*, in which the spinothalamic tract was sectioned to relieve severe pain, failed to provide complete relief and often led only to transient benefit. Loss of pain and temperature appreciation requires a complete anterior hemisection involving both the spinothalamic and spinoreticulothalamic pathways.[75]

Looking back on Brown-Séquard's contributions to the subject, there is a certain irony. His original concepts concerning the sensory pathways in the spinal cord, introduced in his doctoral thesis and expanded by his work in the following decade, were rejected by clinicians and scientists for more than ten years and only gradually gained acceptance after they were confirmed by an independent committee established by the Société de Biologie in Paris. They remain widely accepted even today, having the virtue of simplicity and the merit of seeming to account for various clinical disturbances, such as the contralateral sensory loss, that occur with certain lateralized lesions of the spinal cord. He later modified his original beliefs to account for a number of other clinical sequelae of cord lesions that many observers had preferred to ignore. The hypothesis that Brown-Séquard put forward to account for these confounding clinical observations was intuitively less appealing to most physicians and scientists, if only because of its complexity, and was simply ignored in favor of his (previously rejected) earlier account, which it was intended to complement. It reveals, however, an insight into the operation of the nervous system that was remarkably ahead of its time and is similar in nature to that of modern neuroscientists, most of whom are completely unaware of Brown-Séquard's later views on the subject. Brown-Séquard's observations and their interpretation have profound implications for the rehabilitation of those with spinal injuries, regardless of whether they relate to sensory perception itself or to innate behavioral responses elicited by external stimuli, and help to account for many of the phenomena that clinicians have hitherto held to be inexplicable.

Daily Life

Despite the high academic honors that he had received and the subsequent ridicule to which he was exposed, Brown-Séquard retained the eccentricities that made him such a colorful personality. Until his death, he would jot down ideas on the closest scrap of paper at hand and put the scribbled note in some box or drawer where it would usually be forgotten.[77,78] It is said that he once scribbled on his shirt-cuff while driving in a carriage, forgot to copy the note onto a piece of paper, and put the shirt into a basket of dirty clothes that was sent out to be cleaned. Recalling his casual jotting, he was driven in haste to the laundry where he explained what had happened and offered 100 francs for the return of the shirt with his notes on it. The following day he received a shirt (unfortunately not his own) with some very unscientific scribblings on its cuffs.[79] Regardless of his new-found fame (or infamy), he rarely allowed himself to be photographed. When asked for a picture of himself to be published in a book on famous French physicians,[80] he responded that he did not have any. If he could not avoid being photographed, he usually gave his name as Brown, so that no one would be tempted "to put me on display and sell me!"[78] It seems that he was either superstitious about having his picture taken, concerned that he might be recognized by those he perhaps sought to avoid, or anxious to prevent his name being exploited by others. It is conceivable, however, that his hesitancy related to the unsubstantiated rumor, referred to in Chapter 2, that his mother was either black or partly black. It is unlikely that the truth will ever be known.

The turbulence of his professional life contrasted with the tranquillity and stability of his domestic life with Emma and Charlotte in their apartment at 19 rue François Premier. He disliked social gatherings, hated publicity, but enjoyed debate and discussion. He was always prepared to admit the errors of his ways once convinced that he was indeed in the wrong. When a colleague pointed out the fallacies of a theory that he was espousing, Brown-Séquard subsequently devoted one of his lectures at the Collège to exposing and explaining his own mistake and in praising his colleague.[81]

He came to love and rely more and more on d'Arsonval, his assistant, whom he made an associate editor (for biophysics) of his journal—the *Archives de Physiologie Normale et Pathologique*[U]—along with Albert Dastre (physiology)[V] and François-Franck (pathophysiology).[W] Albert Charrin, one of Brown-Séquard's collaborators, subsequently also became an associate editor of the journal (focusing on microbial physiology) and eventually a professor at the Collège de France. The young d'Arsonval was becoming increasingly prominent in his own right as a biophysicist, studying the effects of high-frequency alternating currents on the body and especially on the nerves and muscles. A deepening relationship developed between Brown-Séquard and Louis Pasteur (1822–1895), the man who showed that the spontaneous generation of life (i.e., from nonliving matter) does not occur, who discovered that certain microorganisms could be destroyed by heat ("pasteurization") or attenuated by other means, and who developed a method of preventing and treating rabies. Indeed, Pasteur himself underwent treatment with testicular extracts

---

[U] Brown-Séquard had originally founded the journal with Vulpian and Charcot, but Vulpian died in 1887 and Charcot moved on to found a new journal of his own, the *Archives de Médecine Expérimentale et d'Anatomie Pathologique*, in 1889.

[V] Albert Dastre (1814–1917), French physiologist and former collaborator of Claude Bernard, became professor of general physiology at the Sorbonne. He is known for his work on diabetes and for his studies on the fibrinogen content of blood (which confirmed the earlier studies of Bernard and Brown-Séquard). He was also interested in the vasomotor system and showed that constriction of blood vessels in the skin and surface tissues is usually accompanied by enlargement of deeper vessels, such as those to the internal organs, i.e., that a regional distribution of blood occurs when necessary. This complemented Brown-Séquard's earlier demonstration of vasomotor reflexes, discussed in Chapter 5.

[W] Charles-Emile François-Franck (1849–1921) French physiologist, and collaborator and successor of Marey at the Collège de France, authored a laboratory manual for cinematographically recording quantitative measurements in physiology so as to accurately record body movements. He studied the cortical localization of function, and his book on the topic was accompanied by a preface written by Charcot; he was also interested in the circulation, pulmonary blood flow, and vasomotor regulation, and introduced sympathectomy (interruption of the sympathetic nervous system) for the relief of pain, a procedure that is still widely used with varying success.

in 1892 and 1893 for reasons of ill health (possibly due to small strokes), apparently with an extremely good result.[82] Other medical friends were Charles Bouchard, Professor of General Pathology at the Faculty of Medicine (and later its dean, as well as president of the Académie des Sciences), who had first documented with Charcot the relationship between saccular aneurysms and cerebral hemorrhage.[X] Much of their correspondence deals with medical politics and attempts to ensure that forthcoming elections for awards and positions favored candidates of their own choosing.[83] Albert Hénocque (1840–1902) was another with whom Brown-Séquard had a close, but at times somewhat stormy, relationship.[84] Hénocque worked with him at the Collège de France but developed his own interest in the changes occurring in the blood with disease and could barely wait for the three-hundred-meter Eiffel Tower to be completed, so that he could study the blood at different altitudes.

He was also very attached to Felix Guyon (1831–1920), a celebrated Parisian urological surgeon who had been born on Reunion, an island neighboring Mauritius, and with whom he therefore had much in common.[Y] He had supported the younger man in his candidacy for various appointments and voted on his behalf.[85] They corresponded frequently, with Guyon writing almost as a son on personal matters. Their letters touched on the merits or otherwise of various candidates for appointment or advancement and express views largely in accord with those of Bouchard and Marey.[86] Particularly interesting is a letter describing Charcot's funeral in 1893—the ceremony had been a simple one, but Bouchard had been there, hidden among a few other faculty members, while Marey had claimed to be too ill to attend; the letter provided an opportunity to suggest that the four of them (Guyon, Brown-Séquard, Marey, and Bouchard) should get together to discuss a successor at the Académie.[87] Brown-Séquard's better-known nonmedical friends included Gustave Eiffel (Hénocque's brother-in-law), whose iron tower, built for the Paris Exhibition of 1889—one hundred years after the storming of the Bastille—was the world's

---

[X] An aneurysm is a localized distension of a blood vessel (or the heart); there is typically a bulging out of the weakened wall, which may rupture. Rupture of a saccular aneurysm (one that pouches out like a sack) in the head is an important cause of hemorrhage and often has a fatal outcome. Saccular aneurysms may develop because of a developmental defect, injury, degenerative vascular disease, infection, or exposure to certain drugs. Modern treatment is to obliterate the connection between the outpouching and the main vessel by surgery or to occlude the aneurysmal lumen by detachable balloons or small coils introduced through an artery in the groin and threaded up to the site of the aneurysm, where they induce clot formation.

[Y] Jean Casimir Félix Guyon (1831–1920), pioneering French urological surgeon who is also well known by neurologists because of his description of a passageway or tunnel about the wrist (now called Guyon's canal) traversed by the ulnar nerve, which supplies various muscles and sensation in parts of the hand.

tallest structure until 1930; Marcel Deprez,[Z] a French electrical engineer whose work focused on transmitting electrical power over long distances; and Ernest Renan,[AA] the administrator of the Collège de France.[88] Brown-Séquard also came to know many titled members of the European aristocracy, politicians and ministers of state, professors, writers, and contemporary intellectuals, with most of whom he does not seem to have been especially close.

His salary provided Brown-Séquard with a sense of financial security that he had lacked during much of the 1870s. Nevertheless, having largely abandoned clinical practice and with no private means of support, he became increasingly strapped financially, as he used his personal income to support his work and to defray the costs of producing the testicular and organ extracts on which he was now focused. He steadfastly refused to seek any gain from the new system of medicine that was evolving around his work. Principles mattered more to him than material reward, even when he was short of funds to support the laboratory staff and young scientists who wanted to work with him.[89] His own personal situation was becoming especially unsettled. When he was almost seventy-three years old, in June 1890, he had to ask d'Arsonval to obtain clarification on his behalf as to whether professors at the Collège could retain until the age of seventy-five or older their title and a portion of their salary if sometimes they did not give lectures,[90] because he had not been a government employee for long enough to earn a pension. Sadly, when Emma died early in 1894, he even had to consider renouncing all that she had bequeathed him because of the death-duties (twenty-five to twenty-eight thousand francs) for which he estimated that he would have been responsible.[91]

An ever-increasing demand for his testicular extracts from physicians around the world led to suggestions, in 1893, that an independent institute be established, similar to that created for Pasteur, supported by friends and wealthy entrepreneurs.[92] D'Arsonval estimated that there would be at least five hundred thousand francs available immediately based on the unsolicited offers of friends and supporters, none of whom were speculators or profiteers.[92] Such a development would have given him financial security but

---

[Z] Marcel Deprez (1843–1918) was said by Brown-Séquard to have invented a means of making a train go ten times as fast as the fastest train then in operation, although at considerable expense [GG Moore. *Society recollections in Paris and Vienna* (pp. 73–75). London: John Long, 1907]. He worked with d'Arsonval to develop a galvanometer consisting of a fixed magnet and movable coil to which was attached a pointer that moved over a calibrated scale. Their galvanometer is the basis of many modern galvanometers.

[AA] Ernest Renan (1823–1892), French scholar and philosopher, was professor of Hebrew at the Collège de France. He was suspended after his inaugural lecture because it was misinterpreted by clerics as denying the divinity of Christ. He is best known for his *Life of Jesus*.

Brown-Séquard adamantly refused to allow it, publishing instead a brochure explaining the manufacturing process[25,93]; others were thus enabled to take advantage of his therapeutic approach for personal profit if they chose. D'Arsonval tried to insist, pointing out that both patients and physicians felt it was a mistake not to maintain the laboratory's monopoly to make the extracts. In allowing its manufacture by industry or the *Assistance publique* (the public hospital system), he held that they would be liable for any accidents or complications that resulted from faulty techniques and there would be added risks for patients. He passed on suggestions that the municipality or *Assistance publique* should be able to provide a grant to cover the cost of added personnel to manufacture, prepare, and deliver the liquid under the laboratory's own label and guarantee, and cited Pasteur's institute as an example to follow.[94] Brown-Séquard refused to budge, believing that they could not be held responsible if others (such as industry) prepared the liquid.[95] Pasteur, very impressed by the benefits from the extracts, which he had experienced at first hand,[82] offered to prepare it at his own institute (the Institut Pasteur).[96] Brown-Séquard's response was swift: "Do not ask the Institut Pasteur to prepare the testicular extracts. If he wants to do it, I would be delighted and would compliment Mr. Pasteur, but I do not want to owe him anything …."[97] And a few days later, "regarding the business of preparing the liquid at the Institut Pasteur. Whose ideas was it? Who is pushing it? What is the plan? … As I wrote previously, you and I should stay out of this movement …. I believe it is the best possible solution to the problem that we want to solve. But I would not want anyone to be able to say that we pushed for it."[98]

Curiously, in late 1892, plans were apparently made to utilize the name "Séquard Institute" without his knowledge by someone unconnected with Brown-Séquard. He discovered by chance that a book on "Force and Health" was to be published by a physician who claimed to be the founder of such an institute, and promptly asked d'Arsonval to seek immediate legal assistance to remove the offending term from the cover and other parts of the book, believing that the threat of litigation would be sufficient, as the profiteer would surely wish to avoid a trial publicizing his unauthorized use of Brown-Séquard's name.[99]

In order to avoid the cold of Paris, Brown-Séquard generally wintered in the south of France, usually staying in Nice at the Villa Mon Plaisir, where he would arrive with some two dozen trunks filled with notes, books, and instruments.[100] He would set up a makeshift laboratory, where he continued his researches, especially on experimentally induced epilepsy and on the biological effects of organic tissue extracts. Summers were spent on the coast in Normandy, and he thus spent only a limited time in the French capital city.

During these absences from Paris, d'Arsonval would run the laboratory and lecture in his place, although he did not receive the formal title of substitute professor (*suppléant*) until 1887.[101]

The expatriate remained loyal to his distant homeland of Mauritius, helping out as he could in times of need, such as when, in 1892, he gave a lecture to the Mauritian colony in Paris in aid of the victims of a devastating cyclone in the island.[102] Visiting Mauritians were always welcome at his home. Judge F. Condé Williams, of the High Court of Mauritius, described such a visit in October 1891:

> "Mauritius" on my card was a passport to the excellent savant's good graces ....
> I found him a gentle, modest, white-haired old man, rather below the middle height, of manners quiet and unassuming, and of a smile full of kindness ....
> He spoke warmly of our little Island ....[103]

An especially intimate friendship developed between Brown-Séquard and the young Eugène Dupuy, another Mauritian, whose father had boarded as a law student with the widow of Captain Brown in Paris many years before, while the young Brown (as he then was) was studying medicine. The younger Dupuy came—in his turn—to Paris as a medical student, worked with Brown-Séquard, became a successful physician and scientist, and cared tenderly for the ailing older man in the days before his death.

Brown-Séquard's own health had been deteriorating for some time. He had suffered with arthritis in his legs for several years and with phlebitis since early in 1891. He injected himself with testicular extract, but the glycerine with which it was mixed caused pain and local inflammation, and ultimately an abscess.[104] Concerned that his wife would find out and worry about him, he begged d'Arsonval not to mention it in his letters.[105] The latter half of 1893 was especially difficult. Arthritis limited his daily activities, and in addition one of his legs became more swollen and painful from the phlebitis, with further worsening early in the new year. Emma, too, became ill and, in January 1894—aged 56—she died while they were in Nice.[106] It was a loss from which Brown-Séquard never recovered. Despite the urging of d'Arsonval and others, he felt the need to get away from the countryside, returning dejectedly to Paris in early March. He hesitated, however, to return to his lonely apartment, preferring to move into the little room adjoining his office. He planned on going to England to settle his wife's estate but was too ill to travel.[107] Emma had made a will there, leaving her estate to Brown-Séquard during his lifetime, with the remainder eventually going to Charlotte and to her own children[108]: "... my family should treat my dear adopted daughter with the same regard as if she were my own child."[109] The will was made under British law, but also had to satisfy the authorities in France because she resided there. French law, however, treated her as a British subject rather than a French citizen. These intricacies of international law required careful consideration, but the will was eventually probated, although by this time Brown-Séquard, too, had died.[108]

Terminal Illness and Death

Within a few weeks of his paper on sensory function of the spinal cord, Brown-Séquard was dead. He provided the details of his own last illness in a letter to Dr. Waterhouse, a friend and relative by marriage,[110] and these have been supplemented by the account give by the devoted Eugène Dupuy, who took care of him.[111] On March 24, he developed sudden loss of vision to the left, accompanied by vertigo and a cognitive disturbance with spatial disorientation and loss of recent memory for several hours. His speech intermittently became thick and slurred, although he had no language difficulty—he was able to find the correct words with which to express himself and could comprehend the speech of others. He was seen by two eminent specialists and also by Dupuy, but little could be done except to provide supportive care. After about four or five days, he was only able to get about the apartment on his hands and knees because of his unsteadiness and visual difficulty, but he would not relax or remain quiet. Nevertheless, he was fully aware of the nature and significance of his symptoms, and discussed them with his visitors as if he were recounting the case history of someone else, attributing them to a probable stroke from a small infarct or hemorrhage. Then, during the night he began to vomit and was found to be mute, with weakness of the right side of the face and the left arm, and deviation outward (abduction) of the right eye. Over the next few hours, he developed a droopy eyelid over the right eye (ptosis). On the following day, he attempted to write but the result was unintelligible except—ironically—for the single word "hyperesthesia." In the early hours of Sunday, April 1, he became comatose, and he died shortly before midnight on that same day. No autopsy was performed, but the clinical picture suggests a brain-stem stroke with involvement also of the right occipital lobe (to account for the visual field deficit) and perhaps also of the right parietal region (to account for the curious cognitive disturbance).

His unexpected death shocked both the scientific community and general public. It seemed that all France suddenly missed him. Pasteur had tears in his eyes when he heard the news. "I cried," he said, "he was a friend and a man. He leaves a great name and a great void."[112] Brown-Séquard had insisted on a simple funeral, without pomp or religious ceremony; he wanted no fuss, speeches, tributes, or other honors. Nevertheless, a magnificent wreath of lilacs, camellias, and roses was delivered to his home from the people of Mauritius,[113,114] and there were also flowers from several friends. After a simple Anglican service, which Brown-Séquard had also not wanted, his coffin was taken to the cemetery of Montparnasse and buried there on 4 April 1894. The funeral procession included representatives of the government, the prefect of police, d'Arsonval, and many of the leading doctors and scientists of the day, with pall bearers representing the Académie des Sciences, Collège de France, Société de Biologie, and the island of Mauritius, as described in Chapter 1.[113–116]

Felix Guyon, the urological surgeon, and Louis Joseph Troost (1825–1911), a distinguished chemist, both professors at the University of Paris, and the loyal d'Arsonval, were named by Brown-Séquard as executors of his will, which he had revised three days before his death.[117] In an earlier will, he had left to Emma all that was permitted under the Napoleonic Code and stated expressly his desire that Charlotte remain in France under the care of the woman who had been the only mother that she had ever known.[118] With Emma's untimely death, he had had to make new arrangements insofar as his own ill health permitted. Charles Bouchard was named guardian of Charlotte, who was still a minor.[117] The French Civil Code safeguards the right of children to inherit from their family, although certain discretionary powers remain to parents in this regard. Brown-Séquard used these powers to favor his adored Charlotte over his granddaughter, Ellen Grace Brown-Séquard, who was the only child of his son by his first marriage and who lived across the ocean in the United States. Thus, he left Charlotte everything except for six thousand francs, which went to Ellen in America. Furthermore, much of the furniture and other possessions in his Paris apartment belonged to Emma and were therefore subject to the terms of her will (which allowed him to use them but left them to Charlotte). He gave to Bouchard the power of deciding with whom Charlotte would live in Paris or England, but emphasized that any demand by his son (her half-brother)[AB] or her maternal family in America to take care of her should be refused.[117]

Obituaries were published in the popular press as well as in the leading medical and scientific journals. He was variably described as British, French, or American depending on the whim of his obituarists, who expressed nationalistic pride in his achievements and scientific stature. In France, the press claimed that he had always regarded himself as French by birth because he

---

[AB] In fact, his son was probably already dead, as discussed in Chapter 8. Father and son had been estranged for years and did not communicate with each other.

refused to recognize British sovereignty over his Mauritian homeland. By contrast, the *St. James's Gazette* (of London) pointed out that many so-called eminent Frenchman of the nineteenth century were actually of different national origins, emphasizing how remarkable it was that France was able to appropriate such men as Bonaparte, Gambetta, and Brown-Séquard for herself.[119] Indeed, to British correspondents, Brown-Séquard's moral courage, pertinacity, and coolness clearly reflected his Anglo-Saxon temperament.[119]

His many obituarists emphasized the numerous advances in medical science for which he could claim credit and referred also to the controversy that surrounded the work of his last years, on treatment with animal extracts. Nevertheless, Brown-Séquard's achievements have largely been forgotten by a busy world, and many of the concepts that he championed against fierce opposition are now taken for granted without recognition of their origin. Doubtless, he would have felt a certain satisfaction in the vindication of his ideas. Yet, there are few public memorials to the man who gave himself so unreservedly to the advance of medicine and physiology, and even those that do exist have not all fared well: the commemorative bust of him that was placed in the Public Gardens in his native city of Port Louis in 1898 was destroyed during a hurricane after several years and had to be replaced with a hardier version by his faithful countrymen.[120] A hospital and street are named after him in the Mauritius, a square in Nice, and a street in Paris, and his picture graced for a time a postage stamp. Nevertheless, human knowledge was advanced by the work of this brilliant eccentric, and the history of science has been enriched by his name.

References and Source Notes

1. Delhoume L. *De Claude Bernard à d'Arsonval* (pp. 227–228). Paris: Baillière, 1939. [Part of the extensive correspondence between d'Arsonval and Brown-Séquard is published in this volume.]
2. Delhoume L. *De Claude Bernard à d'Arsonval* (pp. 251–252). Paris: Baillière, 1939.
3. Brown-Séquard CE. Letter to his wife Emma dated 2 August 1879. MS 979/125. Archives, Royal College of Physicians, London.
4. Vulpian EFA. Séance du 27 Mars 1882. Rapport de M. Vulpian sur les titres de M. Brown-Séquard. Archives, Académie des Sciences, Institut de France, Paris.
5. Vulpian EFA. Prix Lacaze. *C R Acad Sci*, 94:321–323, 1882.
6. Bert P. Prix Lallemand. *C R Acad Sci*, 100:535–537, 1885.
7. Anonymous. The prize awarded to Dr. Brown-Séquard. *Lancet*, 2: 168, 1885.
8. Gosselin L. Proposition de la section de medicine et chirurgie pour le prix biennal de l'Institut. (M. Brown-Sequard.) Rapport de M. Gosselin. Archives, Académie des Sciences, Institut de France, Paris. [Leon Gosselin (1815–1887) was a senior surgeon at the Charité Hospital in Paris and a member of the Académie des Sciences, serving as its president shortly before he died.]
9. Anonymous. Le fait du jour: M. Brown-Séquard. *Le Soir*, 1 July 1885.

10. Anonymous. Le Prix Biennal. *Le Matin*, 30 June 1885.
11. Vulpian EFA. Rapport sur les travaux scientifiques de M. Brown-Sequard. Rapport sur M. Brown-Sequard, candidat de l'Académie des Sciences pour le prix biennal. Archives, Académie des Sciences, Institut de France, Paris.
12. Anonymous. À l'Académie. *Le Gaulois*, 2 July 1885.
13. Anonymous. Beaux-arts, lettres et sciences: à l'Institut. *La France*, 2 July 1885.
14. Child T. The Institute of France. *Harper's New Monthly Magazine*, 78:501–520, 1889.
15. Anonymous. Honorary degrees conferred at Cambridge. *Medical News and Abstract*, 38:635, 1880.
16. Anonymous. The International Medical Congress. *Lancet*, 2:69, 1881.
17. Anonymous. Medicine at the Congress. *Br Med J*, 2:784–785, 1881.
18. Anonymous. The International Medical Congress. *Lancet*, 2:244–246, 1881.
19. Anonymous. The International Medical Congress of 1881. *Br Med J*, 2:290–291, 1881.
20. Anonymous. The festivities of the Congress. *Br Med J*, 2:303–304, 1881.
21. Plan of tables and programme of music, banquet to the president and members of the International Medical Congress, 4 August 1881. MS 999/80. Archives, Royal College of Physicians, London.
22. Anonymous. The International Medical Congress. Section II – Physiology. *Lancet*, 2:326–328, 1881.
23. Brown-Séquard CE. Notes on vivisection (undated). MS 993. Royal College of Physicians, London.
24. Brown-Séquard CE. Des effets produits chez l'homme par des injections sous-cutanées d'un liquide retiré des testicules frais de cobaye et de chien. *C R Soc Biol (Paris)*, 41:415–419, 1889.
25. Hansen B. New images of a new medicine. Visual evidence for the widespread popularity of therapeutic discoveries in America after 1885. *Bull Hist Med*, 73:629–678, 1999.
26. Delhoume L. *De Claude Bernard à d'Arsonval* (pp. 528–530). Paris: Baillière, 1939.
27. Anonymous. Quackery in Paris. *Western Med Reporter*, 16:143, 1894.
28. d'Arsonval A. Letters to Brown-Séquard, dated 11 and 15 December 1891. In: Delhoume L., *De Claude Bernard à d'Arsonval* (pp. 414–416 and 417–418). Paris: Baillière, 1939.
29. Brown-Séquard CE. Letter to d'Arsonval, dated 29 December 1890. In: Delhoume L. *De Claude Bernard à d'Arsonval* (pp. 349–350). Paris: Baillière, 1939.
30. Brown-Séquard CE. Letter to d'Arsonval, dated 9 February 1893. In: Delhoume L. *De Claude Bernard à d'Arsonval* (p. 514). Paris: Baillière, 1939.
31. Anonymous. Obituary [of Brown-Séquard]. *The Daily News (London)*, 3 April 1894.
32. Brown-Séquard CE. Letter to d'Arsonval, dated 10 January 1893. In: Delhoume L. *De Claude Bernard à d'Arsonval* (p. 500). Paris: Baillière, 1939.
33. Charcot JM. *Lectures on the pathological anatomy of the nervous system: Diseases of the spinal cord.* (Translated by Comegys CG; p. 89). Cincinnati: Thomson, 1881.
34. Charcot JM. *Lectures on the pathological anatomy of the nervous system: Diseases of the spinal cord.* (Translated by Comegys CG; pp. 9–10). Cincinnati: Thomson, 1881.
35. Charcot JM. *Lectures on the pathological anatomy of the nervous system: Diseases of the spinal cord.* (Translated by Comegys CG; p. 88). Cincinnati: Thomson, 1881.
36. d'Arsonval A. Letter to Brown-Séquard, dated 6 December 1892. In: Delhoume L. *De Claude Bernard à d'Arsonval* (pp. 474–475). Paris: Baillière, 1939.
37. d'Arsonval A. Letter to Brown-Séquard, dated 11 December(?) 1892. In: Delhoume L. *De Claude Bernard à d'Arsonval* (pp. 480–481). Paris: Baillière, 1939.
38. Brown-Séquard CE. Letter to d'Arsonval, dated 13 December 1892. In: Delhoume L. *De Claude Bernard à d'Arsonval* (pp. 481–482). Paris: Baillière, 1939.

39. Brown-Séquard CE. Letter to d'Arsonval, dated 13 February 1893. In: Delhoume L. *De Claude Bernard à d'Arsonval* (p. 517). Paris: Baillière, 1939.
40. Satran R. Joseph Babinski in the competitive examination (agrégation) of 1892. *Bull N Y Acad Med*, 50:626–635, 1974.
41. Philippon J, Poirier J. *Joseph Babinski: A biography* (pp. 97–114). New York: Oxford University Press, 2009.
42. Bourneville DM. Le concours d'agrégation en médicine. *Prog Med*, 15:223, and 239–240, 1892.
43. Anonymous. Le concours d'agrégation en medicine d'après les journaux politiques. *Prog Med*, 15:248–249, 1892.
44. Anonymous. Le dernier concours d'agrégation de medicine. *Prog Med*, 15:365, 1892.
45. Brown-Séquard CE. Letter to d'Arsonval, dated 26 April 1892. In: Delhoume L. *De Claude Bernard à d'Arsonval* (pp. 438–439). Paris: Baillière, 1939.
46. d'Arsonval A. Letter to Brown-Séquard, dated 7 May 1892. In: Delhoume L. *De Claude Bernard à d'Arsonval* (pp. 443). Paris: Baillière, 1939.
47. Iragui VJ. The Charcot-Bouchard controversy. *Arch Neurol*, 43:290–295, 1986.
48. Anonymous. Special correspondence: Paris. *Br Med J*, 1:678–679, 1892.
49. Brown-Séquard CE. Seconde note sur les effets produits chez l'homme par des injections sous-cutanées d'un liquide retiré des testicules frais de cobaye et de chien. *C R Soc Biol (Paris)*, 41:420–422, 1889.
50. Borell M. Organotherapy, British physiology, and discovery of the internal secretions. *J Hist Biol*, 9:235–268, 1976.
51. Berdoe E. A serious moral question. A letter printed for private circulation and dated 12 July 1889. MS 980/67. Archives, Royal College of Physicians, London.
52. Anonymous. Dr. Brown-Séquard's experiments. *Br Med J*, 2:347, 1889.
53. Anonymous. Obituary: Professor Brown-Séquard. *Lancet*, 1:975–977, 1894.
54. Thompson, Sir H. Letter to Ernest Abraham Hart, dated 17 April 1890. MS 519. Archives, New York Academy of Medicine, New York.
55. Denny-Brown D. The enigma of crossed sensory loss with cord hemisection. In: Bonica JJ, Liebeskind JC, Albe-Fessard DG, eds., *Advances in pain research and therapy* (Vol. 3, pp. 889–895). New York: Raven Press, 1979.
56. Mott FW. Results of hemisection of the spinal cord in monkeys. *Philos Trans R Soc Lond (Biol)*, 183:1–59, 1892.
57. Brown-Séquard CE. Remarques à propos des recherches du Dr. F.W. Mott sur les effets de la section d'une moitié latérale de la moelle épinière. *Arch Physiol Norm Pathol (5th Series)*, 6:195–198, 1894.
58. Brown-Séquard CE. Expériences montrant que l'anesthésie due à certaines lésions du centre cérébro-rachidien peut être remplacée par de l'hyperesthésie, sous l'influence d'une autre lésion de ce centre. *C R Acad Sci*, 90:750–753, 1880.
59. Brown-Séquard CE. Recherches expérimentales et cliniques sur l'inhibition et la dynamogénie. Application des connaissances fournies par ces recherches aux phénomènes principaux de l'hynotisme, de l'extase et du transfert. *Gaz Hebd Med (2nd Series)*, 19:53–55, 1882.
60. Brown-Séquard CE. On certain physiological effects of stretching of the sciatic nerve. *Lancet*, 1:206, 1881.
61. Personal communication from C Vierck, Professor Emeritus, Department of Neuroscience, University of Florida College of Medicine, Gainesville, Florida.
62. Vierck CJ Jr, Greenspan JD, Ritz LA. Long-term changes in purposive and reflexive responses to nociceptive stimulation following anterolateral chordotomy. *J Neurosci*, 10:2077–2095, 1990.

63. Wall PD. The design of experimental studies in the future development of restorative neurology of altered sensation and pain. In: Dimitrijevic MR, Wall PD, Lindblom U, eds., *Recent achievements in restorative neurology* (Vol. 3, pp. 197–205). Basel: Karger, 1990.
64. Fields H. State-dependent opioid control of pain. *Nat Rev Neurosci*, 5:565–575, 2004.
65. D'Mello R, Dickenson AH. Spinal cord mechanisms of pain. *Br J Anaes*, 101:8–16, 2008.
66. Porreca F, Ossipov MH, Gebhart GF. Chronic pain and medullary descending facilitation. *Trends Neurosci*, 25:319–325, 2002.
67. Urban MO, Gebhart GF. Supraspinal contributions to hyperalgesia. *Proc Natl Acad Sci USA*, 96:7687–7692, 1999.
68. Zhuo M, Gebhart GF. Characterization of descending facilitation and inhibition of spinal nociceptive transmission from the nuclei reticularis gigantocellularis and gigantocellularis pars alpha in the rat. *J Neurophysiol*, 67:1599–1614, 1992.
69. Terman GW, Bonica JJ. Spinal mechanisms and their modulation. In Loeser JD, ed., *Bonica's management of pain* (pp. 128–137). Philadelphia: Lippincott Williams & Wilkins, 2001.
70. Benarroch EE. Descending monoaminergic pain modulation: bidirectional control and clinical relevance. *Neurology*, 71:217–221, 2008.
71. Vierck CJ Jr. Tactile movement detection and discrimination following dorsal column lesions in monkeys. *Exp Brain Res*, 20:311–346, 1974.
72. Vierck CJ Jr. Impaired detection of repetitive stimulation following interruption of the dorsal spinal column in primates. *Somatosens Mot Res*, 15:157–163, 1998.
73. Vierck CJ Jr, Cohen RH, Cooper BY. Effects of spinal tractotomy on spatial sequence recognition in macaques. *J Neurosci*, 3:280–290, 1983.
74. Vierck CJ Jr, Hamilton DM, Thornby JI. Pain reactivity of monkeys after lesions to the dorsal and lateral columns of the spinal cord. *Exp Brain Res*, 13:140–158, 1971.
75. Vierck CJ Jr, Luck MM. Loss and recovery of reactivity to noxious stimuli in monkeys with primary spinothalamic cordotomies, followed by secondary and tertiary lesions of other cord sectors. *Brain*, 102:233–248, 1979.
76. Vierck CJ Jr, Light AR. Effects of combined hemotoxic and anterolateral spinal lesions on nociceptive sensitivity. *Pain*, 83:447–457, 1999.
77. Anonymous. Death of Professor Brown-Séquard. *Lancet*, 1:906–907, 1894.
78. Dauriac J. Necrologie: Brown-Séquard. *Le Progrès Médical*, 19:270–271, 1894.
79. Anonymous. Courrier de Paris. Newspaper article, source not cited. MS 1000/88b. Royal College of Physicians, London.
80. Bianchon H. *Nos grands médicins d'aujourdhui*. Paris: Société d'Editions Scientifiques, 1891.
81. Anonymous. Brown-Séquard. *Le Petit Centre de Limoges*, 4 April 1894.
82. Brown-Séquard CE. Letter dated 25 March 1893. *Revue Historique et Litteraire de l'Ile Maurice*, 16 July 1894.
83. Bouchard C. Letters to Brown-Séquard. Archives, Académie des Sciences, Paris.
84. Brown-Séquard CE. Letter to d'Arsonval, dated 26 December 1892. In: Delhoume L. *De Claude Bernard à d'Arsonval* (pp. 493–494). Paris: Baillière, 1939.
85. Brown-Séquard CE. Letter to Jean Casimir Felix Guyon, undated. MS BROWC/994/3. Archives, Royal College of Physicians, London.
86. Guyon F. Letters to Brown-Séquard. Archives, Académie des Sciences, Paris.
87. Guyon, JCF. Letter to Brown-Sequard dated 19 August 1893. MS BROWC/980/79. Archives, Royal College of Physicians, London.
88. Renan JE and/or CE. Letters to Dr. or Mrs. Brown-Séquard, 1885–1894. MS 981/119–127. Archives, Royal College of Physicians, London.

89. d'Arsonval A. Letter to Brown-Séquard, dated 14 December 1889. In: Delhoume L. *De Claude Bernard à d'Arsonval* (pp. 306–308). Paris: Baillière, 1939.
90. Brown-Séquard CE. Letter to d'Arsonval, dated 19 January 1890. In Delhoume L. *De Claude Bernard à d'Arsonval* (pp. 312–313). Paris: Baillière, 1939.
91. Brown-Séquard CE. Letter to d'Arsonval, dated 23 March 1894. In: Delhoume L. *De Claude Bernard à d'Arsonval* (pp. 560–562). Paris: Baillière, 1939.
92. d'Arsonval A. Letter to Brown-Séquard, dated 20 February 1893. In: Delhoume L. *De Claude Bernard à d'Arsonval* (p. 519). Paris: Baillière, 1939.
93. d'Arsonval A. *Note sur la préparation de l'extrait testiculaire concentré.* Paris: Masson, 1893.
94. d'Arsonval A. Letter to Brown-Séquard, dated 16 December 1892. In: Delhoume L. *De Claude Bernard à d'Arsonval* (pp. 484–486). Paris: Baillière, 1939.
95. Brown-Séquard CE. Letter to d'Arsonval, dated 17 December 1892. In: Delhoume L. *De Claude Bernard à d'Arsonval* (pp. 486–487). Paris: Baillière, 1939.
96. d'Arsonval A. Letter to Brown-Séquard, dated 25 December(?) 1892. In: Delhoume L. *De Claude Bernard à d'Arsonval* (pp. 490–491). Paris: Baillière, 1939.
97. Brown-Séquard CE. Letter to d'Arsonval, dated 26 December 1892. In: Delhoume L. *De Claude Bernard à d'Arsonval* (pp. 493–494). Paris: Baillière, 1939.
98. Brown-Séquard CE. Letter to d'Arsonval, dated 30 December 1892. In: Delhoume L. *De Claude Bernard à d'Arsonval* (pp. 494–495). Paris: Baillière, 1939.
99. Brown-Séquard CE. Letter to d'Arsonval, dated 13 December 1892. In: Delhoume L. *De Claude Bernard à d'Arsonval* (pp. 482–483). Paris: Baillière, 1939.
100. Binet L. Discours. Cérémonie en l'honneur de C.E. Brown-Séquard. *La Presse Médicale*, 13 August 1938.
101. Delhoume L. *De Claude Bernard à d'Arsonval* (p. 269). Paris: Baillière, 1939.
102. Tomel G. La colonie mauricienne. *Le Figaro*, 17 June 1892.
103. Condé Williams F. In memoriam: C.E. Brown-Séquard. In: Rouget FA. *Brown-Séquard et son oeuvre. Esquisse biographique* (pp. 153–155). Ile Maurice: General Printing & Stationery Co., 1930.
104. Brown-Séquard CE. Letter to d'Arsonval, dated 26 February 1891. In: Delhoume L. *De Claude Bernard à d'Arsonval* (pp. 368–369). Paris: Baillière, 1939.
105. Brown-Séquard CE. Letter to d'Arsonval, dated 27 March 1891. In: Delhoume L. *De Claude Bernard à d'Arsonval* (pp. 382–383). Paris: Baillière, 1939.
106. Ville de Nice. Extrait du Registre des Actes de Décès, tenu à la Mairie de Nice pour l'année 1894.
107. Brown-Séquard CE. Letter to d'Arsonval, dated 23 March 1894. In: Delhoume L. *De Claude Bernard à d'Arsonval* (pp. 560–562). Paris: Baillière, 1939.
108. Anonymous. Mrs. Brown-Séquard. Probate of her will after a discussion on a delicate point of law. *New York Herald*, 1 May 1894.
109. Manuscript by Emma Brown-Séquard (Doherty). MS 999/78a. Archives, Royal College of Physicians, London.
110. Brown-Séquard CE. Extracts from letters written to Dr. W.D. Waterhouse. *Lancet*, 1:977, 1894.
111. Ogle JW. Further remarks on Dr. Brown-Séquard's last illness. *Lancet*, 1:1391, 1894.
112. Anonymous. Brown-Séquard. Quelques notes intimes sur le célèbre physiologiste. *L'Eclair*, 4 April 1894.
113. Anonymous. Obsèques de M. Brown-Séquard. *La Presse*, 5 April 1894.
114. Anonymous. Obsèques du Docteur Brown-Séquard. *Le Gaulois*, 5 April 1894.
115. Anonymous. Les obsèques du Doctor Brown-Séquard. *La Presse*, 5 April 1894.
116. Anonymous. Les obsèques de M. Brown-Séquard. *Le Figaro*, 5 April 1894.

117. Brown-Séquard CE. Last will, dated 29 March 1894. MS 999/90. Archives, Royal College of Physicians, London.
118. Brown-Séquard CE. Draft of will, undated but with a correction by Brown-Séquard dated 3 October 1886. MS 999/89. Royal College of Physicians, London.
119. Anonymous. The late Professor Brown-Séquard. Anecdotes of a great physiologist. *St. James's Gazette (London)*, 4 April 1894.
120. Editorial. Brown-Séquard. *Lancet*, 2:753–754, 1930.

13

A New System of Medicine

HORMONES ARE CHEMICAL substances released into the blood to influence the function of other parts of the body, but the term is customarily restricted to substances that have more specific functions than simply subserving the general metabolic requirements of the body. Some of the tissues that secrete hormones are referred to as *endocrine glands*, but other hormone-secreting structures are customarily categorized with reference to the primary anatomical system of which they are a part. In consequence, the hormonal functions of such organs or tissues as the brain,[A] kidney,[B] gastrointestinal

---

[A] The hypothalamus secretes a number of hormones that regulate the release of hormones from the pituitary gland. It also secretes *hypocretins,* which are involved in regulating sleep–wake cycles and food intake. The pituitary gland releases growth hormone (controlling metabolism, protein synthesis, and growth), thyroid-releasing hormone (that stimulates the thyroid gland), adrenocorticotrophic hormone (stimulating the release of certain steroid hormones from the cortex of the adrenal glands), prolactin (regulating milk production by the breasts), luteinizing and follicle-stimulating hormones (regulating aspects of reproductive function), antidiuretic hormone (that affects the excretion of water by the kidneys), and oxytocin (that affects uterine contraction and other reproductive and sexual functions). The pineal gland secretes melatonin, which affects circadian (daily) rhythms and aspects of reproduction.

[B] The formation of renin in the kidney is stimulated by a decline in blood pressure or a low blood volume. Renin induces the formation (from a precursor in the blood) of angiotensin, a powerful constrictor of the blood vessels, thereby raising the blood pressure. Angiotensin also stimulates the adrenal cortex to secrete the hormone aldosterone, which causes the kidneys to retain more sodium and water. This, in turn, increases the blood volume, which leads to a further increase in blood pressure.

tract,[C] adipose (fatty) tissues,[D] and heart[E] are less well recognized than those of the endocrine glands themselves.

Chemical or humoral mechanisms have a major role in the integrative actions of the body, but this has been recognized only relatively recently. Chemical neurotransmitters, it is now widely known, are involved in the direct communication that occurs between nerve cells or between nerve cells and effector cells, such as muscle fibers. Other chemical messengers pass to their target cells in the interstitial fluid rather than in the bloodstream.

Organotherapy consists of the administration for medical purposes of tissues derived from the body. The term *opotherapy* has sometimes been used when such substances are administered in the form of extracts. Organotherapy flourished for centuries before Christ, and Pliny the Elder later documented more than two hundred and fifty remedies involving the administration of tissues of human and animal origin.[1] Its use for most of this time was without any scientific foundation and based upon superstition and mysticism. In certain cultures, however, the consumption of portions of the body, such as the liver or brain, for purposes other than nutrition remained a common practice until recently. In 1873, the hearts of British soldiers killed in battle during the Ashanti campaign were eaten by an enemy intent on acquiring the bravery of their luckless former owners.[1] As late as the middle of the twentieth century, ritual cannibalism was customary among certain tribes of New Guinea, in order to embody the spirit of recently deceased relatives.

The French physician Théophile de Bordeu (1722–1776), court physician of Louis XV, is generally credited with first formulating, in 1775, the concept that the individual organs give off substances ("emanations") that influence the body as a whole,[2] and he stressed the possible role in this regard of the testicles and ovaries. Neither his writings nor the speculative comments of other eighteenth-century authors stimulated any attempts to establish the veracity

---

[C] These hormones include gastrin (secreted by the stomach and small intestine; it stimulates the secretion of gastric acid and influences gastric motility), cholecystokinin (which is secreted by the small intestine and leads to release of enzymes from the pancreas and bile from the gall bladder to aid in the digestion of fat and proteins, as well as signaling satiety to the nervous system), secretin (which stimulates the secretion of bile from the liver and of water and bicarbonate from the pancreas when excess acid enters the small intestine from the stomach), ghrelin (an appetite stimulant that is secreted by the stomach), and motilin (which is released by the small intestine and affects gastrointestinal motility).

[D] Leptin is a hormone produced primarily by fatty tissues that controls appetite and energy expenditure by its effects on certain parts of the brain (primarily the hypothalamus).

[E] Atrial natriuretic factor, released by the heart, has several effects but, in particular, influences fluid and electrolyte balance and relaxes blood vessels, thereby increasing cardiac output and reducing blood volume.

of such concepts.[1] In 1849, however, Arnold Adolph Berthold (1803–1861), a German physiologist working in Göttingen, perhaps inspired by the similar but largely unknown, earlier work of John Hunter (1728–1793),[3] gave a talk at the Göttingen Royal Scientific Society and then published a remarkable paper that demonstrated the effect of the testicles on distant parts of the body and, in particular, on the secondary sexual characteristics.[4] Cockerels that were castrated at the age of two or three months developed into fat and docile capons, unable to crow, unwilling to fight, uninterested in hens, and without the combs, wattles, and spurs of normal cocks. By contrast, castrated cockerels in which a testicle was reimplanted in the abdominal cavity, at a site where it could regain a blood supply, subsequently developed into normal, strutting, combative cocks with a healthy interest in hens. At autopsy, Berthold noted that the grafted testicle was revascularized but had no nerve supply. He therefore concluded that the testicles acted through the blood (rather than through the nervous system, as had previously been supposed) to influence the animals and their behavior. This experimental work was simply ignored by Berthold's contemporaries, in part because it could not be replicated,[3] and there were no further developments of note until Brown-Séquard turned to this topic some years later.

Claude Bernard and Brown-Séquard are clearly the founders of the conception of the internal secretions.[1] Bernard showed that the liver manufactures sugar from a substance stored within it (glycogen) and secretes it directly into the blood. Such internal secretions, he believed, served to maintain the composition of the blood. Bernard initiated modern concepts of carbohydrate metabolism and formulated the concept of an internal environment that is kept constant by the interaction of different processes in the body. Perhaps surprisingly, however, relatively little contemporary interest was aroused by his work. Brown-Séquard, by contrast, concluded that the various glands and other tissues influence the activity of other parts of the body by secreting chemicals into the blood and thereby maintain the normal state of the organism. He stimulated the medical and scientific community to look closely at organs and tissues from a new perspective, and his work led directly to the development of modern endocrinology and hormone replacement therapy. Indeed, his belief in humoral integrative mechanisms was a logical extension of his earlier views concerning the integrative action of the nervous system and the functional processes subserving this role. Further, his work on the use of organ extracts really marks the beginning of gerontology (the science of ageing), led to recognition that ageing is a medical problem, and put sexual disturbances such as erectile dysfunction into the clinical arena.

Organ Extracts in the Treatment of Human Disease

In lectures that he delivered in Paris and elsewhere in 1869, Brown-Séquard first advanced the belief that "all glands, with or without excretory ducts, give to the blood, by an internal secretion, principles which are of great importance if not necessary."[5] This belief led him, in 1875, to undertake certain grafting experiments in dogs while at Nahant, near Boston, but the results were equivocal. In 1888, he returned to the topic, experimenting on rabbits with sufficient success that he decided to pursue the work using himself as an experimental subject. Reference was made in Chapter 12 to the remarkable—electrifying—communication that Brown-Séquard subsequently delivered on 1 June 1889, to the Société de Biologie in Paris, in which he suggested that the testicles of animals contain an invigorating substance that can be extracted and injected into humans.[6-8] He reminded his audience of what was then the generally accepted, contemporary view that intellectual and physical activity is impaired in eunuchs and in men prone to sexual excesses or masturbation. He then declared his belief that the weaknesses of elderly men depend on both "a natural series of organic changes and the gradually diminishing action of the spermatic glands." In other words, he believed that a diminution of testicular function was partly responsible for some of the changes that occur in the elderly.[F]

The seventy-two-year-old professor had noted various changes in himself over the previous decade—he had become more frail, tired easily, slept badly, and suffered with worsening constipation. The power of his forearm flexor muscles, which he had measured serially over the years, had diminished: he had been able to move a weight of 50 kg in the years between 1860 and 1862, but could now move no more than 38 kg. He therefore decided to inject himself with testicular extracts to determine their effects, and accordingly prepared a solution in distilled water of testicular blood, seminal fluid, and testicular extract derived from healthy dogs and guinea pigs. After filtering it, he injected himself subcutaneously with this solution on several occasions over a two-week period. His mental concentration and physical endurance

---

[F] It is now known that the testes (or "spermatic glands"), in addition to producing sperm, do indeed manufacture several hormones (androgens) that are secreted into the blood stream, including testosterone. Testosterone, first isolated and synthesized in 1935, is responsible for the development of the male genitalia and secondary sexual characteristics, such as a deep voice, muscular frame (that is, an increased muscle mass), a characteristic distribution of facial and body hair, and other features that reflect what is taken for masculinity. Testosterone levels do, in fact, decline with advancing years but the clinical significance of this decline remains controversial.

increased, his bowel habits became more regular, he was able to walk without having to rest, and the flexor muscles of his forearm became stronger, so that he could move weights that were six or seven kilograms heavier than before. He had measured his urinary stream before and after the first injection, under similar circumstances, and noted that the average length of the jet of urine during the ten days preceding injection was 25 percent less than in the twenty days following injection.

The old man's initial communications were made in the hope that others would be motivated to undertake similar self-experimentation. He was well aware that the changes that he had observed in himself might reflect some personal idiosyncrasy or the effects of suggestion, and for this reason did not try his injections on patients, preferring to wait for more evidence of their efficacy.[6,8] Others were not so cautious. A certain Dr. Variot tried the same approach, without Brown-Séquard's advice or agreement, on three elderly men with similar results,[9] leading Brown-Séquard to believe that the observed effects were real.[10] He therefore suggested that the injected material was able to influence the function of many parts of the body and that, at the very least, the subject merited further study.[7,8] He also suggested to some of his patients that sexual excitement (as by masturbation) without ejaculation might increase their general vigor, presumably because seminal retention might lead to renewed vigor if debility was indeed the result of seminal loss.[11,12]

An awkward, even embarrassed, response followed his initial reports, which some regarded as evidence for " ... the necessity of retiring professors who have attained their threescore years and ten."[13] Brown-Séquard was undeterred and returned repeatedly to the topic over the following months, especially when a number of confirmatory reports were published by others.[5,14] William Hammond, retired Surgeon-General of the United States Army (see footnote A, Chapter 8, p. 122), used testicular extracts of a young ram in ten cases (one being himself), and reported beneficial effects on pain, lumbago, impotence, the residual effects of a cerebral hemorrhage, "rheumatism," cardiac failure, and a variety of other disorders. He spoke scathingly of the reaction of the popular press to the new therapeutic approach[15,16]:

> It is only the sensational newspapers that speak of it [the testicular juice] as an "elixir of life" or as an agent capable of making an old man permanently young again. It seems to be the chief object of some of these mediums for communicating intelligence to distort the truth, not only by the use of sensational headings printed in large letters of a grossly misleading character, but to misinterpret, misconstrue, and misquote the medical information given them at their solicitation. The venerable originator of the method of treating certain

infirmities and diseases to which this paper relates has been abused, not only by an irresponsible press, but by physicians who ought to have exhibited more consideration and decency than they have shown ....[16]

The editors of some of the more influential medical journals were also skeptical, adopting a censorious attitude and attempting to limit information on the topic. Indeed, the *British Medical Journal*, in its account of 22 June 1889 concerning Brown-Séquard's initial communication to the Société de Biologie, pointed to the unfortunate attention already attracted in the public press, emphasized that his statements "recall the wild imaginings of mediaeval philosophers in search of *elixir vitae*," and concurred with the opinions of certain other physicians that the findings required rigid testing and confirmation by others.[17] It chose not to mention Brown-Séquard's own plea that other investigators examine the question objectively.[6,8] Over the following weeks, the editors of the *British Medical Journal* commented on Dr. Variot's reported success,[18] and then on a claim from Indianapolis that "a decrepit old man" had been invigorated by Dr. Brown-Séquard's "rejuvenating fluid."[19] The tone of their commentary remained skeptical, however, and this antagonism may have been colored by antivivisectionist sentiment and Victorian disquiet about the sexual undertones of Brown-Séquard's work,[20,21] as well as by more intellectual and methodological concerns. The boldness of Brown-Séquard's assertions with regard to the sexual climate of the time cannot be overestimated. Sexual excess and impropriety was held to predispose to insanity, and even lascivious ruminations were regarded as harmful. Masturbation was considered sinful as well as medically hazardous by many because of the resulting loss of precious bodily fluids that occurs in men and because women were not supposed to find sexual activity pleasurable. In fact, of course, Brown-Séquard's belief that the retention of seminal fluid would have an invigorating effect actually accorded with the belief that loss of these fluids had deleterious effects.

Reaction in the United States, as elsewhere, was ambivalent. The views there concerning masturbation and sexuality were as rigid as in Europe, particularly among zealous reformers. For example, Sylvester Graham (1794–1851) a dietary reformer, regarded all excitement as hazardous to the health (and thus invented the bland Graham cracker), but sexual excitement as especially troublesome and masturbation as a cause of insanity. John Preston Kellogg (1852–1943), chief medical officer of the Battle Creek Sanitarium and a health-food fanatic who developed peanut butter, co-founded a breakfast cereal company, and wrote prolifically on lifestyles, believed that masturbation caused physical, moral, and mental decay, a host of medical disorders, and much of the boorish behavior of adolescents, and went so far as to advise circumcision, with its attendant discomfort, to discourage or halt it temporarily. A paper summarizing Brown-Séquard's experience and experiments was published in the *Scientific American Supplement* of 10 August 1889 with predictable consequences.[22] A one-paragraph accompanying editorial exclaimed sardonically:

> The number of elderly people who are anxious to be made young and happy again is almost countless, and there is likely to be an epidemic desire among them to try the new medicine. A golden harvest seems to be in view for the doctors.[23]

And the New York correspondent of *The Lancet*, in January 1890, concluded in a more serious vein:

> There is always a class of medical men who are ready at once to test the value of any new remedy, and during the past month the newspapers have been filled with experiments made in various parts of the country. It is surprising at the first blush to note the different results obtained as reported. In the hands of one experimenter the paralysed immediately walk, the lame throw aside canes and crutches, the deaf hear, and the blind see. The same experiments failed altogether in the practice of another.[24]

The two satirical American magazines *Puck* and *Judge* (whose editor went on to found the *New Yorker*) did not fail to take note of the new method. Although some were skeptical, many physicians and the lay-public were quick to adopt the approach, leading Brown-Séquard to complain that

> In the United States especially ... several physicians or rather the medicasters and charlatans have exploited the ardent desires of a great number of individuals and have made them run the greatest risks ....[14,25]

The procedure was indeed not without risk, especially of infection at the injection site, which sometimes led to local abscess formation until sterile commercial preparations were developed. Nevertheless, the demand for treatment with testicular extracts increased rapidly although, as mentioned in Chapter 12, Brown-Séquard refused all opportunities to profit from it. Instead, he spent much of his own money to make the extracts available to others[26] and proceeded to publish a detailed account of how the extract should be prepared, as his own laboratory was not able to produce sufficient amounts of extracts to meet the demands for it. Not surprisingly, then, a number of less scrupulous physicians and charlatans exploited his work for their own gain, making extravagant and unjustified claims for the so-called Elixir of Life, which became the title of a book edited by Newell Dunbar and published in the United States.[27]

Whether Dunbar's aim was to profit from a best-seller or to promote the new therapeutic approach is unclear, but he took the liberty of freely quoting Brown-Séquard, provided his biographical details, and summarized his bibliography, thereby giving the impression that Brown-Séquard was its author or at least had acquiesced in its publication.

The reader should not assume that women were ignored. Shortly after his initial publication, Brown-Séquard suggested that the ovaries produced secretions[G] with similar effects on women as those of the testicles on men.[11] Soon after, he reported that a midwife in Paris had taken with benefit a liquid made from pigs' ovaries, and that an American, Dr. Augusta Brown, had given several elderly women filtered guinea pig ovaries, with an apparently beneficial response in cases of hysteria, various uterine disorders, and senescent debility,[28] although any benefit was subsequently disputed.[29] I have, however, been unable to verify the suggestion that he reportedly prescribed two sheep's ovaries in a sandwich of unleavened bread for the treatment of hot flushes.[30]

The method of preparing testicular extracts was described in full,[H] including details of the filtration process:

> We procure testicles of bulls at the slaughter-house. Just after the killing of the animal a ligature is placed as high as possible on the whole mass of the spermatic cord, so as to get at least a certain amount of the blood contained in the veins. When the organs reach the laboratory their coverings are at once cut away with scissors sterilised by heat. The organs are then washed in Van Swieten's liquor, and afterwards in recently boiled water. That being done, each of the testicles is cut in four or five slices, which, with the piece of cord, are placed in a glass vase, in which is thrown, for each kilogramme of the organs used, one litre of glycerine marking 30°. The vase is covered, but it is essential, during the next 24 hours, to turn over a good many times the slices and other pieces of organs. At the end of that period an addition of 500 cubic centimeters

---

[G] The ovaries are now known to secrete estrogens, which affect the development of the female genitalia and secondary sexual characteristics (such as breasts and widened hips and a characteristic distribution of body hair and fat). They also regulate the changes that occur with menstruation and pregnancy and affect behavior. Other female sex hormones also exist, and the interested reader should consult standard medical texts for further information.

[H] The methodological details were updated periodically to inform professional colleagues of technological advances. The details quoted here were from 1893, but several earlier accounts were published. See, for example, Brown-Séquard CE, d'Arsonval A. Préparation des extraits liquides provenant des différents organes de l'économie animale destinés aux injections sous-cutanées thérapeutiques. *Arch Physiol Norm Pathol (5th Series)*, 3:593–597, 1891. See also Brown-Séquard CE, d'Arsonval A. Nouveaux modes de préparation du liquide testiculaire pour les injections sous-cutanées. *Arch Physiol Norm Pathol (5th Series)*, 4:164–167, 1892.

of freshly boiled water, containing 25 grammes of pure chloride of sodium, is made. The liquid so obtained is then made to pass through a paper filter .... [T]he paper filter and the glass funnel in which it is placed must be thoroughly washed with boiling water. The filtered liquid is slightly rose-coloured. To hasten the filtration it is well to raise the temperature of the glyceric solution to 40° C. (104° F.) .... Of the various means we have made use of to obtain a liquid absolutely free from microbes or other dangerous pieces of solid matter, the most important is the sterilising d'Arsonval filter ....[5]

Brown-Séquard had suspected for more than fifteen years that if the internal secretions of a gland from a living animal could be introduced into the blood of humans suffering from a lack of that secretion, "important therapeutic effects would thereby be obtained."[5] He believed and stated publicly that the internal secretions of specific organs might be identified by the response of specific diseases to treatment with them and that, if certain conditions could indeed be treated by an organ extract, it was probable that the condition was caused by impaired production of that secretion.[12] Over the years, he had expanded this concept to suggest that not merely the glands, but all tissues,[I] contribute internal secretions to the blood supply, thereby influencing the activity of other parts of the body.[31,32] To his satisfaction, then, his beliefs stimulated a number of reputable physicians, and his laboratory was soon inundated by requests to prepare extracts of different organs for therapeutic trials,[33] in keeping with his philosophy.

International interest in Brown-Séquard's approach increased in the early 1890s, and even the skeptics became less hostile. Encouraging reports of the beneficial effects of testicular extracts, in particular, were received from physicians in Russia, Poland, Rumania, Austria, and Italy,[34] as well as from colleagues in France, England, and the United States, and the approach almost certainly influenced work proceeding in England on the treatment of hypothyroidism (myxedema).[J]

[I] Although there is no evidence that every tissue secretes chemical messengers into the blood, an increasing number of organs and tissues do, in fact, communicate by humoral means.

[J] Hypothyroidism is a common disorder resulting from insufficient thyroid hormone. It may occur as a consequence of inflammation (Hashimoto's thyroiditis) or destruction of the thyroid gland by surgery, treatment with radioactive iodine (for example, in patients with thyroid cancer or benign enlargement of part or all of the gland), or exposure to radiation for other reasons. Symptoms include some combination of fatigue, weight gain, coarse hair and dry skin, hair loss, hoarse voice, weakness, weight gain, cold intolerance, depression, constipation, muscle and joint pain, irritability and memory changes, slowed thinking, reduced libido, menstrual changes, and a slowed heart-rate. Untreated, it may eventually lead to coma and even a fatal outcome. Treatment is with thyroid replacement therapy.

The function of the thyroid gland was unknown, but an enlarged gland (goiter) or the congenital absence of thyroid tissue had come to be associated with a distinct clinical disorder that also followed total operative removal of the gland, as noted by surgeons in Switzerland (Reverdin and Kocher). Victor Horsley, the British neurosurgeon, had at one time explored experimentally the effects of surgical removal of the thyroid gland, as had Moritz Schiff[K] many years earlier. He now returned to the subject by suggesting (as Schiff had previously) the grafting for therapeutic purposes of thyroid tissue into patients with hypothyroidism. George Redmayne Murray (1865–1939), Horsley's protégé and former student, proposed in 1890 the injection of thyroid extract for treating the disease,[35] and it seems probable that this idea related directly to the studies then in progress concerning the therapeutic use of testicular extracts.[12] Nevertheless, when Murray, in July 1891, reported his successful treatment of hypothyroidism with subcutaneous injections of thyroid extract, he made no mention of Brown-Séquard.[36] Murray undoubtedly deserves great credit for his achievement, but it must be viewed in the context of the concept of internal secretions and the related therapeutic role for organ extracts that Brown-Séquard had advanced so tenaciously, and in the setting of the previous work of Schiff, Horsley, Reverdin, and Kocher. Indeed, Theodor Kocher (1841–1917) was awarded the Nobel Prize in 1909 for his work on the pathology of the thyroid gland. In his Nobel lecture, he generously mentions Brown-Séquard and his work: "Brown-Séquard has directed attention to the great importance of the internal secretions and has sought to turn those of the sex organs to therapeutic account."[37]

[K] Moritz Schiff (1823–1896), German physiologist, studied under François Magendie in Paris. He served as a military surgeon in the revolutionary army during the 1848 uprising in Germany, was captured, condemned to death, escaped, and went to Switzerland, where he accepted a professorship in anatomy at the University of Bern (1854–1863). He then became professor of physiology at the Istituto di Studii Superiori in Florence (until 1876), and finally professor of physiology at the University of Geneva, where he died in 1896. Among his accomplishments, he showed early in his career that dogs died after removal of the thyroid gland and later that death was prevented by injections of thyroid extracts. He subsequently used thyroid extracts successfully to treat humans. He also showed the importance of the brainstem in controlling the circulation and studied the sensory pathways in the spinal cord. Like Brown-Séquard, Schiff was pursued by the antivivisectionists for his animal experiments and had to abandon his laboratory in Florence and flee to Switzerland because of them. His interests were similar to those of Brown-Séquard, and the chair in Geneva that he finally occupied was the one that Brown-Séquard originally accepted but then declined (Chapter 9, p. 149). Short in stature, with long hair and a flowing white beard, he was an unmistakable character, with a great sense of fun but entirely devoted to his work. For relaxation, he would simply turn form one topic in his work to another.

It is legitimate to question whether Brown-Séquard's approach did indeed influence the treatment of hypothyroidism, as seems very likely, or whether the approach to the treatment of an underactive thyroid gland was reached independently. Brown-Séquard had corresponded with Victor Horsley and sent him extracts and details of the production method.[38] Horsley, in turn, was in close contact with Murray, his ex-student, who credited him with the idea of injecting thyroid extracts into hypothyroid patients. The contemporary medical establishment also viewed thyroid extracts as an example of Brown-Séquard's organotherapy, as did Brown-Séquard himself.[5] Indeed, in his correspondence with d'Arsonval, his faithful assistant, he even provides specific instruction on how to treat thyroid disease.[39] Thus, it seems reasonable to recognize his contribution to the development of a successful treatment for that disorder.[40]

In 1893, Brown-Séquard reviewed his experience in an article in the *British Medical Journal*, emphasizing the innocuity of parenterally administered extracts of organ tissue when prepared in accordance with his guidelines.[5] He discussed the experience with extracts of kidney pancreas, liver, thymus, adrenal glands, spleen, pituitary gland, bone, brain, muscle, thyroid, and various other tissues, as well as with the testicles. Since he had offered (in 1892) to provide his organ preparations to physicians at no charge if they would simply furnish him the case histories and response to therapy of patients whom they had treated, some 1,200 practitioners had accepted the offer and more than 1,600 cases had been treated by testicular extracts.[5] Many nonspecific symptoms (such as malaise, lassitude, fatigue, cachexia, poor appetite, and insomnia) of several different disorders including cancer, locomotor ataxia,[L] and pulmonary tuberculosis seemed to be relieved or diminished, and such benefit was attributed by Brown-Séquard to a nonspecific tonic effect. He made no claims concerning the response of the underlying pathology itself; indeed, he stressed that any tumor remained unchanged. In his own words:

> We reserve the question of cure of organic diseases. All that we have just stated applies to the cessation of morbid manifestations.[5]

This must be clearly understood, because it has often been claimed, without justification, that Brown-Séquard made extravagant claims for cures, when this was not the case. Experiments on animals (guinea pigs or pigeons) with

---

[L] Locomotor ataxia, more commonly now known as *tabes dorsalis*, is a form of tertiary neurosyphilis characterized by sensory deficits, spontaneous stabbing pains, and impaired coordination of movement, especially in the legs, so that the gait becomes unsteady. Symptoms may not develop for years after the initial infection.

lesions in the central nervous system also suggested that the resulting neurological deficits (but not the lesions themselves) were improved by treatment with testicular extract.[5]

In view of his work on the adrenal glands in the 1850s (see pp. 91–93), it was only to be expected that Brown-Séquard would try to treat patients with Addison's disease by the administration of aqueous extracts of these glands. The results were disappointing,[5] even though he obtained encouraging results in preliminary studies in guinea pigs.[41] Indeed, attempts to treat Addison's disease with adrenal extracts were futile until extracts were made with fat solvents in the 1930s, when therapeutic success was finally achieved.[42] Brown-Séquard and others also used extracts of a number of different tissues—as mentioned earlier—for certain other diseases, with mixed results.[5] He nevertheless concluded that

> when a morbid state, as myxoedema [hypothyroidism], or a series of symptoms such as we see in cases of deficiency of the internal secretion of any gland, exists, it is very easy to understand how the cure is obtained when glandular liquid extracts are used: we simply give to the blood the principle or principles missing in it .... The great movement in therapeutics as regards the organic liquid extracts, has its origin in the experiments I made on myself in 1889, experiments which were at first so completely misunderstood.[5]

The editors of the *British Medical Journal* were circumspect. In their response, they at first seemed contrite. They acknowledged that many had originally sneered at Brown-Séquard, and accepted the fact that his beliefs had steadily gained support, especially since the successful use of thyroid extract. Thus, they no longer questioned the conceptual basis of his work but only its uncritical application by medical practitioners, something that Brown-Séquard himself had tried to avoid. They continued, however, to question many of the cures claimed for organ extracts, pointed to the cottage industry that had developed for producing such extracts by manufacturing chemists, and suggested that benefit often resulted from suggestion.[43]

> Physiologists have recently been making a number of observations, which show that many organs do more than what was formerly regarded as their functions. The experiments ... have led to the introduction of the expression "internal secretions." We think that this term is a rather unfortunately chosen one; but it, nevertheless, expresses that the organs in question have some action on the blood, and through it on the tissues generally, which influences their metabolic changes .... But the precise *modus operandi* is in all these cases still a sealed book. The composition of the internal secretion, where it exists, is unknown.

It is, however, presumed that an extract of the fresh organ must contain the active substances .... There can be little doubt that these substances are of a complex organic nature, substances which call on the resources of the organism to manufacture for itself. We can, therefore, hardly be surprised that if these substances are administered to a debilitated person unable to make them for himself, some amount of temporary stimulant effect is produced; and in one instance at least—that of myxedoema [hypothyroidism]—the curative result has justified the method used. Fully granting this, we still feel compelled to doubt many of the so-called other cures ... we may hope that we are now not to suffer an epidemic of universal injections. Manufacturing chemists are making extracts not only of thyroid, but of nearly every organ in the body .... We find medical men writing of these ideas and of the cures achieved in the most sanguine strain, and often upon no better evidence than quacks produce for their "cures."[43]

The reservations and disquiet expressed in respected medical journals were reasonable in the circumstances, if only because the uncritical acceptance of various extravagant but unfounded claims by certain practitioners was liable to mislead the public and result in unrealistic expectations for the future, and to bring the profession into disrepute. Indeed, many of Brown-Séquard's own specific therapeutic claims failed to stand the test of time; the manner of preparation of his extracts probably resulted in a loss of biological activity, and the doses administered and absorption characteristics of the injected extracts undoubtedly varied in different studies. The responses described by him and others are now generally regarded as reflections of a placebo effect—they believed that the testicular and other organ extracts would lead to benefit and so, at least for a while, they did—but whether there may also have been a true humoral effect to account for some of his findings is less clear.

Regardless of the uncertainty that surrounded their utility, it is not surprising that, shortly after their introduction, therapeutic organ extracts were taken in an attempt to enhance athletic performance. In 1889, the Irish-American baseball pitcher for Pittsburgh, Jim Galvin—nicknamed "Pud" because of his ability to reduce opposing batsmen to pudding—supposedly used them to enhance his game. A little later, in 1896, the Austrian physiologists Oskar Zoth (1864–1933) and Fritz Pregl (1869–1930; later a Nobel laureate in chemistry) used Brown-Séquard's approach to investigate whether testicular extracts would improve athletic performance. They injected themselves with extracts of bovine testicles and then recording their strength. Benefit was found, but may well have been a placebo effect.[44]

It has been strangely difficult to obtain a definitive statement from reproductive scientists as to whether the testicular extracts promoted by

Brown-Séquard could have had any true biological activity, but a report published in the *Medical Journal of Australia* in 2002 suggests that they did not. Andrea Cussons and her colleagues obtained testicles from five healthy dogs undergoing routine castration and kept them at 4°C until processed by Brown-Séquard's original method.[45] One testicle from each dog was mixed with distilled water in a quantity of up to twice the volume of the testicle and crushed with a mortar and pestle. The solution was then filtered and the testosterone concentration (see footnote, p. 238) was measured. (Other androgens such as dihydrotestosterone were not measured, as these are present in much smaller quantities in the testicles.) The mean testosterone concentration in the extracts was equivalent to 112 micrograms per liter (a microgram is one-millionth of a gram), and the five injections, each of 1 ml, of dog testicles that Brown-Séquard gave himself would have thus been equivalent to 112 nanograms of testosterone per injection or 186 nanograms per day (a nanogram is one-billionth of a gram). Testosterone secretion in healthy men is about 6 milligrams (a milligram is one-thousandth of a gram) daily. Thus, the dose of testosterone administered through canine testicular extracts is dramatically less than is required for testosterone replacement in hypogonadal men.[M] These results are consistent with what is now known about testicular physiology, because testosterone is mainly secreted as it is made rather than being stored to any major extent in the testicles. Furthermore, because it is largely insoluble in water, testosterone is unlikely to be present in significant concentrations in testicular extracts dissolved in water.[45]

Subsequent Work on Rejuvenation in the Early Twentieth Century

Over the following years, many physicians, scientists, and charlatans continued to exploit Brown-Séquard's work and name in a vain search for some means of rejuvenating the elderly or arresting the human frailties that develop with time. This work by others was undertaken after he had died, and some of it seemed scientifically reasonable and a logical extension of his efforts. The reason for the heightened interest in rejuvenation procedures, as opposed to transplantation in general, is uncertain, although such interest commonly occurs in cycles. David Hamilton, in his book,[46] speculates that social factors, such as the declining birth rate and the death of so many young men during

---

[M] Brown-Séquard also gave himself several injections of extracts from guinea-pig testicles over the subsequent eighteen days, but the testosterone concentration in these extracts is also likely to have been very low.

World War I, may have been responsible in part. In 1919, for example, the main topic of conversation in Paris related to rejuvenation rather than politics, the war, or the Peace Conference.[46]

Eugen Steinach (1861–1944),[N] a Viennese physiologist, having shown that grooming, an interest in the opposite sex, and the other physical and behavioral sexual characteristics of small animals such as rats and guinea pigs depend on the production of testicular and ovarian hormones, began by manipulating the sexual hormones in order to treat certain conditions then regarded as abnormal. In 1918, he removed the tuberculous testicle of a homosexual man, replacing it with an undescended testicle that needed to be removed from a heterosexual donor. Shortly thereafter, the patient began to have erotic dreams and then sought the services of a lady of the night; within a year he was married.[47] Others, however, were unable to replicate Steinach's findings in homosexuals, and the approach fell into disrepute.[48] Steinach then examined the effects on rejuvenation of tying off the vas deferens (i.e., of a vasectomy) in the hope of stimulating the production of male hormones in older animals. Such a procedure would also prevent the exit of sperm from the testicle and should therefore have an invigorating effect. His senile, listless, and underweight rodents became more active, sexually interested, and sleek. In 1920, believing that tying off the duct on one side was effective in increasing hormone production, he began operating on the tired elderly or middle-aged patients who could afford his procedure. Attempts were also made to graft testicular tissue into the abdominal muscles for the same reason.[49] Within two or three years, all the major European and American cities boasted of vasectomy specialists. Among the patients so treated were Sigmund Freud, then aged 66 and suffering with oral cancer, and the Irish poet and Nobel laureate William Butler Yeats (1865–1939), whose literary and sexual abilities were in decline. Both his general physical and sexual energy were restored, and cognitive and creative functions also improved. Women also supposedly benefited by various related procedures, such as irradiation of the ovaries to increase their production of hormones after it had been observed that "remarkable rejuvenation" occurred following such irradiation for benign conditions.[50,O] Such procedures soon fell into disrepute, however, and although ovarian transplantation was

---

[N] In his book *Sex and Life* (New York: Viking Press, 1940), Steinach, who was a devotée of Brown-Séquard, refers to 1 June 1889—the date of the famous presentation to the Société de Biologie—as "the birthday of the theory on internal secretion, and of the science of endocrinology."

[O] The popular American novelist Gertrude Atherton (1857–1948) claimed to feel thirty years younger after undergoing this procedure, and her best-selling novel, *Black Oxen*, published in 1923, is based on her experience.

also attempted in a few instances, the limited supply of human organs restricted the approach. Steinach's published account of his accumulated experience over many years remains of historical interest.[51]

Serge Voronoff (1866–1951), a Parisian surgeon who was the son of a Russian vodka manufacturer, took a somewhat different approach in the 1920s. In the belief that ageing resulted from testicular exhaustion, he began grafting testicular tissue from chimpanzees and baboons into elderly men—he was prohibited from using human testicles by French law and, in any event, young men were understandably hesitant about relinquishing one of their testicles—in what came to be referred to as the "monkey-gland operations." He believed that this would be more effective that simply administering a liquid extract, along the lines of Brown-Séquard. The operation seemed to be an enormous success and earned him a fortune. Voronoff, a man of great charm, received the Legion of Honor from the French government for his work after World War I, eventually took charge of a special section on grafting at the military hospital in Cannes, and went on to marry several times, his second wife conveniently being an heiress who helped finance his work and his last wife being an attractive Viennese girl almost fifty years his junior.[52] Many eminent surgeons on both sides of the Atlantic took up his procedure, although this was conveniently forgotten later when the operations were discredited.

Opinions varied as to the legitimacy of this approach, although some of its early advocates soon became disillusioned. Ernest Starling[p] in his Harveian Oration on hormones to the Royal College of Physicians of London in 1923, remarked on the results of the Steinach operation that

> these authors [Steinach and others] claim to have produced an actual rejuvenation in man, and thus to have warded off for a time senility with its mental and corporeal manifestations. Further experiments and a longer period of observation are necessary before we can accept these results without reserve, but it must be owned that they are perfectly reasonable and follow, as a logical sequence, many years' observations and experiments in this field.[53]

Some of the contemporary literature bears witness to these attempts at rejuvenation: Aldous Huxley's *Brave New World* is a world without old age; Conan Doyle's *The Adventure of the Creeping Man* portrays a rejuvenated

---

[p] Ernest Henry Starling (1866–1927), British physiologist, Jodrell Professor of Physiology at University College, London, and subsequently Foulerton Research Professor of the Royal Society, investigated the production of lymphatic fluid, the factors controlling the movement of fluid across capillary walls, the motility of the intestine, and the control of pancreatic secretion (by the hormone secretin), but he studied especially the cardiovascular system using a heart–lung preparation. His close collaborator was his brother-in-law, William Bayliss.

professor who begins to behave like a monkey, such as by climbing trees; and Dorothy L. Sayers refers to Voronoff's work in *The Unpleasantness at the Bellona Club*.

Unfortunately, similar experimental work was conducted in a much more troublesome manner by others and would not have met with Brown-Séquard's approval or acceptance, as it failed to conform to his ethical beliefs or scientific principles, and the personal profits made by some of those concerned would have offended him. Leo Stanley (1886–1976), physician until 1954 at the penitentiary at San Quentin near San Francisco, published his experience of one thousand testicular grafts into six hundred fifty-six human subjects using recently executed prisoners or—more often—various animals as donors and, for the most part, prisoners as recipients. Beneficial results were claimed in diverse medical disorders such as acne, asthma, diabetes, "rheumatism," senility, and neurasthenia,[Q] and the spontaneous pains (but not the disease itself) of locomotor ataxia (see footnote, p. 245) were said to be eased; no ill effects were reported, although in occasional cases sloughing of the transplanted material occurred.[54]

Another person involved with rejuvenation was John Brinkley (1885–1942), a drunken fraud who purchased rather than earned his medical diploma, injected colored distilled water as a rejuvenating agent for twenty-five dollars per treatment, and then went on to perform thousands of transplant procedures using testicles from goats, the first (in 1917) being undertaken several years before Voronoff's initial case. Described as a genius by some,[55] he went on to make a fortune, but a number (variously estimated as up to several hundred) of his patients died as a result of his surgery. Among his satisfied patrons, however, was Harry Chandler, the owner of the *Los Angeles Times* newspaper. The state of Kansas attempted to revoke his license for immorality and unprofessional conduct at the insistence of the American Medical Association, and eventually succeeded based on his fraudulent medical qualifications. The Federal Radio Commission shut down the radio station that he had built and operated[R] on the grounds that it was promoting fraud. He twice campaigned

---

[Q] Neurasthenia, a disorder described by the American neurologist George Beard in 1869, is supposedly characterized by nonspecific symptoms such as fatigue, lassitude, headache, anxiety, depression, aches and pains, disturbed sleep, and diverse other complaints. It is doubtful whether it is a distinct diagnostic entity.

[R] One of the most powerful radio stations in the United States, its call letters were KFKB, standing for Kansas First, Kansas Best. It broadcast programs by singers, orchestras, and preachers, and—most importantly—folksy medical lectures by Brinkley that included exhortations to restore waning male virility by his transplantation method. He thereby attracted many new patients to his clinic.

unsuccessfully to become governor of Kansas, but died bankrupt and disgraced after being sued for malpractice and back taxes.

The equation of clinical endocrinological practice with charlatanism for many years undoubtedly relates to such questionable activities. Indeed, even in the early 1920s, no less an authority than Harvey Cushing[s] is said to have referred to the uncritical followers of Brown-Séquard as "endocriminologists."[56] It was to take several years before it came to be realized that the approaches of Brown-Séquard, Steinach, and Voronoff were not the answer to advancing age or declining sexual activity, and that administration of sex hormones in pure form did not have the desired effects—many other systems are involved in sexual behavior. In particular, the eventual isolation of testosterone from the testicle—more than forty years after Brown-Séquard had declared that it contained an active principle—led to the demonstration that it influenced the development and presence of the so-called secondary sexual (male) characteristics but did not retard ageing or the sexual decline that occurs with advancing years. Thus, efforts at rejuvenation based on testicular extracts or grafting came to an end, to be replaced by a new approach called *cellular therapy*.

Paul Niehans (1882–1971), a Swiss physician, reported in the 1930s and 1940s that he could cure illnesses through injections of live cells obtained from healthy animal organs. He believed that adding new tissue stimulated rejuvenation and recovery, and his main emphasis was in preventing the effects of ageing. Among the rich and famous who reportedly came knocking at the door of his clinic in Switzerland were the writers Somerset Maugham and Thomas Mann, several politicians (including Winston Churchill, Charles de Gaulle, and Konrad Adenauer), and certain actors and actresses (Charlie Chaplin, Merle Oberon, and Gloria Swanson). He is said to have cared for members of the British royal family and also to have treated Pope Pius XII for diverse symptoms with subcutaneous injections of fetal brain cells from sheep and monkeys (which the Pontiff survived), following which he was nominated to the Vatican Academy of Science. Unfortunately, however, there is no valid evidence that such an approach confers any benefit. Cells from one species generally cannot replace cells from another, and attempts to do so lead simply to immunological rejection.

---

[s] Harvey Williams Cushing (1869–1939), pioneer American neurosurgeon, devised many new operative techniques and introduced routine blood pressure measurement into the United States. He reported a hormonal disorder caused by a malfunction of the pituitary gland (Cushing's disease), described various neurological syndromes and the clinical signs of increased intracranial pressure, and received a Pulitzer Prize for his biography of Sir William Osler.

Although the possibility of rejuvenation still arouses hopes and expectations in those with increasing infirmity, such dreams are yet to be realized and—at least for the present—remain the unrealized prize of an endless quest. In the meantime, fortunes are spent on purported agents—pills, potions, food supplements, diets—and various lifestyle modifications that, it is claimed, may stop the clock.

Brown-Séquard's Achievements

Brown-Séquard clearly forecast many concepts that are now widely accepted concerning the presence and action of male hormones. He recognized correctly that, in addition to their function in procreation, the testicles had other functions and manufactured substances that are secreted internally, with important biological effects on many parts of the body. It was several decades later, however, before the gonadal steroid hormones (such as the male hormone, testosterone) were isolated. Brown-Séquard made no claim that aging resulted solely from a decline in testicular function, but held that this was perhaps one contributory factor. In fact, the production of testosterone does gradually decline with age, as well as in certain disease states. Certain symptoms, such as fatigue, malaise, weakness, reduced muscle mass, loss of bone density, depression, and sexual difficulties (e.g., reduced potency and libido) may also occur in elderly men, but whether because of declining testosterone levels is unclear. Modern medical authorities remain undecided as to whether a male menopause occurs, but hormone replacement therapy (with testosterone) is generally not advised because its benefits are unclear and it is associated with certain risks, although not all would agree with this approach.[57] The work undertaken by Brown-Séquard on testicular extracts involved the study of ageing, and in this regard his work marks the beginning of the science of gerontology and led to greater public awareness of the sexual, physical, and psychological changes that occur with advancing age.

Brown-Séquard also anticipated by his speculations the importance of chemical mediators or messengers—hormones and neurotransmitters—in integrating the diverse functions that maintain the integrity of the organism. His work directed medical and public attention to the therapeutic potential of organ extracts, with important consequences. The advances that occurred in the treatment of hypothyroidism have already been mentioned, but there are other examples, such as the discovery that adrenal extracts led to a marked increase in blood pressure[58,59] (Chapter 6), an observation that led within a few years to the purification of epinephrine (adrenaline), and then to its synthesis in the laboratory. In 1904, the similarity between the effects of injected epinephrine and stimulating the sympathetic nerves led T.R. Elliott[T] to propose that these nerves release epinephrine at their terminations. Later, it was shown that the inhibitory effects on the heart of vagal nerve stimulation are also chemically mediated—by acetylcholine—and this provided further support for the notion that chemical substances are released by (or in) the various bodily tissues and coordinate their activity with that of the organism as a whole.

Brown-Séquard died in 1894, before his concept of chemical integrative mechanisms was vindicated and before the subsequent development of hormone replacement therapy. He died at a time when many of his contemporaries still doubted the value of organ extracts and attributed to him the unrealistic public expectations that resulted from his work and the exploitation of these expectations by an unethical medical and pharmaceutical minority for which Brown-Séquard was not responsible. Thus, an editorial in the *Journal of the American Medical Association* characterized his work on organ extracts as "the vagary of an old man, undergoing senile cerebral changes" and urged that his friends "blot out from the record that last act in the drama of his life, whereby he very nearly caused his professional brethren of the entire world to palm off on the public a pretentious fraud."[60] In fact, he was not senile and—as evidenced by his experimental work and writings in other areas, but especially on the sensory system—he retained his remarkable ability to conceive and formulate new concepts of biological relevance until the very end. With time, the general principles that underpinned his work have been substantiated, and organotherapy led directly to the development of modern endocrinology as a distinct clinical specialty, even though the specific therapeutic benefits that Brown-Séquard claimed have failed to gain general acceptance. The fact that the nostrums of his clinical contemporaries were equally ineffective seems to have been overlooked by his critics. Much of Brown-Séquard's work was based on intuition and few can doubt that he

---

[T] Thomas Renton Elliott (1877–1961) British physician and physiologist, worked on the chemical transmission of nerve action. His work and that of others led to the concept of chemical neurotransmission. He was not yet 30 years old when he emphasized the similar effects of sympathetic nerve stimulation and adrenal gland extracts, and showed that chemical transmission by epinephrine (adrenaline) must occur between sympathetic nerves and smooth muscle at sympathetic nerve terminals. The role of neurotransmitter chemicals in enabling the nerve impulse to cross the synapse to activate another neuron or an effector (e.g., muscle) cell with which it connects was contested for some years but is now widely accepted. Elliott also worked on the nerve supply of the bladder and other bodily organs. He became professor of medicine at University College Hospital Medical School (University of London), where Victor Horsley was also on the staff, and remained there for his entire professional career, except for military service during World War I.

had remarkable insight, but his insight sometimes overshadowed the more limited conclusions that his experimental work justified and brought on him the chilling disapproval of the academic community.

The Judgment of History: His Legacy

The emerging specialty of clinical endocrinology, launched by Brown-Séquard's concepts of internal secretions and by his use of organ extracts in various contexts, had a difficult childhood. Indeed, Herbert Evans[U] remarked that endocrinology "suffered obstetric deformation in its very birth by the extravagant claim of the septuagenarian Brown-Séquard that he had magically restored his youth with testicular substance."[61] Others were also scathing, suggesting that a "drought descended upon the field of clinical endocrinology which persisted, with but a few scattered refreshing contributions, for almost thirty years."[62] These assessments are not entirely fair. The field of clinical endocrinology arguably did not exist prior to Brown-Séquard who, at the very least, aroused interest in the subject among both the medical profession and general public. There is wide agreement that Brown-Séquard deserves credit for the good, as well as some of the responsibility for the more unfortunate consequences of his sensational report of 1889, even though he was not to blame for them. He was aware, and indeed warned, about the power of auto-suggestion, although his concerns appear to have been mollified by the uncontrolled reports of many others for success with his testicular extracts.[40] At that time, clinical trials were not placebo controlled and the danger of subconscious self-delusion to obtain the desired results was very real (and remains so today, even with the more rigorous methodology now employed in clinical trials).

On the one hand, in the years that followed Brown-Séquard's famous presentation to the Société de Biologie in 1889, therapeutic extracts were made from a variety of different organs, the active ingredients or hormones in these extracts were isolated and prepared in pure form, and their use to cure or ameliorate disease became commonplace. Even when a specific organ extract appeared to be therapeutically unhelpful, attempts were made to identify any contained active ingredients that might be present. Thus, although early attempts (including those by Brown-Séquard and d'Arsonval) to treat diabetes by pancreatic extracts (as opposed to pancreatic grafts, which were effective in

---

[U] Herbert McLean Evans (1882–1971), American anatomist who studied human nutrition, endocrinology, embryology, and histology. Among his accomplishments were the isolation of human growth hormone and the co-discovery of vitamin E.

animals with diabetes induced experimentally by removal of the pancreas) were without success, an effective treatment subsequently emerged with the isolation in 1922 of insulin from the pancreas. The early observation of therapeutic benefit from thyroid extracts in patients with hypothyroidism, the recognition in 1902 of secretin, a hormone produced by the duodenum that stimulates pancreatic secretion (see footnote C, p. 236), and the identification of the active agent in extracts of the adrenal glands (1901) boosted these developments and led to clinical advances and scientific respectability. On the other hand, the use of organotherapy in a frivolous and thoughtless manner by persuasive charlatans, to their own financial benefit, led only to public deception and a general distrust of physicians. Yet, it sometimes seemed as if the one helped the other. Henry Harrower (1893–1934), for example, an expatriate Englishman living in the United States, trained as a physician, developed an interest in alternative medicine, became a major fan of organotherapy, and discussed it in detail in his book *Practical Hormone Therapy,* as well as in many other publications.[63] Establishing his own clinic in Glendale, California, he proceeded to make a fortune by using extracts of every conceivable part of the body to treat a diversity of disease. More tellingly, he encouraged the use of multiglandular mixtures in the belief that the body would somehow be able to use just what it needed to restore itself and harmlessly rid itself of the remainder. This implied that overtreatment could not occur, a reassuring belief for patients and practitioners alike. Ironically, Harrower had a major role in founding the Society of Internal Secretions in 1916 (now the much-respected Endocrine Society) and served briefly as first editor of its official new journal, *Endocrinology.*[64]

In 1895, Edward Schäfer[V]—in a famous address to the British Medical Association—spoke about the internal secretions, defining them as secreted materials that are "returned to the blood" rather than being poured out upon an external surface. He emphasized that it was not only the ductless glands "which possess the property of furnishing internal secretions, for it is clear, according to our definition, that this will apply to any organ of the body."[65]

[V] Edward A. Schäfer (1850–1935), later Sir Edward Albert Sharpey-Schäfer (the name of his teacher, Sharpey, being added to his own in 1918 to avoid contemporary anti-German sentiment), was professor of physiology at University College London and subsequently at Edinburgh University. He was probably best known for his method of artificial respiration in the prone position, but his early work was on muscle histology. He subsequently collaborated with George Oliver to demonstrate the effects on the blood pressure of adrenal extracts, thereby becoming engaged in work on the endocrine system. He was also known for his short temper, as must have been in evidence during his famous lecture on the internal secretions—he could not use the lantern slides with which he had intended to illustrate his talk (the lecture hall was not suited for this purpose) and instead had to trace imaginary curves with his finger to illustrate results.

As the historian Merriley Borell has pointed out,[12] this is precisely the sense in which Brown-Séquard and d'Arsonval generalized the concept of internal secretions in 1891. Schäfer was prepared to stress the importance of the internal secretions because physiological evidence now existed to support the concept that Brown-Séquard had advanced without adequate experimental justification and that had so hastily been dismissed by his professional colleagues. Curiously, Schafer did not accept Brown-Séquard's belief that the sex glands produce internal secretions, and he hardly referred to them in his lecture except to attribute to the nervous system the changes that develop in other parts of the body following their removal, a belief that is clearly incorrect. Whether this was a reflection of his intellectual beliefs, related to "an Englishman's subconscious dislike of focusing the limelight on sex,"[66] or resulted from concern with Brown-Séquard's approach remains purely conjectural. In any event, he subsequently changed his mind and came to regard their effects as being mediated chemically rather than through the nervous system.[67] Moreover, he credited Brown-Séquard for his contribution:

> The first attempts—at any rate, in modern times—to determine the physiological effects of tissue extracts and juices appear to be those of Brown-Séquard, who investigated upon himself and others the effects of subcutaneous injections of the expressed juices of the ovaries and testicles of animals .... That the internal secretions and extracts of these glands contain hormones, which influence the development of other generative organs and of secondary sexual characters is, as we have seen, more than probable ....[67]

While recognizing that clinical observation is clearly important in guiding physiological research, Schäfer went on to put the study of internal secretions on a rigorous scientific footing by making and encouraging the use of objective measurement of physiological changes resulting from the administration of animal extracts, rather than relying on subjective clinical impressions. For this, he deserves enormous credit.

In December 1934, Professor Holmgren of the Karolinska Institute in Stockholm, in announcing that George Minot and William Murphy of Harvard Medical School and George Whipple of the University of Rochester were the winners of the Nobel Prize in Physiology or Medicine,[W] reflected on the

---

[W] The prize was awarded for their work showing that the anemia described by Thomas Addison (p. 91), now known as Addisonian pernicious anemia, responds to the consumption of large quantities of liver. At the time of the award, it was unclear whether the beneficial effects of liver were due to a hormone, a vitamin, or something else. It is now known that it results from vitamin B_{12}, which is stored in the liver.

history of organotherapy, now known as hormone replacement therapy. Patients in whom some organ is not functioning normally are required, he said, to consume portions of the organ or to be injected with preparations made from it. Such an approach "is not so absolutely new as many people may think. Thus, we may recall that a French physiologist, Brown-Séquard, as long ago as 1889, carried out investigations, which aroused great astonishment at the time, as to the effect of an injection into the body of testicular juice, got from the male genital glands. He gave himself injections of testicular juice and observed considerable rejuvenating effects both physically and mentally. That constituted the first achievement in the direction in question that science accomplished. Hence, it is Brown-Séquard who laid the foundation of organotherapy."[68]

References and Source Notes

1. Rolleston HD. *The endocrine organs in health and disease with an historical review* (pp. 1–22). London: Oxford University Press, 1936.
2. de Bordeu T. *Recherches sur les maladies chroniques, leurs rapports avec les maladies aigues, leurs periodes, leur nature: et sur la manière dont on les traite aux eaux minerales de Bareges, et des autres sources de l'Aquitaine.* Paris: Ruault, 1775.
3. Benedum J. The early history of endocrine cell transplantation. *J Mol Med*, 77: 30–35, 1999.
4. Berthold AA. Transplantation der Hoden. *Arch Anat Physiol Wissensch Med*, 42–46, 1849. [Translated by Quiring DP. The transplantation of testes. *Bull Hist Med*, 16:399–401, 1944.]
5. Brown-Séquard CE. On a new therapeutic method consisting in the use of organic liquids extracted from glands and other organs. *Br Med J*, 1:1145–1147 and 1212–1214, 1893.
6. Brown-Séquard CE. Des effets produits chez l'homme par des injections sous-cutanées d'un liquide retiré des testicules frais de cobaye et de chien. *C R Soc Biol (Paris)*, 41: 415–419, 1889.
7. Brown-Séquard CE. Expérience démontrant la puissance dynamogénique chez l'homme d'un liquide extrait de testicules d'animaux. *Arch Physiol Norm Pathol (5th Series)*, 1:651–658, 1889.
8. Brown-Séquard CE. Note on the effects produced on man by subcutaneous injections of a liquid obtained from the testicles of animals. *Lancet*, 2:105–107, 1889.
9. Variot G. Trois expériences sur l'action physiologique du suc testiculaire injecté sous la peau, suivant la méthode de M. Brown-Séquard. *C R Soc Biol (Paris)*, 41:451–454, 1889.
10. Brown-Séquard CE. Remarques à l'occasion du travail de M. Variot, sur les injections de liquide testiculaire chez l'homme. *C R Soc Biol (Paris)*, 41:454–455, 1889.
11. Brown-Séquard CE. Seconde note sur les effets produits chez l'homme par des injections sous-cutanées d'un liquide retiré des testicules frais de cobaye et de chien. *C R Soc Biol (Paris)*, 41:420–422, 1889.
12. Borell M. Organotherapy, British physiology, and discovery of the internal secretions. *J Hist Biol*, 9:235–268, 1976.
13. Hamilton D. *The monkey gland affair* (p. 10). London: Chatto & Windus, 1986.
14. Brown-Séquard CE. Du role physiologique et thérapeutique d'un suc extrait de testicules d'animaux d'après nombre de faits observés chez l'homme. *Arch Physiol Norm Pathol (5th Series)*, 1:739–748, 1889.
15. Hammond WA. The elixir of life. *N Am Rev*, 149:257–264, 1889.

16. Hammond WA. Experiments relative to the therapeutical value of the expressed juice of the testicles when hypodermically introduced into the human system. *NY Med J*, 50:232–234, 1889.
17. Editorial. The pentacle of rejuvenescence. *Br Med J*, 1:1416, 1889.
18. Anonymous. Dr. Brown-Séquard's hypodermic fluid. *Br Med J*, 2:29, 1889.
19. Anonymous. The new elixir of youth. *Br Med J*, 2:446, 1889.
20. Berdoe E. A serious moral question. A letter printed for private circulation and dated 12 July 1889. MS 980/67. Archives, Royal College of Physicians, London.
21. Anonymous. Dr. Brown-Séquard's experiments. *Br Med J*, 2:347, 1889.
22. Brown-Séquard CE. Note on the effects produced on man by subcutaneous injections of a liquid obtained from the testicles of animals. *Sci Am*, 28(Suppl 710):11347–11348, 1889.
23. Anonymous. Dr. Brown-Séquard's recent experiments. *Sci Am*, 61:80, 1889.
24. Anonymous. Dr. Brown-Séquard's "Elixir of Life." *Lancet*, 1:57–58, 1890.
25. Borell M. Brown-Séquard's organotherapy and its appearance in America at the end of the nineteenth century. *Bull Hist Med*, 50:309–320, 1976.
26. Anonymous. Obituary: Professor Brown-Séquard. *Lancet*, 1:975–977, 1894.
27. Dunbar N, ed. *The elixir of life: Dr. Brown-Séquard's own account of his famous alleged remedy for debility and old age, Dr. Variot's experiments, and contemporaneous comments of the profession and the press. To which is prefixed a sketch of Dr. Brown-Séquard's life, with portrait.* Boston: Cupples, 1889.
28. Brown-Séquard CE. Remarques sur les effets produits sur la femme par des injections souscutanées d'un liquide retiré d'ovaire d'animaux. *Arch Physiol Norm Pathol (5th Series)*, 2:456–457, 1890.
29. Andrews HR. The internal secretion of the ovary. *J Obstet Gynaecol*, 5:448–465, 1904.
30. Sturdee DW. Newer HRT regimens. *Br J Obstet Gynaecol*, 104:1109–1115, 1997.
31. Brown-Séquard CE, d'Arsonval A. Recherches sur les extraits liquides retirés des glandes et d'autres parties de l'organisme et sur leur emploi, en injections sous-cutanées, comme méthode thérapeutique. *Arch Physiol Norm Pathol (5th Series)*, 3:491–506, 1891.
32. Brown-Séquard CE, d'Arsonval A. De l'injection des extraits liquides provenant des glandes et des tissues de l'organism comme méthode thérapeutique. *C R Soc Biol (Paris)*, 43: 248–250, 1891.
33. d'Arsonval A. Letter to Brown-Séquard dated 24 March 1891. In: Delhoume L. *De Claude Bernard à d'Arsonval* (pp. 377–380). Paris: Baillière, 1939.
34. Brown-Séquard CE. Exposé de faits nouveaux montrant la puissance du liquide testiculaire contre l'affaiblissement dû à certaines maladies et en particulier la tuberculose pulmonaire. *Arch Physiol Norm Pathol (5th Series)*, 3:224–229, 1891.
35. Paget S. *Sir Victor Horsley: A study of his life and work* (pp. 65–66). London: Constable, 1919.
36. Murray GR. Note on the treatment of myxoedema by hypodermic injections of an extract of the thyroid gland of a sheep. *Br Med J*, 2:796–797, 1891.
37. Kocher ET. Concerning pathological manifestations in low-grade thyroid diseases. Nobel Lecture, 11 December 1909. In: *Nobel lectures, physiology or medicine 1901–1921* (pp. 330–383). Amsterdam: Elsevier, 1967.
38. Brown-Séquard CE. Four letters to d'Arsonval dated 17 to 22 February 1893. In: Delhoume L. *De Claude Bernard à d'Arsonval* (p. 365). Paris: Baillière, 1939. [That d'Arsonval did as requested by Brown-Séquard and sent samples of the fluids to Horsley and others is documented in his letter to Brown-Séquard, 25 February 1891. In: Delhoume L. *De Claude Bernard à d'Arsonval* (pp. 366–367). Paris: Baillière, 1939.]
39. Brown-Séquard CE. Letter to d'Arsonval dated 27 March 1891. In: Delhoume L. *De Claude Bernard à d'Arsonval* (pp. 383–384). Paris: Baillière, 1939.
40. Wilson JD. Charles-Edouard Brown-Séquard and the centennial of endocrinology. *J Clin Endocrinol Metab*, 71:1403–1409, 1990.

41. Brown-Séquard CE. Influence heureuse de la transfusion de sang normal après l'extirpation des capsules surrénales chez le cobaye. *C R Soc Biol (Paris),* 45:448–449, 1893.
42. Young FG. The evolution of ideas about animal hormones. In: Needham J, ed., *The chemistry of life* (pp. 125–155). Cambridge: Cambridge University Press, 1970.
43. Editorial. Animal extracts as therapeutic agents. *Br Med J,* 1:1279, 1893.
44. Hoberman JM, Yesalis CE. The history of synthetic testosterone. *Sci Am,* 272:76–81, 1995.
45. Cussons AJ, Bhagat CI, Fletcher SJ, Walsh JP. Brown-Séquard revisited: a lesson from history on the placebo effect of androgen treatment. *Med J Aust,* 177:678–679, 2002.
46. Hamilton D. *The monkey gland affair* (pp. 27–30). London: Chatto & Windus, 1986.
47. Sengoopta C. *The most secret quintessence of life: Sex, glands, and hormones, 1850–1950* (pp. 78–82). Chicago: University of Chicago Press, 2006.
48. Schmidt G. Allies and persecutors: science and medicine in the homosexuality issue. *J Homosex,* 10: 127–140, 1985.
49. Schultheiss D, Denil J, Jonas U. Rejuvenation in the early 20th century. *Andrologia,* 29:351–355, 1997.
50. Del Regato JA. Guido Holzknecht. *Int J Rad Oncol Biol Phys,* 2:1201–1208, 1977.
51. Steinach E. *Sex and life: Forty years of biological and medical experiments.* New York: Viking Press, 1940.
52. Romm S. Rejuvenation revisited. *Aesth Plast Surg,* 7:241–248, 1983.
53. Starling EH. Hormones. *Nature,* 112:795–798, 1923.
54. Stanley LL. An analysis of one thousand testicular substance implantations. *Endocrinology,* 6:787–794, 1922.
55. Herman JR. Rejuvenation: Brown-Séquard to Brinkley. *NY State J Med,* 82:1731–1739, 1982.
56. Fulton JF. *Selected readings in the history of physiology,* 2nd ed. (pp. 410–411). Springfield: Thomas, 1966.
57. Morley JE. The politics of testosterone. *J Sex Med,* 4:554–557, 2007.
58. Oliver G, Schäfer EA. The physiological effects of extracts of the suprarenal capsules. *J Physiol,* 18:230–276, 1895.
59. Dale H. Accident and opportunism in medical research. *Br Med J,* 2:451–455, 1948.
60. Editorial. The death of Brown-Séquard. *JAMA,* 22:516, 1894.
61. Evans HM. Present position of our knowledge of anterior pituitary function. *JAMA,* 101:425–432, 1933.
62. Lisser H. The Endocrine Society: The first forty years (1917–1957). *Endocrinology,* 80: 5–28, 1967.
63. Harrower HR. *Practical hormone therapy: A manual of organotherapy for general practitioners.* London: Baillière, Tindall & Cox, 1914.
64. Schwartz TB. Henry Harrower and the turbulent beginnings of endocrinology. *Ann Intern Med,* 131:702–706, 1999.
65. Schäfer EA. Address in physiology: On internal secretions. *Lancet,* 2:321–324, 1895.
66. Medvei VC. *The history of clinical endocrinology* (p. 186). Carnforth (UK): Parthenon, 1993.
67. Schäfer EA. The hormones which are contained in animal extracts: their physiological effects. *Pharm J,* 79:670–674, 1907.
68. Holmgren I. Presentation speech. The Nobel Prize in physiology or medicine 1934. In: *Nobel lectures, physiology or medicine 1922–1941.* Amsterdam: Elsevier, 1965.

14

Scenes from the World of a Scientist

IT IS REMARKABLE that Brown-Séquard was able to explore experimentally so many different aspects of medicine and physiology. His papers—written in French or English and numbering more than five hundred—are widely disseminated in the medical and scientific literature (see Appendix). Some are difficult to digest, filled as they are with claims and counterclaims over priority, the contradictory observations of different observers, and interpretative comments of uncertain significance. It is clear, however, that much of his work is fragmentary and was not followed up by him. Some of it was important, has stood the test of time, but has been forgotten because he documented it inadequately or because his many other scientific contributions overshadowed it. Other work was clearly not correct but is of historical interest. Appraisal of these various studies, which were peripheral to his major contributions, is difficult because it is not always clear whether some of his statements related to his experimental observations or to his unsubstantiated beliefs. Nevertheless, this work is considered further in the present chapter to give the reader an appreciation of the broad range of Brown-Séquard's interests and the importance of many of his observations.

The breadth of his interests was such that it included studies on the ear and the eye. He made the observation, not pursued further, that irrigation of the ear with cold water leads to "a kind of vertigo, and ... it is difficult to walk straight for some time after this irritation."[1] It was subsequently found by others that nystagmus—an involuntary jerky movement of the eyes—was induced by irrigation of the ear canals with water. This eventually led to the development of the *caloric test*, in which the ears are irrigated with warm and cold water, to investigate disorders of balance. For this and related work on the physiology and pathology of the vestibular apparatus, Robert Bárány was awarded the Nobel Prize for Medicine or Physiology in 1914 (when he was a Russian prisoner-of-war, having been captured while serving as a civilian with the Austrian army). In his studies on the vertebrate eye, Brown-Séquard found that the iris of batrachians and fish showed autonomous excitability, with light having a direct effect on it. Thus, pupillary constriction (i.e., contraction of the iris) occurred in response to light in frogs that were dead or had received various toxins in fatal concentrations. When the eye was enucleated, illumination of the iris but not of the retina (through the pupil) led to contraction.[2-4] Experiments involving colored glass as a filter revealed that light of long wavelength was more effective than short-wavelength light. These observations continue to be confirmed and referenced as recently as the beginning of this century, more than one hundred and fifty years after Brown-Séquard first made them, thus attesting to their relevance and originality.

Sleep was another topic that caught his attention early on, when he published a short paper on torpidity in the tenrec.[5] Such a report on a small mammal living in Mauritius and neighboring areas may seem irrelevant or inconsequential to the modern scientist but, as pointed out by the late Julius Comroe, founding director of the world-famous Cardiovascular Research Institute at the University of California in San Francisco, it "provided proof that even an animal living in the tropics could be made to hibernate in its winter months by relatively small decreases in body temperature and paved the way for hypothermia of patients during cardiac surgery."[6]

The cause and purpose of sleep have puzzled philosophers and scientists over the centuries. Four types of theory have been advanced with regard to its cause.[7] Vascular theories held that sleep occurred because blood flow to the brain decreased (leading to a lack of blood) or increased (filling the brain and causing congestion) relative to the rest of the body. Although the congestive hypothesis was most popular in the early nineteenth century, the "anemic" concept of insufficient cerebral blood flow had among its advocates such eminent physician-scientists as William Hammond (p. 122) in America and Franciscus Donders (p. 201) in Europe. Brown-Séquard showed experimentally that the vascular concept was untenable: rabbits, guinea pigs, cats, and dogs sleep normally after interruption in the neck of the sympathetic nerves that pass to the blood vessels in the head and control their caliber.[8] By the end of the century, then, vascular concepts for the basis of sleep had fallen into disfavor. Instead, neural theories attempted to explain sleep on the basis of changes in the shape of neurons, usually alterations in the nerve cell processes that supposedly either limited the transfer of information from one cell to another or, conversely, allowed sleep-inducing impulses to pass more easily between cells. These theories also became discredited although, in the early twentieth century, modifications in neurotransmitter and synaptic function briefly replaced changes in cell morphology as the hypothetical basis of sleep. In the latter half of the nineteenth century, chemical (humoral) theories of sleep gained favor for a period, it being suggested that oxygen deprivation or the accumulation of carbon dioxide or other toxic metabolites related to activity was responsible.

A variety of behavioral theories were also advanced to explain the reason for sleep, and they gained increasing support. Among these, the most popular was the inhibition theory of Brown-Séquard, who attributed sleep—somewhat vaguely—to an inhibitory effect of one or more regions of the brain on higher cerebral ("intellectual" or "psychic") function,[8] based in part on earlier work in animals showing that removal of parts of the brain was followed by an intermittent sleep-like state. The inhibitory theory came to be supported by the experimental work of Emil Heubel at Kiev University, in the Ukraine, who related sleep to the loss of peripheral sensory stimulation,[9] and then by the work of Pavlov[A] in the early part of the twentieth century.[10] More recently, however, the emphasis has been on the role of the brainstem in stimulating animals to remain awake through an ascending reticular activating system and then on the existence of a sleep-generating system in the hypothalamus, just above the brainstem.

Brown-Séquard had more morbid interests as well. In the 1840s and 1850s, he investigated the relationship between rigor mortis, putrefaction, and muscle activity prior to death,[11–16] and he later summarized his findings—in his Croonian Lecture to the Royal Society of London in 1861—that in rested, cold, or paralyzed muscle, rigor mortis or postmortem rigidity was delayed in onset but persisted for longer before the beginning of putrefaction compared to muscles that had been violently exercised prior to death.[17] Such conclusions are widely accepted and have major implications for forensic pathologists trying to establish the time of death of their luckless subjects. He also pointed

---

[A] Ivan Petrovich Pavlov (1849–1936), professor at the Military Medical Academy and Director of the Institute for Experimental Medicine in St. Petersburg, Russia, is renowned for his work on conditioned reflexes. He showed that the sight, smell, or taste of food stimulated salivation and the flow of gastric juices as an unconditioned reflex, and that if a specific preceding external stimulus such as a musical note comes to be associated with the food, it too will elicit secretory responses in anticipation of the forthcoming food, but as a conditioned reflex. In 1904, he received the Nobel Prize for Physiology or Medicine for his work on the physiology of digestion.

out that soldiers who died in battle sometimes maintained their body and limbs in the same posture as at the moment of death, presumably because of the immediate onset of rigidity. In a later article, he went into more detail, referring to the occasional persistence after sudden and violent death of facial expressions or certain postures of the body and limbs, so that a raised limb did not drop or a man standing or on horseback did not fall over after death.[18] A dramatic example was the corpse of a soldier found near Sedan in 1870. The soldier was half-seated on the ground and was holding a tin cup directed toward a mouth that no longer existed, a cannonball having taken off most of his head. Several other examples were given from battles such as those at Magenta and Solferino (Second Italian War of Independence), Inkermann (Crimean War), and Antietam (American Civil War). Brown-Séquard believed that the abnormal posture resulted from a tonic persistent muscle contraction because—as he correctly pointed out—its instantaneous onset excluded rigor mortis. As with so many of his papers, however, he failed to give an adequate explanation for its basis but simply stated: "Some experiments that I cannot here give the details of have shown me that it is a fixed contraction ...."[18] Perhaps this was not altogether surprising in this instance, as the precise cause of such instantaneous rigidity is unknown, but the phenomenon remains of considerable importance to forensic scientists. Brown-Séquard also noted the interesting occurrence of rigidity within three minutes after respiration had ceased and while the heart was actually still beating in a patient with typhoid fever; that is, in a patient who was technically still alive.[15,17]

A number of his experimental studies, such as those in which he grafted the tail of a cat, dog, or other animal on the comb of a cock, hold a certain exotic fascination but were undertaken for uncertain reasons. These bizarre experiments, performed in the early 1850s in France[19] and Virginia,[20] seemed always to come to an untimely end, with the deformed cock being attacked by its outraged companions. Equally bizarre was the work that he undertook in June 1851, when he arranged for blood to be withdrawn from his own arm, whipped it to make it less liable to clot, and then infused it into the arm of a 20-year-old man who had been guillotined some 13 hours earlier.[21,22] Rigor mortis disappeared from the irrigated limb, and all but two of the nineteen muscles that he studied regained their contractile properties, as discussed later in this chapter.

Self-Experimentation

The dramatic claims made by Brown-Séquard after he injected himself with testicular extracts from animals were discussed in detail in Chapters 12 and 13.

Unfortunately, such observations were marred by the subjective nature of the changes that he claimed had resulted from the injections, a problem that he himself recognized and commented on specifically in his very first communication on the subject.[23] There were many other instances in which he used himself as an experimental subject, going back to his student days, when he swallowed sponges attached to a string to absorb his gastric juices and then withdrew them to analyze their content. For years afterwards, he felt embarrassed about eating in company because of flatulence and the bovine tendency of regurgitating his food. As the opportunity to report his own symptoms was irresistible, Brown-Séquard later described in detail the condition of a patient whom he allegedly encountered in 1851, but who is undoubtedly himself. The report is particularly interesting because of the description provided of his way of life. At the time, he was suffering from postprandial abdominal distension, flatulence, heartburn, and gastric regurgitation, as well as general malaise and lassitude to such an extent that he was unable to work, but a careful dietary regime in restful surroundings helped him to regain his vigor.[24]

> The first patient I submitted to this plan was a scientific man, 34 years old ... reduced from several causes to a lamentable state of health .... For about eight years, he had been working very hard, taking no exercise, and living almost all the time in a vitiated atmosphere. He slept very little, and usually passed 18 or even 19 hours a day writing, reading, or experimenting. His diet was miserable, and, with the object of avoiding the need of much food, he took a great deal of coffee .... His digestion ... had gradually become very bad. He suffered greatly from pyrosis, and a feeling of great distress, and gastric distention after each meal. Acid eructations and gas were frequently thrown up into his mouth, and when he did not vomit he found that his food remained on his stomach so long, that in the morning he frequently rejected things eaten the previous day .... His emaciation and weakness and dyspeptic symptoms increased, and his friends decided to have him removed to the country .... After a few days, finding that he had not improved, I decided to try a radical change of his alimentation, as regards the quantity of food to be taken at a time. Instead of *three* meals a day I made him take *sixty* or more. Every twelve or fifteen minutes he took two or three mouthfuls of solid food, chiefly meat and bread .... On the very first day this mode of alimentation was begun, his digestive troubles (one of the symptoms which had preceded the others—merycism, persisted, and has remained ever since, being now as before of daily occurrence) disappeared, and within a week he was so well that he returned to Paris ... he continued this same mode of alimentation for about three weeks, and then gradually diminished the number of his homeopathic meals, and increased the

amount taken at each of them, until in about 8 or 10 days he came to eat only three times a day, and a full meal at each time.[24]

Some of the other, sometimes seemingly inconsequential, experiments that he performed on himself have also been alluded to in earlier chapters but, for the reader's convenience, are summarized here. In 1854, for example, while treating the victims of a cholera epidemic in Mauritius, he reputedly swallowed the vomit of patients and—feeling symptoms of cholera developing in himself—took laudanum in an attempt to demonstrate the utility of this form of treatment. In fact, in his enthusiasm, he took such large doses of this opiate that he had to be resuscitated with coffee.[25] In Virginia, shortly afterward, he nearly died on one occasion when he was found unconscious on the floor after he had covered himself all over with flypaper varnish while studying the functions of the skin.[26] The precise reason for the experiment is unclear, but it was probably based on an attempt to prevent the skin from secreting what he supposed to be a toxic substance, so that it would be absorbed by the blood.[27] One of his students saved his life by removing the varnish with alcohol or, as one story has it, with sandpaper.

No opportunity was lost. He is said to have crossed the Atlantic some sixty times, but the time was not wasted. On one voyage, he used the occasion to examine the temperature of his own urine on more than thirty occasions (and also that of "ten strong sailors") and showed that it tended to be higher than the sublingual temperature and was relatively constant regardless of the varied external conditions.[28] For years, he measured (with a dynamometer) and recorded the strength of certain muscles in his arms, and this data was useful when he later studied on himself the effect of testicular extracts of dogs and guinea pigs (Chapters 12 and 13). He even made observations on the graying of his own beard, concluding that individual hairs may become white overnight,[29] and on his tendency to facial sweating while eating.

Frey's syndrome, named after Lucja Frey of the University of Warsaw,[B] is the eponym for a disorder characterized by gustatory sweating, that is, the tendency to sweat and flush on one side of the face after eating spicy foods. Such symptoms typically develop some weeks or more after an injury to the parotid salivary gland or to the cervical sympathetic nerves. Although credit for the original description of this disorder has been given in the past to others,[30] many of the early cases clearly did not have the syndrome as it is

---

[B] Lucja Frey-Gottesman (1889–1942), Polish physician. Because she was Jewish, she was transported during World War II to a ghetto and is believed to have perished there or in a Nazi death camp.

currently defined. Frey not only provided (in 1923) an accurate clinical account, but related it to the innervation of the salivary glands and the skin.[31] Damage to the nerve leads to regeneration of nerve fibers, but some of the fibers are misrouted and grow in the wrong direction, passing to the sweat glands in the skin instead of to the salivary glands. Thus, sweating occurs instead of salivation in response to the sight, smell, or taste of food. Brown-Séquard did not have Frey's syndrome, but he reported in 1849 his tendency to sweat profusely when eating spicy foods,[32] and this may well have helped later authors understand the nature of the moisture appearing on the face in similar circumstances but after facial injury.

Work on the Respiratory System

It is not necessary to review every facet of Brown-Séquard's work on the respiratory system and related areas, which included studies to compare in different animal species the resistance to asphyxia[33] and the duration of survival after ablation of the medulla at the base of the brain.[34] The main areas on which he focused were important, however, and merit examination.

Pulmonary Edema

Pulmonary edema—the presence of fluid in the lungs—is a serious medical disorder that interferes with gas exchange between the atmosphere and the body. It arises most often in patients with heart or lung disease. Its manifestations may include cough, shortness of breath, rapid shallow breathing, wheezing, chest tightness or discomfort, frothy pink sputum, cyanosis, cold extremities, an increased heart rate, and low blood pressure. Deterioration may occur rapidly, and a fatal outcome sometimes follows. The sudden development of pulmonary edema and congestion within a few minutes or hours of damage to the central nervous system is called *neurogenic pulmonary edema*.

In the 1870s, Brown-Séquard described the clinical phenomenology and pathology of neurogenic pulmonary edema in humans and studied it experimentally in animals. He stressed specifically that death in patients with certain neurological disorders could result from inflammation or edema of the lungs.[35]

> I found, a year ago, that one of the most frequent causes of death, when it does not occur immediately or very soon after wounds of the brain, in guinea pigs especially, was pneumonia .... The results obtained were startling; in almost all

cases of injuries by crushing or section of the pons Varolii ecchymoses [bruising and bleeding] were found in the lungs. Sometimes the whole lung was crowded with effused blood, and real pulmonary apoplexy existed .... A haemorrhage is not the only immediate effect that can be observed after an irritation of the base of the brain by crushing or cutting: an anaemic condition, oedema, and emphysema can also be produced. Some small parts of the lungs are found perfectly white, and, according to the examination of a distinguished micrographer, M. Ranvier, who has kindly helped me in some of these researches, absolutely deprived of blood, no doubt through a spasm of the blood vessels having emptied them of their contents. This may occur after injuries of almost all the parts of the base of the brain, but especially the pons Varolii. Not so as regards oedema, which principally appears after an injury to the medulla oblongata ... in man, diseases of or injuries to the brain very frequently produce organic alterations in the lungs.[36]

His observations received little or no notice. The importance of severe (often fatal) pulmonary edema after major head injuries or other acute intracranial lesions only came to be appreciated during the twentieth century, and the contributions and detailed descriptions of earlier investigators are generally overlooked by those studying the phenomenon.

Thus, it was almost forty years after the publication of Brown-Séquard's work that Shanahan, in 1908, reported the occurrence of acute pulmonary edema after generalized convulsions in several patients, four of whom died; autopsies in two were confirmatory.[37] Two years later, Ohlmacher reported on a large series of patients who died after one or more convulsions with clinically evident pulmonary edema, confirmed in some instances by postmortem examination.[38] Its occurrence in this context has since come to be widely accepted and may account for some of the cases of sudden unexplained death that occur in patients with epilepsy.[39] Moutier subsequently reported the occurrence of neurogenic pulmonary edema among soldiers with head wounds sustained in the trenches during World War I,[40] and it is now known that it may also develop abruptly after subarachnoid or intracranial hemorrhage, stroke, tumors, increased intracranial pressure, or other acute intracranial pathology, as well as after spinal trauma.[41,42] Moutier postulated that it was caused by a massive release of epinephrine due to stimulation by the brain,[40] and subsequent experimental and clinical work has provided support for this view.

Clinical and experimental evidence suggests that neurogenic pulmonary edema relates to involvement of the brainstem, in particular, the medulla, just as Brown-Séquard had forecast. Among patients with cerebral hemorrhage in various locations, for example, those with brainstem hemorrhage are most likely to develop pulmonary edema, and among patients with bulbar poliomyelitis, those with medullary involvement are most prone to it.[43] Within the medulla, the critical area may be the so-called nucleus tractus solitarius, a structure that receives input for the vagus nerves (which supply sensory input from the heart and lungs and from the pressure sensors—baroreceptors—in certain major blood vessels).

The underlying cause of neurogenic pulmonary edema is uncertain. One view is that it results from a primary increase in permeability of the capillaries in the lungs that may occur independently of any increase in pressure in the pulmonary blood vessels. The other view relates it to a direct hydrostatic mechanism, such as an increase in pulmonary arterial pressure or marked pulmonary venoconstriction. A massive sympathetic discharge from the brain, and in particular from the hypothalamus, is said to lead to peripheral vasoconstriction, an increase in systemic blood pressure, and thus a diversion of blood to the low-resistance pulmonary circulation, causing an increase in pulmonary vascular pressure and a leakage of fluid from the capillaries into the lungs. In fact, both mechanisms may operate, as a sudden rise in pulmonary vascular pressure may itself lead to increased capillary permeability.

His experimental studies in animals had led Brown-Séquard to suggest that neurogenic pulmonary edema depends on the integrity of the sympathetic (or vasomotor) system,[36,44] and this view has been vindicated and is reflected by the manner in which it is now treated. Its importance came to be appreciated during the latter half of the twentieth century, and measures to block the related pathological sympathetic discharge (with alpha-adrenergic blockers) then became important in its management.[45]

Breathing (Ventilation)

Legallois[C] is generally credited with first suggesting, in 1812, that a region responsible for the regulation and rhythm of respiratory movements existed in the medulla, at the base of the brain. This concept was advanced further by

---

[C] Julien Jean César Legallois (1770–1814), French experimental physiologist who was the first to localize a center for respiration and was reportedly the first to show by experiment that a region within a major part of the brain had a specific function of its own. He emphasized the importance of the central nervous system in the functioning of the heart and lungs and believed that artificial (extracorporeal) circulation could enable parts of the body to be preserved and retain their function. His work on the circulation and respiration in fetuses and the newborn was not published until some six years after he first made it known because he was "more careful in ascertaining the facts than eager to publish them."

Flourens (see footnote G, Chapter 10) in the middle of the nineteenth century, when he localized the respiratory center (or *noeud vital*) to a discrete region (the size of the head of a pin) in the medulla by lesion experiments.[46] Since then, the medullary location of the generator of respiratory movements has been accepted widely, although how it operates and its connectivity have remained unsettled. During the latter part of the nineteenth century, two views emerged regarding the control of respiratory movements. One held that this control was primarily through neural connections, with input passing from the muscles of breathing to the medulla, from which the respiratory center influenced the activity of these muscles. The other view emphasized the influence of chemicals, especially carbon dioxide, on the activity of the medullary respiratory center.[47] It is now known, of course, that both neural and chemical mechanisms are operative.

Brown-Séquard was one of the few physiologists contemporaneous with Flourens who questioned his conclusion that respiratory movements depend solely on the respiratory center in the medulla, claiming that he had sometimes observed rhythmic respiratory movements in decapitated birds, kittens, and puppies (in whom the influence of any medullary centers would have been abolished) and implying that other central structures must therefore *also* be capable of generating the rhythmic pattern characteristic of respiration.[48] Such inconvenient observations were ignored, misunderstood by some who suggested that he had described respiratory centers in the spinal cord,[49] or explained away by others who claimed, for example, that all he had observed were terminal asphyxial movements.[50]

A number of studies have confirmed Brown-Séquard's observations that rhythmic respiratory activity may occur for a variable period in certain decapitated animals, including young mammals. To explain such findings, it has been suggested that the respiratory generator in the medulla may extend into the upper segments of the spinal cord or that a spinal generator does exist, distinct from that in the brainstem, and, under certain circumstances, permits a rhythmic respiratory movement to occur in animals whose spinal cord has been transected completely in the upper cervical region.[51-53]

Brown-Séquard's concept of the neural regulation of breathing also receives some support from more recent work. Most authors have used the designation "respiratory center" to refer to a discrete structure that is presumed to coordinate and integrate the various excitatory and inhibitory pathways that influence respiratory movements, thereby matching the respiratory pattern to the ongoing metabolic and behavioral demands. The ongoing metabolic (chemical) drive and behavioral demands may, however, be integrated in the spinal cord at a segmental level to determine the final output of respiratory motor neurons and thus the respiratory pattern.[54,55] Inputs to the motor neurons that innervate inspiratory or expiratory muscles converge on the spinal cord from different regions of the brain, including the cerebral cortex and brainstem (where neurons driving inspiration and expiration are located especially in the medulla) and also from the periphery. These inputs pass to an interneuronal network in the spinal cord, such that when the inspiratory motor neurons are to be excited, the expiratory neurons are reciprocally inhibited, and vice versa, as detailed elsewhere.[54-56] Such a view is not entirely dissimilar to that contemplated by Brown-Séquard, who concluded, on the basis of his own experiments, a review of the previously published work of others, and his clinical experience of patients with brainstem hemorrhage that

> the respiratory movements do not depend only upon the medulla oblongata … [they] depend upon all the incito-motory parts of the cerebro-spinal axis, and on the gray matter which connects those parts with the motor nerves going to the respiratory muscles … excitations coming from all parts of the body, as shown by Volkmann and Vierordt, and also direct irritations of the base of the encephalon and of the spinal cord, almost constantly taking place, contribute to the production of respiratory movements.[48]

Toxicity of Expired Air

In the latter half of the nineteenth century, increasing evidence seemed to suggest that the expired air contained toxic substances that were detrimental to health. Expired air does, of course, contain carbon dioxide, but it was not on this—but on something additional—that attention was focused in the scientific laboratories of several European countries. Brown-Séquard and d'Arsonval investigated this possibility in guinea pigs and rabbits because of concern that it may be relevant in patients with pulmonary tuberculosis, who often seemed to live in poorly ventilated, overcrowded conditions.[57] They attempted to concentrate the suspected toxins by washing the pulmonary mucous membranes with distilled water or collecting the liquid condensed by cold from the breath.[58-60] These solutions containing the supposed toxins were then injected subcutaneously or directly into the circulation. The animals developed signs of respiratory difficulty, with labored breathing, and died soon after in obvious distress; the duration of survival declining as the dose was increased[61]; the liquid retained its toxicity even after boiling, so an infective cause seemed unlikely.[59] Brown-Séquard and his faithful assistant also made animals breathe air contaminated by the expired gases of other animals.[62] They arranged a series of boxes or cages, each containing a rabbit or some other small animal;

a continuous current of air was then passed through the boxes so that it became more "toxic" as it left each box. In other words, the animal in the first box was exposed to fresh air, but those in the succeeding boxes were exposed to increasingly impure or "toxic" air. The experiment was such that the carbon dioxide content of the air in the last boxes was kept constant.[62] Nevertheless, the rabbits in the last boxes in the series nearly all died rapidly with similar symptoms. If, however, the current of air was passed over pumice stone soaked in sulfuric acid to absorb any organic matter (without change in oxygen and carbon dioxide content) before it was passed into the last boxes, the animals survived. They therefore concluded that the expired air did indeed contain a volatile toxin.

Others were unable to replicate these findings. Haldane[D] and Smith, in England, performed comparable experiments using both the injection technique and the ventilation method, but found no "disturbance of health" attributable to a toxin in expired air. They therefore were unable to confirm Brown-Séquard's conclusions, whose findings remain difficult to explain.[63] One possibility is that the observed toxic effects were related to ammonia derived from the fecal and urinary excretions of the animals used in the experiments, although Brown-Séquard considered this possibility and claimed to have excluded it.[64] In any event, this work is now largely forgotten although, at the time, it seemed to have important implications for public health.

Reflex Paraplegia

In his lectures of 1859, Brown-Séquard marshalled clinical evidence in support of the concept of reflex paraplegia, a speculative diagnosis that was widely accepted in the early and middle of the nineteenth century, but discarded in the 1880s and thereafter.[65] Many of his illustrious predecessors and contemporary colleagues (including Graves, Gull, Stokes, Rayer, Cruveilhier, Chomel, Charcot, and Romberg) had published accounts of the disorder. It was

---

[D] John Scott Haldane (1860–1936), Scottish physiologist, was in the words of his obituarist in the *Canadian Medical Association Journal*, "...a super-man and a member of a super-family. The late Professor Sir John Burdon Sanderson was his uncle; Viscount Haldane of Cloan and Sir W.S. Haldane, W.S., were brothers; Miss Elizabeth Haldane, C.H., was a sister; J.B.S. Haldane, F.R.S., professor of genetics in the University of London, is his son; and Mrs. Naoli Mitchison, a well-known novelist, is his daughter." He studied the control of respiration and the role of carbon dioxide in its regulation. He also investigated mine disasters, studied the toxicity of carbon monoxide, and introduced the canary to detect dangerous levels of the gas in mines. He invented the prototype of the gas mask used by British troops in World War I.

characterized by weakness or paralysis of the legs occurring in relation to disease of various organs (such as the uterus, urethra, bladder, prostate, kidneys, bowels, or lungs) or to a variety of other circumstances, without any evidence of a lesion directly affecting the spinal cord, which was typically normal at autopsy. In contrast to cases with more definite evidence of cord involvement, there was usually little or no pain, sensory disturbance, sphincter impairment, or muscle wasting. The concept did not originate with Brown-Séquard, who simply tried to find an explanation for it and came to believe that a reflex constriction affected the blood vessels to the cord and perhaps also those to the nerves or muscles.

Reflex paraplegia is no longer regarded as a diagnostic entity. Some cases may have been examples of polyneuritis,[66] whereas in others any association of leg weakness with external factors was probably coincidental. Almost certainly, the diagnosis was often made to account for otherwise inexplicable cases of paraplegia, some of which today would probably be attributed to ischemic or inflammatory involvement of the spinal cord. On reviewing the published cases, however, it is difficult to escape the conclusion that in most instances the cause of the weakness was nonorganic, as suggested by the lack of any objective neurological signs other than weakness and by the rapidity with which recovery accompanied cure of the primary condition, regardless of whether it was uterine prolapse, a bladder infection, or some external irritation.[65]

The reason that Brown-Séquard upheld the existence of an entity lacking any convincing scientific foundation is uncertain. It may be that it appealed to him because it brought together his views on the importance of reflex actions and on the neural control of blood vessels, but the degree to which he championed this notion remains surprising.

Pyramidotomy

The cerebral cortex and certain other regions of the brain influence the activity of the spinal cord, affecting both the sensory input that passes from the periphery to the brain or is processed in the spinal cord, and also the motor or efferent output of the spinal cord to the muscles and other effector structures. The motor fibers descending from the brain to the spinal cord traverse the brainstem. A major component—derived predominantly if not exclusively from the motor and other areas of the cerebral cortex—passes through the protruding columns (or pyramids) at the front of the medulla. These fibers constitute the "pyramidal" or corticospinal fibers. Most are "crossed"; that is, they pass from one side to the other in the medulla, to travel in the lateral funiculus of the spinal cord. Thus, corticospinal fibers from the right hemisphere pass mainly (but not exclusively) to the left side of the spinal cord to influence the activity of the left side of the body. Some corticospinal fibers descend without crossing, however, and these travel mainly in the anterior funiculus of the spinal cord.

It was Brown-Séquard—in 1889—who first performed pyramidotomies in animals.[67,68] He cut the pyramids on both sides in the medulla, leaving the rest of the brainstem largely intact, and found that stimulation of the cerebral cortex elicited limb movements almost as powerful as before the transection. He thus showed that some motor fibers must take other routes to the spinal cord, and these fibers came to make up what was subsequently called the *extrapyramidal system*. His experimental approach has been widely used by others to study the anatomy of the motor pathways and to determine the clinical consequences of discrete central lesions destroying them. The distinction between the pyramidal and extrapyramidal systems is somewhat artificial, however, because they operate in concert and are interconnected. Nevertheless, it has been useful clinically and is now hallowed by tradition. Clinical neurologists thus speak of a "pyramidal lesion," that is, a lesion involving the corticospinal fibers or their cells of origin (which are erroneously believed to be restricted to the motor cortex) or of a "pyramidal deficit" (the supposed neurological consequences of a pyramidal lesion). The clinical features of a pyramidal deficit typically include stiffness (spasticity), weakness, brisk muscle stretch reflexes, and a Babinski sign[E] on the affected side. In fact, this is a convenient fiction, as these clinical stigmata reflect lesions involving many other structures in the central nervous system than simply the pyramidal tract. Moreover, the pyramidal tract is not a homogeneous system although, unlike other connections between the cerebral cortex and spinal cord, it is a direct nonstop pathway without synaptic interruption and thus allows more immediate control by the cortex on spinal mechanisms.[69] The attempt to relate specific symptoms and signs to lesions in isolated parts of the nervous system has been somewhat misleading, and it was something that Brown-Séquard warned against when he opposed the doctrine of cortical localization of function (Chapter 10), even though he too fell into exactly the same trap when he wrote about the functional consequences of lesions or injuries to particular parts of the nervous system.

[E] See footnote P, Chapter 12.

Perfusion Experiments

Brown-Séquard's famous—or, as some would say, infamous—perfusion experiments have fascinated many people, perhaps because of their grisly nature and because they attempted to answer questions that few people dared pose. Can a head, separated from a body, think and feel emotions if its circulation is maintained? Can a part of an otherwise dead body be kept alive by irrigating it with fresh blood? Brown-Séquard's work on this topic was important because it had some bearing on the later development of cardiopulmonary bypass procedures and the management of patients with traumatic amputation of a limb or digit.

His initial experiments revealed that perfusing the extremity of a recently killed animal with fresh blood (so as to restore an effective circulation) led to reversal of rigor mortis and the return of mechanical responses to stimulation of muscles or their motor nerves.[21] His initial approach was to connect one animal to the circulatory apparatus in another.

> On the body of a rabbit, in which cadaveric rigidity had already existed for 10, 20, and in one case, 33 minutes, I divided the aorta and the vena cava in the abdomen [i.e., the main artery taking blood from the heart, and main vein returning blood to the heart] .... By means of small tubes, a communication was established between ... [them] and the corresponding vessels divided in a living rabbit. The blood of this living animal circulated immediately in the posterior [hind] limbs of the dead one. After about six, eight, or ten minutes, rigidity disappeared, and, a few minutes afterwards, movements took place when I excited the muscles or the muscular nerves.[21]

He took to injecting blood into the regional circulation of limbs separated from the body of rabbits and found that he was able to reverse rigor mortis and maintain the muscles in an excitable state. However,

> It is nearly indifferent in these experiments whether we use venous or arterial blood; but it is absolutely necessary to employ red blood, i.e. oxygenated blood .... I have tried, sometimes, arterial blood rendered black by the substitution of nitrogen or hydrogen for a great part of its oxygen, and I have found that such blood was unable to reproduce the vital properties of nerves and muscles .... Oxygen is necessary ....[21]

He undertook similar experiments in humans, working on the bodies of executed criminals. In June 1851, for example, he infused blood into the arm of a 20-year-old man who had been guillotined some thirteen hours earlier.[21,22] He wished to inject human blood and, because he could not obtain it from a hospital because of the lateness of the hour, he used his own blood. About "half a pound" of his blood was taken and immediately beaten vigorously and then filtered through a cloth to remove any clots. By beating the blood in this way, he both ensured it was oxygenated and prevented it from clotting any further by defibrinating it. It was injected at room temperature rather than at normal body temperature. The arm had been severed from the body and the injection was made over about ten minutes into the radial artery just above the wrist. As the blood flowed out from the severed vessels, it was collected and reinjected, so that the total perfusion time was about forty-five minutes. Ten minutes later, rigor mortis had disappeared from the irrigated hand and all but two of its nineteen muscles had regained their contractile properties.

He experimented on another guillotined criminal, but this time used fresh blood from a dog. Again, rigor mortis disappeared and muscles became excitable. Subsequent experiments were designed to determine how long a limb, separated from the body of an animal, may be kept alive by irrigating it with blood. He was able to maintain "local life in one of the limbs of a rabbit [for] more than 41 hours."[21] He also showed that perfusion with serum, milk, or the albumen of eggs had no effect.

Finally, he examined the effect of injecting oxygenated blood into the four major arteries carrying blood to the head of a decapitated dog in which all movement had ceased.[70,71] Two or three minutes later, movements of the eyes and muzzle returned and looked volitional in nature.

It is clear, at least today, that the tissues of the body do not all die at the same time, and that the brain is particularly sensitive to arrest of the circulation or a lack of oxygen. Brown-Séquard found that when the circulation of oxygenated blood to the brain was interrupted in dogs by compressing the four arteries to the head, the animals died; restoration of the circulation within two to four minutes, but not after five minutes, allowed the dogs to recover.[70]

Vulpian (see footnote A, p. 85), then an associate professor, in his textbook of physiology, referred to Brown-Séquard's experiment in which he perfused the isolated head of a dog with oxygenated blood and obtained the return of eye and facial movements. He went on to comment

> If a physiologist were to attempt this experiment on the head of a guillotined person, several moments after death, he would perhaps take part in a great and terrible spectacle. Perhaps he could return to the head the functions of its brain, and return to its eyes and facial muscles movements which, in humans, are provoked by their feelings and thoughts ....[72]

The work also had an impact on the science fiction of the period. In George Eliot's complicated novella, *The Lifted Veil*, published in 1859, Charles Meunier, a scientist modeled on Brown-Séquard,[73] perfuses a dead maid with his own blood so that she briefly comes back to life and accuses her mistress of a plot to poison her husband. Weir Mitchell (see Chapter 8), the eminent neurologist, writer, and friend of Brown-Séquard, was also taken by the idea in a short story—"Was He Dead?"—published in the *Atlantic Monthly* in January 1870. The corpse of a criminal is revived by pumping blood through his brain, and the dead man then confesses to the brutal murder of a woman for which an innocent man has already been executed.

Nevertheless, Brown-Séquard's work on perfusion did not receive immediate or general acceptance when first it was published, and its gruesome nature caused a certain revulsion and anger among the general public.[74] It was, however, among several other notable contributions that were cited by the committee of the Académie des Sciences that recommended the award to him of the prestigious Prix Lacaze in 1881.[75] Indeed, he had made several important observations, namely that the viability of tissue can be maintained by extracorporeal circulation, that the blood used to perfuse it has to be oxygenated, and that the blood does not need to be at body temperature. These were essential concepts, for which he deserves great credit, with regard to the later development of cardiopulmonary bypass procedures.[76] From then on, it was clear that ensuring an adequate supply of oxygen to the blood was necessary for perfusion to be successful, and this was to be a difficult problem when a cardiopulmonary bypass device came to be constructed.

Work similar to that of Brown-Séquard's was subsequently undertaken on humans by Jean Baptiste Vincent Laborde,[F] who tried in 1884 to revive the heads of guillotined convicts by perfusing them with blood. It is said that one of his objectives was to determine whether guillotined heads were aware, if only transiently, of their bodiless situation.[77,78] Apparently, no signs of consciousness appeared, although some movements occurred about the face. A more systematic study was attempted by the French physician, Paul Loye (1861–1890), who guillotined a number of dogs and studied their responses, but with similar results. There appeared to be no signs of canine consciousness, despite some activation of the facial muscles. There matters rested until the 1920s, when Brukhonenko, a respected Soviet physiologist, maintained the isolated head of a dog alive for some three hours using a heart-lung

---

[F] Jean Baptiste Vincent Laborde (1831–1903), French physician and physiologist, developed a method of resuscitating asphyxiated persons by rhythmical pulling on the tongue and was also a strong advocate of temperance.

machine that he had developed for total body perfusion.[G] The head apparently reacted to the environment, licked its lips, opened its mouth, and even swallowed some cheese placed within it.[76] People were excited or appalled by the experiment. George Bernard Shaw, the playwright, is said to have imagined this as a means of preserving the brains of brilliant professors whose bodies are beginning to fall apart and even to have mused, one hopes ironically, about the temptation "to have my own head cut off so that I can continue to dictate plays and books without being bothered by illness, without having to dress and undress, without having to eat, without having anything else to do ...."[78]

Other work was not so successful. It included the transplantation of a head onto an intact animal, which therefore ended up with two heads, or the transplantation of both the head and upper torso onto an intact animal.[H] The resulting grotesque monsters generated a certain horrified fascination, but the transplanted brain was almost certainly either dead or badly damaged by ischemia or anoxia. Then, in the early 1970s, Robert White and his associates in the neurosurgery department at the Cleveland Metropolitan General Hospital reported the successful transplantation of the isolated head of one monkey onto the headless body of another, with "normalization of cerebral function"— in three to four hours, each transplanted head showed what they regarded as evidence of external awareness by accepting and attempting to chew food placed in the mouth and tracking with the eyes objects placed in the visual fields.[79,80] Although the possibility of extending such work to humans was raised, the public outcry that followed its announcement limited its further development. Moreover, it raised many ethical and moral issues, including those relating to the nature of personal identity. In the future, head transplants might be of more clinical relevance if and when the technology is developed to repair the resulting damage to the spinal cord, so that the new brain is functionally connected to the rest of the body.

[G] Sergei Sergeevich Brukhonenko (1890–1960) designed one of the first heart-lung machines and was the first to perform a total body perfusion with the heart of the animal isolated from the circulation. An account of his work can be found in Konstantinov IE, Alexi-Meskishvili VV. Sergei S. Brukhonenko: the development of the first heart-lung machine for total body perfusion. *Ann Thorac Surg*, 69: 962–966, 2000.

[H] Among those who undertook such work was the French experimental surgeon Alexis Carrel (1873–1944), who went on to receive the Nobel Prize for Medicine or Physiology in 1912 for his work on the transplantation of tissues and organs and on the anastomosis (joining together) of blood vessels.

References and Source Notes

1. Brown-Séquard CE. *Course of lectures on the physiology and pathology of the central nervous system* (pp. 195–196). Philadelphia: Collins, 1860.
2. Brown-Séquard E. Recherches expérimentales concernant l'action de la lumière et celle d'un changement de température sur l'iris, dans les cinq classes d'animaux vertébrés. *C R Acad Sci*, 25:482–483, and 508, 1847.
3. Brown-Séquard E. Note complémentaire d'un mémoire sur l'action de la lumière et d'un changement de température sur l'iris. *C R Acad Sci*, 25:508–510, 1847.
4. Brown-Séquard E. Recherches expérimentales sur l'influence excitatrice de la lumière, du froid et de la chaleur sur l'iris, dans les cinq classes d'animaux vertébrés. *J Physiol*, 2:281–294, 1859.
5. Brown-Séquard E. On the causes of the torpidity of the tenrec, (*Erinaceus ecaudatus*, Linn.). *Med Exam (Philadelphia)*, 8:549–550, 1852. [*Experimental researches applied to physiology and pathology* (pp. 25–26). New York: Bailliere, 1853.]
6. Comroe JH Jr. Retroscope: Feet on the ground?? *Am Rev Respir Dis*, 112:251–253, 1975.
7. Thorpy MJ. History of sleep medicine. In: Aminoff MJ, Boller F, Swaab DF, eds., *Handbook of clinical neurology*, in press.
8. Brown-Séquard C. Le sommeil normal, comme le sommeil hypnotique, est le résultat d'une inhibition de l'activité intellectuelle. *Arch Physiol Norm Pathol (5th Series)*, 1:333–335, 1889.
9. Heubel E. Ueber die Abhangigkeit des wachen Gehirnzustandes von ausseren Erregungen. *Pfluger's Arch*, 14:158–210, 1876.
10. Pavlov IP. Internal inhibition and sleep as one and the same process with regard to their intimate mechanism. Lecture XV. In: Pavlov IP, *Conditioned reflexes: an investigation of the physiological activity of the cerebral cortex* [Trans. Anrep GV]. London: Oxford University Press, 1927.
11. Brown-Séquart [sic]. Recherches sur la rigidité cadavérique et la putréfaction. *C R Soc Biol (Paris)*, 1:39–40, 1849.
12. Brown-Séquard E. Influence de l'électro-magnétisme et de la foudre sur la durée de la rigidité cadavérique. *C R Soc Biol (Paris)*, 1:138–140, 1849.
13. Brown-Séquard E. Sur la mort par la foudre et par l'électro-magnétisme. *C R Soc Biol (Paris)*, 1:154–156, 1849.
14. Brown-Séquard E. Des rapports qui existent entre l'irritabilité musculaire, la rigidité cadavérique et la putréfaction. *C R Soc Biol (Paris)*, 1:173–174, 1849.
15. Brown-Séquard E. Apparition de la rigidité cadavérique avant la cessation des battements du coeur. *C R Soc Biol (Paris)*, 2:194–195, 1850.
16. Brown-Séquard E. Recherches sur les lois de l'irritabilité musculaire, de la rigidité cadavérique et de la putréfaction. *C R Acad Sci*, 45:460–464, 1857.
17. Brown-Séquard CE. On the relations between muscular irritability, cadaveric rigidity, and putrefaction. [The Croonian Lecture.] *Proc R Soc Lond*, 11: 204–214, 1861.
18. Brown-Séquard CE. Attitudes after death. *Knowledge*, 6:115–117, 1884.
19. Brown-Séquard E. On a singular case of animal graft. *Med Exam (Philadelphia)*, 8:560–561, 1852. [*Experimental researches applied to physiology and pathology* (p. 36). New York: Bailliere, 1853.]
20. Taylor WH. Old days at the old college. *Old Dominion J Med Surg*, 17:57–100, 1913.
21. Brown-Séquard E. Influence of red blood on muscles and nerves deprived of their vital properties. *Med Exam (Philadelphia)*, 9:280–288, 1853. [*Experimental researches applied to physiology and pathology* (pp. 88–95). New York: Bailliere, 1853.]
22. Brown-Séquard E. Recherches sur le rétablissement de l'irritabilité musculaire chez un supplicié. *C R Acad Sci*, 32:897–902, 1851.

23. Brown-Séquard CE. Des effets produits chez l'homme par des injections sous-cutanées d'un liquide retiré des testicules frais de cobaye et de chien. *C R Soc Biol (Paris)*, 41:415–419, 1889.
24. Brown-Séquard CE. On a new mode of treatment of functional dyspepsia, anaemia, and chlorosis. *Arch Sci Pract Med (NY)*, 1:30–33, 1873.
25. Rouget FA. *Brown-Séquard et son oeuvre. Esquisse biographique* (pp. 15–20). Port-Louis, Ile Maurice: General Printing & Stationery Co., 1930.
26. Taylor WH. Old days at the old college. *Old Dominion J Med Surg*, 17:57–100, 1913.
27. Brown-Séquard E. On the influence of poisons upon animal heat as a cause of death. *Med Exam (Philadelphia)*, 8:550–553, 1852. [*Experimental researches applied to physiology and pathology* (pp. 26–28). New York: Bailliere, 1853.]
28. Brown-Séquard E. On the normal degree of the temperature in man. *Med Exam (Philadelphia)*, 8:554–556, 1852. [*Experimental researches applied to physiology and pathology* (pp. 30–32). New York: Bailliere, 1853.]
29. Brown-Séquard CE. Expériences démontrant que les poils peuvent passer rapidement du noir au blanc, chez l'homme. *Arch Physiol Norm Pathol*, 2:442–443, 1869.
30. Dulguerov P, Marchal F, Gysin C. Frey syndrome before Frey: the correct history. *Laryngoscope*, 109:1471–1473, 1999.
31. Frey L. Le syndrome du nerf auriculo-temporal. *Rev Neurol*, 2:92–104, 1923.
32. Brown-Séquard CE. Production de sueur sous l'influence d'une excitation vive des nerfs du goût. *C R Soc Biol (Paris)*, 1:104, 1849.
33. Brown-Séquard CE. On the influence of the temperature of a warm-blooded animal upon the duration of its life when it is asphyxiated. *Med Exam (Philadelphia)*, 8:617–626, 1852. [*Experimental researches applied to physiology and pathology* (pp. 45–54). New York: Bailliere, 1853.]
34. Brown-Séquard CE. On the persistence of life in animals deprived of their medulla oblongata. *Med Exam (Philadelphia)*, 8:565–569, 1852. [*Experimental researches applied to physiology and pathology* (pp. 40–45). New York: Bailliere, 1853.]
35. Brown-Séquard CE. Faits demontrant que la mort, dans les affections cérébrales, peut être due à ce qu'elles ont produit des lésions pulmonaires. *C R Soc Biol (Paris)*, 23:101–102, 1871. [This is the subject matter, as documented by Brown-Séquard and shown in the Appendix, of a presentation by him that has no formal published title.]
36. Brown-Séquard CE. On the production of haemorrhage, anaemia, oedema, and emphysema in the lungs by injuries to the base of the brain. *Lancet*, 1:6, 1871.
37. Shanahan WT. Acute pulmonary oedema as a complication of epileptic seizures. *NY Med J*, 87:54–56, 1908.
38. Ohlmacher AP. Acute pulmonary oedema as a terminal event in certain forms of epilepsy. *Am J Med Sci*, 139:417–422, 1910.
39. Terrence CF, Rao GR, Perper JA. Neurogenic pulmonary edema in unexpected, unexplained death of epileptic patients. *Ann Neurol*, 9:458–464, 1981.
40. Moutier F. Hypertension et mort par oedème pulmonaire aigu, chez les blessés cranio-encéphaliques. *Presse Med*, 26:108–109, 1918.
41. Simon RP. Breathing and the nervous system. In: Aminoff MJ, ed., *Neurology and general medicine* (4th ed., pp. 1–21). Philadelphia: Elsevier, 2008.
42. Paine R, Smith JR, Howard FA. Pulmonary edema in patients dying with disease of the central nervous system. *JAMA*, 149:643–646, 1952.
43. Brown RH Jr, Beyerl BD, Iseke R, Lavyne MH. Medulla oblongata edema associated with neurogenic pulmonary edema. *J Neurosurg*, 64:494–500, 1986.
44. Brown-Séquard CE. Faits nouveaux contre l'opinion que c'est par une action du nerf vague que se produisent les ecchymoses pulmonaires dans les lésions cérébrales.

C R Soc Biol (Paris), 24:181, 1872. [This is the subject matter, as documented by Brown-Séquard and shown in the Appendix, of a presentation by him that has no formal published title.]

45. Norris JW. Cardiovascular manifestations of acute neurological lesions. In: Aminoff MJ, ed., *Neurology and general medicine* (pp. 159–167). New York: Churchill Livingstone, 1989.
46. Olmsted JMD. Historical note on the noeud vital or respiratory center. *Bull Hist Med*, 16:343–350, 1944.
47. Allen GE. J.S. Haldane: the development of the idea of control mechanisms in respiration. *J Hist Med Allied Sci*, 22:392–412, 1967.
48. Brown-Séquard CE. *Course of lectures on the physiology and pathology of the central nervous system* (pp. 187–192). Philadelphia: Collins, 1860.
49. Evans CL. *Starling's principles of human physiology*, 6th edition. Philadelphia: Lea & Febiger, 1933.
50. Olmsted JMD. *Charles-Édouard Brown-Séquard. A nineteenth century neurologist and endocrinologist* (pp. 114–115). Baltimore: Johns Hopkins Press, 1946.
51. Viala D, Freton E. Evidence for respiratory and locomotor pattern generators in the rabbit cervico-thoracic cord and their interactions. *Exp Brain Res*, 49:247–256, 1983.
52. Coglianese CJ, Peiss CN, Wurster RD. Rhythmic phrenic nerve activity and respiratory activity in spinal dogs. *Resp Physiol*, 29:247–254, 1977.
53. Aoki M, Mori S, Kawahara K, Watanabe H, Ebata N. Generation of spontaneous respiratory rhythm in high spinal cat. *Brain Res*, 202:51–63, 1980.
54. Sears TA. Spinal integration of the command for respiratory movements. *Exp Brain Res Suppl*, 9:86–94, 1984.
55. Sears TA. Central rhythm generation and spinal integration. *Chest*, 97:45S–51S, 1990.
56. Aminoff MJ, Sears TA. Spinal integration of segmental, cortical and breathing inputs to thoracic respiratory motoneurones. *J Physiol*, 215:557–575, 1971.
57. Brown-Sequard CE, d'Arsonval A. Recherches sur l'importance, surtout pour les phtisiques, d'un air non vicié par des exhalaisons pulmonaires. *C R Acad Sci*, 105:1056–1060, 1887.
58. Brown-Sequard CE, d'Arsonval A. Nouvelles recherches sur les phénomènes produits par un agent toxique très puissant qui sort sans cesse des poumons de l'homme et des mammifères, avec l'air expiré. *C R Acad Sci*, 106:165–169, 1888.
59. Brown-Sequard CE, d'Arsonval A. Nouvelles recherches démontrant que les poumons sécrètent un poison extrêmement violent qui en sort avec l'air expiré. *C R Soc Biol (Paris)*, 40:33–37, 1888.
60. Brown-Séquard CE, d'Arsonval A. Recherches démontrant que l'air expiré par l'homme et les mammifères, à l'état de santé, contient un agent toxique très puissant. *C R Acad Sci*, 106:106–112, 1888.
61. Brown-Sequard CE, d'Arsonval A. Sur quelques points importants relatifs à la durée de la survie des lapins après l'injection sous-cutanée du liquide contenant le poison de l'air expiré. *C R Soc Biol (Paris)*, 40:151–153, 1888.
62. Brown-Sequard CE, d'Arsonval A. Description d'un appareil permettant de faire respirer à plusieurs animaux de l'air libre et pur quant à ses proportions d'oxygène et d'acide carbonique, mais contenant des quantités considérables du poison de l'air expiré. *C R Soc Biol (Paris)*, 40:110–111, 1888.
63. Haldane J, Smith JL. The physiological effects of air vitiated by respiration. *J Path Bact*, 1:168–186, 1892.
64. Brown-Séquard CE, d'Arsonval A. Recherches montrant que la mort par inhalation du poison que contient l'air expiré n'est pas activée par les émanations de vapeurs

provenant de l'urine et des matières fécales des animaux soumis à cette inhalation. *C R Acad Sci*, 108:1294–1296, 1889.
65. Brown-Séquard E. *Lectures on the diagnosis and treatment of the principal forms of paralysis of the lower extremities* (pp. 5–56). Philadelphia: Collins, 1861.
66. Spillane JD. *The doctrine of the nerves: Chapters in the history of neurology* (pp. 331–332). Oxford: Oxford University Press, 1981.
67. Albanese A. Extrapyramidal system and extrapyramidal disorders. In: Rose FC, ed., *Neuroscience across the centuries* (pp. 97–109). London: Smith-Gordon, 1989.
68. Brown-Séquard CE. Expériences montrant combien est grande la dissémination des voies motrices dans le bulbe rachidien. *Arch Physiol Norm Pathol (5th Series)*, 1:606–608, 1889.
69. Brodal A. *Neurological anatomy in relation to clinical medicine* (2nd ed., pp. 151–254). New York: Oxford University Press, 1969.
70. Brown-Sequard CE. Recherches expérimentales sur les propriétés physiologiques et les usages du sang rouge et du sang noir, et de leurs principaux éléments gazeux, l'oxygène et l'acide carbonique. *J Physiol (Paris)*, 1:95–122, 353–367, and 729–735, 1858.
71. Brown-Sequard CE. Recherches expérimentales sur les propriétés et les usages du sang rouge et du sang noir. *C R Acad Sci*, 45:562–566, 1857.
72. Vulpian A. *Leçons sur la physiologie générale et comparée du système nerveux faites au Muséum d'Histoire Naturelle* (pp. 458–460). Paris: Baillière, 1866.
73. Flint K. Blood, bodies, and *The Lifted Veil*. *Nineteenth Century Lit*, 51:455–473, 1997.
74. Janin J. Monstrueuse enterprise d'un docteur en médecine, etc. Feuilleton *du Journal des Debats*, du 7 Juillet 1851. MS 985. Archives, Royal College of Physicians, London.
75. Vulpian EFA. Prix Lacaze. *C R Acad Sci*, 94:321–323, 1882.
76. Konstantinov IE, Alexi-Meskishvili VV. Sergei S. Brukhonenko: the development of the first heart-lung machine for total body perfusion. *Ann Thorac Surg*, 69:962–966, 2000.
77. Roach M. *Stiff: The curious lives of human cadavers* (p. 202). New York: Norton, 2003.
78. Boese A. *Elephants on acid and other bizarre experiments* (pp. 12–14). Orlando: Harcourt, 2007.
79. White RJ, Wolin LR, Massopust LC, Taslitz N, Verdura J. Cephalic exchange transplantation in the monkey. *Surgery*, 70:135–139, 1971.
80. White RJ, Albin MS, Verdura J, Takaoka Y, Massopust LC, Wolin LR, Locke GE, Taslitz N, Yashon D. The isolation and transplantation of the brain. An historical perspective emphasizing the surgical solutions to the design of these classical models. *Neurol Res*, 18:194–203, 1996.

15

A Backward Glance and a Reckoning

THE WORLD WAS stunned by the sudden death of the larger-than-life figure of Brown-Séquard during the night of 1 April 1894. But after all was said and done, when the eulogies and obituaries were over, his name soon came to be forgotten. Many of the ideas that he had spawned or championed were taken over by others who—in providing experimental validation for them—were assumed to have been their originator. Other concepts that had been greeted by incredulity when first he conceived of them gradually gained such wide acceptance that they were taken as self-evident and their origin forgotten.

There are other factors that doubtless contributed to his later obscurity. He had no great personal following, and left no school of disciples, perhaps in consequence of his lifestyle, with his erratic wandering from one place of learning to another. There was no personal identity to which others could relate—his idiosyncratic refusal to having his likeness portrayed photographically, and the separation of his private and professional life did not help—and he lacked. the easy charm, wit, and social style that are so important in a natural leader (but are often a useful camouflage for those without true ability). His relations with others must also have been influenced by his dramatic mood swings from apathy, lack of interest, poor concentration, and a sense of being overwhelmed (i.e., from depressive episodes) to exuberance, boundless energy, pressure of speech, irritability, anxiety, and unrealistic grandiosity (which are features of manic or hypomanic episodes), and by his tendency to simply pack up and flee when personal tragedy struck. Given this behavior and that of his son, it seems likely that he suffered from bipolar disorder (see p. 133), for which no adequate treatment then existed but which can be very disruptive of personal relationships. Further, his career was troubled. He seemed to be incapable of coping with success until his later years, resigning from enviable appointments as he became successful in London, Boston, and Paris, until eventually his career was in ashes and he was almost destitute. It is remarkable that he was able to weather the crises that followed and make a professional "come-back." Finally, he was not really the right man to personify the image that scientists seek to portray of themselves to the outside world. The disturbing overtones of an impulsive but erratic experimentalist cast a shadow over the measured calm of the reasoned investigator to which scientists aspire. The ridicule that replaced respect after he announced his work on testicular extracts placed a heavy burden on his reputation and tarnished his memory.

The question thus emerges as to whether Brown-Séquard was a jewel in the crown of international science or a trinket that deceived the eye. What is his rightful place in history? He was appointed to positions of enormous prestige and power in the upper reaches of academic society but that, in itself, does not signify much, even though he attained these positions despite being an outsider without benefit of money or family connections. More to the point is whether he really mattered—is there something that sets him apart from the many others who have contributed in large or small ways to the advance of medicine and science? In order to consider these questions and his legacy, it is important that his life, work, and achievements are placed in perspective. The aim is not to efface the contradictions in his life and work but, rather, to highlight them.

The experiences and ideals of the man inevitably color the motivation and achievements of the professional. Brown-Séquard, foreign and fatherless, was a man of principle who remained faithful throughout his life to the socialist ideals of his youth. He lived frugally, was generous to others, did not accept the exorbitant fees offered by the well-to-do for his medical advice (instead requesting no more than his customary charge), and refused to profit from the organ extracts that he developed, instead using his own limited resources to subsidize their production and restricting their distribution to medical practitioners.

He was a man of unquestionable professional as well as personal integrity, despite the ill-founded claims that behind the façade of a scientist was the bluster of a self-serving charlatan who made extravagant claims for, and huge profits from the organ extracts that came to bear his name. In fact, he made no such claims, being particularly careful regarding the benefits he attributed to these extracts and constantly reminding his readers that any claims of benefit required careful scrutiny and validation. He certainly made no profits, refusing to allow others to establish an institute in his name and distributing without charge, often at his own expense, the testicular extracts that were manufactured in his laboratory. He had the intellectual rigor to challenge the scientific pieties of the day—for example, concerning the course of the sensory pathways in the spinal cord—and later refused to be seduced by emerging and popular or fashionable hypotheses, such as those on the cortical localization of various cerebral functions. He eventually came to be regarded as an out-of-date crank, and his credibility and reputation slipped to a low point. Regardless, he championed concepts of neurological function that involved the interaction and integration of excitatory and inhibitory influences at multiple levels and sites within the central nervous system through the operation of functional or task-specific networks, anticipating in many ways concepts that have gained favor especially in the last forty years. Furthermore, his suggestion of and belief in chemical (hormonal) integrative mechanisms was a logical extension of his views concerning the integrative action of the nervous system and the functional processes subserving this role, and he is rightly regarded by many as the father of experimental endocrinology (based on his work on the adrenal glands) and the founder of hormone replacement therapy and clinical endocrinology by his work with tissue extracts

It must sometimes have seemed, even to his colleagues, that he was building castles in the air, because his work was based on inspired intuition. Individual projects may have failed, and certain of his hypotheses may not have withstood the test of time, but his concepts were nevertheless profoundly influential for the later development of clinical medicine and neuroscience. To many, he seemed to have so many interests that he was regarded as a dilettante rather than as someone to be taken seriously, especially as he was almost too eager to rush into print with some observation or other. But his work must be viewed in the context of the times. It was common in the nineteenth century for learned men to excel in multiple areas. Thus, a urological surgeon such as Guyon (p. 222) would write knowledgeably about the nervous system, and an explorer such as Galton (p. 112) would also achieve fame as a meteorologist, statistician, and eugenicist. Brown-Séquard was no exception in the multiplicity of his interests.

That said, it must nevertheless be remarked that a common thread ran through much of his work. He tried to grasp the complex relationship that existed between different parts of the body, between the different components of living organisms, and the neurological and chemical (hormonal) means by which they are integrated into a functioning unit. In this regard, he seemed to have an amazing instinct for understanding the operation of the intact organism. Further, much of his work—not just that on organ extracts—captured the imagination of the public, provided a scientific underpinning to aspects of clinical practice, and elicited widespread interest in the biological sciences.

His concept of sensory anatomy and processing within the central nervous system evolved with time. His original views, published in his doctoral thesis and in subsequent papers while he was in his thirties and forties, met with such opposition that it required independent scrutiny by a scientific committee before they gained wide acceptance. Ironically, the facts that they embodied are now standard teaching. And yet, when in his seventies, the weary scientist not only lauded a challenge to his work but went further, showing by experiment that his own earlier interpretation failed to provide an adequate explanation of certain sensory phenomena that result from spinal cord lesions. Just a few weeks before he died, he published a short paper—regarded by some as one of the most important in neurology—in which he developed a new but widely ignored explanation that is so modern in its outlook and so important in its implications that it merits the attention of all neuroscientists interested in the physiology of sensation and pain. Indeed, recent concepts of the anatomy of pain involve just the sorts of inhibitory and excitatory influences from the brain and periphery on the spinal segmental apparatus that he envisioned. This remarkable man, ridiculed by his colleagues over his unorthodox views concerning tissue extracts, nevertheless had the humility and grace to reject in part the work on which his own reputation had originally depended and—in response to the challenge of a junior and as-yet unknown colleague—put forth a new concept, based on further experimentation that led him to view the nervous system as a system of dynamic processes rather than hard-wired structures. The ability to conceive of such a concept, and in this way to foresee much of the work that occupied neuroscientists almost a century later, attests to his intuitive understanding of the manner of operation of the nervous system.

Brown-Séquard's work profoundly changed clinical medicine, leading to recognition of a new branch of medicine—endocrinology—and to a new system of treatment—hormone replacement therapy—as well as to a better understanding of the nervous system and its operation in health and disease. His work on the neural control of the circulation, on the interactions between the respiratory and nervous systems, on rigor mortis and related phenomena, and on the perfusion of tissues with fresh or oxygenated blood to maintain their viability, had important and lasting consequences that add to his legacy. His work on the physiological changes that occur with age and his use of organ extracts led to recognition that ageing is in itself a medical problem and that the study of ageing—gerontology—constitutes a science of its own, and it brought sexual disturbances such as erectile dysfunction into the clinical arena. He provided new insights to several different areas of scientific enquiry, sometimes without adequate experimental justification—but it was the ideas themselves that were important, and his capacity for such insight that marks him as a genius. Yet, the work of this unpretentious maverick aroused the antagonism of large segments of the population: the antivivisectionists for his treatment of animals as objects for experimentation, the religious for the sexual implications of his work on testicular extracts, the establishment because he was always somewhat of an outsider, and many members of the medical and scientific community for the unorthodoxy of his views. Indeed, the professional colleagues most hostile to his views were generally those who were more likely to test the scientific concepts and hypotheses of others than to come up with original views of their own. This implacable antagonism from so many quarters must surely have contributed to the chilling neglect to which he has been subjected.

But Brown-Séquard also had his failings. He was a brilliant observer, but his reasoning was sometimes convoluted and tortuous, lacking the clarity of some of his scientific contemporaries with whom he came into conflict. Unfortunately, he sometimes provided no reasons at all for accepting a particular belief, instead asking the reader to take his views on trust. Thus, a number of his papers contain statements such as "Some experiments that I cannot here give the details of have shown me that ...." All too often, the details were never provided. Science does not always advance by ordered and logical steps. Instead, an observation is often made by chance, and reasons are then found to justify the experiment that led to it and explain the observation. When the advance of science is in seemingly unconnected fits and starts, some starts will come to be forgotten, even if they generate new concepts that ultimately have wide validity, because they occurred too soon, deviated too broadly from accepted beliefs, or could not meet every objection raised by a skeptical community. Many of Brown-Séquard's concepts and hypotheses indeed came too soon and were too unorthodox to allow their easy acceptance, and they were sometimes buttressed inadequately by the experimental findings. His experimental approach in his early years, as detailed, for example, in his initial work on the sensory pathways in the spinal cord, on the vasomotor nerves, and on the adrenal glands was exacting and of a high standard, with "controls" to ensure that the observations made were not explicable by means other than those he reported. By contrast, his approach in later years, for example with regard to the development of organ extracts—a fundamental innovation to the treatment of disease—was often sloppy, ill-considered, and illogical, and in this respect he must be considered a failure. It is unlikely that the scales ever fell from his eyes—he probably never understood that the inadequacy of his experimental observations or his failure to document them must have contributed to the opposition that he met from the scientific establishment to the concepts that he advanced. But he was a man whose experimental studies did not truly match the grandeur of his ideas, and in his intuitive grasp of concepts and principles of biological importance, he was truly exceptional. Furthermore, by his ability to suggest new concepts and hypotheses, he aided the advance of the biosciences by stimulating others to devise experiments for testing and extending them and to develop new approaches to understanding the functioning of the organism. The fact that many of his views later turned out to be correct is a testimony to his visionary genius.

An imperfect experimenter, an unfocused investigator who seemed unable to follow an object of study to its logical conclusion, he was—improbable as it may have seemed—able to grasp the wider issues facing biologists and conceive of the manner in which the various activities of an organism are integrated to allow that organism to function as a unit. His remarkable insight anticipated many later developments in neurology and endocrinology even when, at times, he was led to conclusions that were difficult to justify and were difficult for his contemporaries to accept. Although some felt unable to move forward with him, they were equally unable to step back and ignore his work, which was of consequence because it set medicine and neuroscience on a new course. Simply put, he was the originator of new beliefs and fundamental concepts that are his legacy and forever changed the face of medicine, widening its horizons.

General Biographical References

Aminoff MJ. *Brown-Séquard: A visionary of science*. New York: Raven Press, 1993.

Aminoff MJ (ed). Special issue: Brown-Séquard centennial. *J Hist Neurosci*, 5:3–42, 1996.

Anonymous. Obituary: Charles Edouard Brown-Séquard. *Nature*, 49:556–557, 1894.

Anonymous. Obituary: Professor Brown-Séquard. *Lancet*, 1:975–977, 1894.

Anonymous. Death of Professor Brown-Séquard. *Lancet*, 1:906–907, 1894.

Anonymous. The late Professor Brown-Séquard. Anecdotes of a great physiologist. *St. James's Gazette (London)*, 4 April 1894.

Berthelot M. Notice sur la vie et les travaux de M. Brown-Séquard. Paris: Institut de France, 1898.

Binet L. *Médecins, biologistes, et chirurgiens* (pp. 117–125). Paris: Segep, 1954.

Binet L. *Figures de savants français* (pp. 37–70). Paris: Vigot, 1946.

Brown-Séquard CE. Autobiographic details provided in a letter dated 17 December 1852, and addressed to Lady Blanche [Ellen Fletcher] who was to become his first wife. MS 977/1. Archives, Royal College of Physicians, London.

Brown-Séquard CE. *Notice sur les travaux scientifiques du Docteur C-E Brown-Séquard, Professeur de Medicine au Collège de France*. Paris: Masson, 1886.

Bowditch HP. Memoir of Charles Edouard Brown-Séquard, 1817–1894. *Biographical Memoirs Natl Acad Sci USA*, pp. 93–97. Read before the National Academy, April 1897.

Carmichael EB. Charles Edouard Brown-Séquard—physician, endocrinologist, neurologist, physiologist. *Alabama J Med Sci*, 9:224–237, 1972.

Damrau F. *Pioneers in neurology* (pp. 9–17). St. Louis: Dios Chemical Co., 1937.

Dupuy E. Biographies scientifiques. Brown-Séquard. *Rev Scientifique*, 2:737–743, 1894.
Francis SW. Biographical sketches of distinguished living New York physicians. V. C.E. Brown-Séquard, M.D., F.R.S., etc. *Med Surg Reporter (Philadelphia)*, 15:169–172, 1866.
Gooddy W. Some aspects of the life of Dr. C.E. Brown-Séquard. *Proc R Soc Med*, 57:189–192, 1964.
Gooddy W. Charles Edward Brown-Séquard. In: Clifford Rose F, Bynum WF, eds., *Historical aspects of the neurosciences* (pp. 371–378). New York: Raven Press, 1982.
Gmrek MD. Brown-Séquard, Charles-Édouard. In: Gillispie CC, ed., *Dictionary of scientific biography* (Vol. 2, pp. 524–526). New York: Scribner's Sons, 1970.
Koehler PJ, Aminoff MJ. The Brown-Séquard syndrome. In: Koehler PJ, Bruyn GW, Pearce JMS, eds., *Neurological eponyms* (pp. 200–206). Oxford: Oxford University Press, 2000.
Major RH. Charles Edouard Brown-Séquard. In: *Essays in biology: In honor of Herbert M. Evans* (pp. 371–377). Berkeley: University of California Press, 1943.
Olmsted JMD. Charles-Edouard Brown-Séquard: A nineteenth-century neurologist and endocrinologist. Baltimore: Johns Hopkins Press, 1946.
Ott I. Dr. Brown-Séquard. *Med Bull*, 18:361–366, 1896.
Putnam JJ. Charles Edouard Brown-Séquard. *Proc Am Acad Arts Sci*, 30:589–592, 1894–1895.
Rengachary SS, Colen C, Guthikonda M. Charles-Edouard Brown-Séquard: an eccentric genius. *Neurosurgery*, 62:954–964, 2008.
Role A. La vie etrange d'un grand savant: Le professeur Brown-Séquard. Paris: Plon, 1977.
Rouget FA. *Brown-Séquard et son oeuvre. Esquisse biographique*. Ile Maurice: General Printing and Stationery Co., 1930.
Ruch TC. Charles Edouard Brown-Séquard (1817–1894). *Yale J Biol Med*, 18:227–238, 1946.
Tyler HR, Tyler KL. Charles Edouard Brown-Séquard: Professor of physiology and pathology of the nervous system at Harvard Medical School. *Neurology*, 34:1231–1236, 1984.
Williams H. The healing touch (pp. 221–270). Springfield, IL: CC Thomas, 1951.
Wilson JD. Charles-Edouard Brown-Séquard and the centennial of endocrinology. *J Clin Endocrinol Metab*, 71:1403–409, 1990.

Appendix

The Scientific Works of Brown-Séquard

IN THIS APPENDIX, Brown-Séquard's publications and scientific presentations are divided into three parts. The first, covering his career up to 1878, is based on the bibliography that he prepared to support his application for the chair of medicine at the Collège de France. His work was listed in chronological order, subdivided by subjects, and accompanied by an analysis of its importance, and published as *Notice sur les Travaux Scientifiques de M. Brown-Séquard* (Masson: Paris, 1878). The second part is based on the summary that he prepared to support his successful candidacy for the chair vacated by Vulpian in the Académie des Sciences, which listed with annotations his publications in physiology and medicine from 1878 to 1886. This was published as *Notice sur les Travaux Scientifiques du Docteur C-E Brown-Séquard, Professeur de Medicine au Collège de France* (Masson: Paris, 1886) and incorporated the earlier *Notice*.

The bibliography listed in these first two parts of this Appendix has been checked for accuracy; a number of citation errors have been corrected, and more complete information has been provided to enable the reader to locate articles of interest. In a few instances in which it was not possible to verify an article because its location was cited erroneously by Brown-Séquard, the incorrect citation has been omitted if the paper was published in more than one journal; it is otherwise reproduced, but with a note indicating that the correct location of the publication could not be verified. The commentary on these publications provided by Brown-Séquard has been omitted for brevity, but his grouping and numbering of these works have been retained. In a number of instances, he listed several articles in the same entry when a single body of work was published in multiple parts or in several journals. A few articles omitted by him from the original bibliographies have been included, placed in the appropriate group, marked by an asterisk, and listed in chronological order, but without altering the original numbering sequence. Many of the citations to the *Comptes Rendus* of the Société de Biologie refer to official accounts of presentations and commentaries by Brown-Séquard at meetings, rather than to formal abstracts or papers. I have nevertheless felt it important to include these because the experimental findings briefly recounted are sometimes not detailed elsewhere and because they reveal the evolution of Brown-Séquard's views on particular topics. In such instances, the title used to designate these works is that given by Brown-Séquard in his bibliographies of 1878 and 1886. The third part of the Appendix covers the period from 1886 to 1894, and is based on a literature search by the present author.

The entire Appendix appeared in my earlier (now out-of-print) biography of Brown-Séquard and is republished here for the convenience of readers and scholars.

Part 1: Work to 1878

A. Physiology and Pathology of the Nervous System

1. Recherches et expériences sur la physiologie de la moelle épinière. *Thèse de doctorat*, Paris, 3 janvier 1846.
2. Note sur la durée de la vie des grenouilles, en automne et en hiver, après l'extirpation de la moelle allongée et de quelques autres portions du centre nerveux cérébro-rachidien. *C R Acad Sci*, 24:363 and 688, 1847.
3. Recherches critiques et expérimentales sur les propriétés et les fonctions de la moelle épinière et de la moelle allongée, et sur les rapports de ces fonctions avec celles des muscles et du système nerveux ganglionnaire. *C R Acad Sci*, 24:849, 1847.
4. Recherches anatomiques, physiologiques et pathologiques sur les fonctions due système nerveux cérébro-spinal. *C R Acad Sci*, 24:889, 1847.
5. Recherches expérimentales sur les résultats de la destruction des centres nerveux, et particulièrement de la moelle allongée dans les cinq classes de vertébrés. *C R Acad Sci*, 26:413, 1848.

6. Des rapports qui existent entre la lésion des racines motrices et des racines sensitives. *C R Soc Biol (Paris)*, 1:15, 1849.
7. Expériences sur les plaies de la moelle épinière. *C R Soc Biol (Paris)*, 1:17, 1849.
8. De la force nerveuse dans la moelle épinière. *C R Soc Biol (Paris)*, 1:18, 1849.
9. L'action de téter est indépendante du cerveau. *C R Soc Biol (Paris)*, 1:60, 1849.
10. Production de sueur sous l'influence d'une excitation vive des nerfs du goût. *C R Soc Biol (Paris)*, 1:104, 1849.
11. Tubercule comprimant la moelle cervicale chez un lapin. *C R Soc Biol (Paris)*, 1:122, 1849.
12. Du tournoiement et du roulement consécutifs à l'arrachement du nerf facial. *C R Soc Biol (Paris)*, 1:133, 1849.
13. Sur les altérations pathologiques qui suivent la section du nerf sciatique. *C R Soc Biol (Paris)*, 1:136, 1849.
14. Cas de régénération complète du nerf sciatique. *C R Soc Biol (Paris)*, 1:137, 1849.
15. Recherches sur la physiologie de la moelle allongée. *Bull Soc Philomatique Paris (5th Series)*, 14:117, 1849.
16. Cas de méningite rachidienne chronique très-ancienne; méningite cérébrale aigue; tubercules à la face convexe du lobe cérébrale gauche; ramollissement des cordons postérieurs de la moelle à la région cervicale—paralysie des mouvements volontaires des membres; conservation de la sensibilité; atrophie, contracture et flexion ou adduction des quatre membres. [With M. Tailhé.] *C R Soc Biol (Paris)*, 1:160, 1849.
17. Recherches sur un moyen de mesurer l'anesthésie et l'hyperesthésie. *C R Soc Biol (Paris)*, 1:162, 1849.
18. Sur le siége de la sensibilité et sur la valeur des cris comme preuve de perception de douleur. *C R Acad Sci*, 29:672, 1849.
19. Des différences d'énergie de la faculté réflexe, suivant les espèces et suivant les âges, dans les cinq classes d'animaux vertébrés. *C R Soc Biol (Paris)*, 1:171, 1849.
20. De la transmission des impressions sensitives par la moelle épinière. *C R Soc Biol (Paris)*, 1:192, 1849.
21. Régénération des tissus de la moelle épinière. *C R Soc Biol (Paris)*, 2:3, 1850.
22. De l'arrêt passif des battements du coeur par l'excitation galvanique de la moelle allongée et par la destruction subite du centre cérébro-rachidien. *C R Soc Biol (Paris)*, 2:26, 1850.

23. De la conservation de la vie sans trouble apparent des fonctions organiques, malgré la destruction d'une portion considérable de la moelle épinière, chez des animaux à sang chaud. *C R Soc Biol (Paris)*, 2:28 and 49, 1850; *C R Acad Sci*, 30:828, 1850.
24. De la transmission croisée des impressions sensitives par la moelle épinière. *C R Soc Biol (Paris)*, 2:33, 1850.
25. De l'influence des nerfs vagues sur les battements du coeur. *C R Soc Biol (Paris)*, 2:45, 1850.
26. De la persistance de la faculté réflexe malgré des altérations considérables de la moelle épinière. *C R Soc Biol (Paris)*, 2:46, 1850.
27. Explication de l'hémiplégie croisée du sentiment. *C R Soc Biol (Paris)*, 2:70, 1850.
28. Troubles survenant dans la nutrition de l'oeil, par suite de la section d'une moitié latérale de la moelle épinière, au dos. *C R Soc Biol (Paris)*, 2:134, 1850.
29. D'une action spéciale qui accompagne la contraction musculaire, et de l'existence de cette action dans certains cas pathologiques et dans ce que M. Magendie a appelé sensibilité récurrente. *C R Soc Biol (Paris)*, 2:171, 1850.
30. De la conservation partielle des mouvements volontaires, après la section transversale d'une moitié latérale de la moelle épinière. *C R Soc Biol (Paris)*, 2:195, 1850.
31. De l'innocuité de la mise à nu de la moelle épinière. *C R Soc Biol (Paris)*, 2:202, 1850.
32. Mémoire sur la transmission des impressions sensitives dans la moelle épinière. *C R Acad Sci*, 31:700, 1850.
33. Déviation et contracture permanente des membres après l'écrasement de la moelle épinière. *C R Soc Biol (Paris)*, 3:15, 1851.
34. De la survie des batraciens et des tortues après l'ablation de leur moelle allongée. *C R Soc Biol (Paris)*, 3:73, 1851.
35. Des actes de la génération chez des animaux atteints de paraplégie incomplète. *C R Soc Biol (Paris)*, 3:75, 1851.
36. Expérience nouvelle sur la voie de transmission des impressions sensitives dans la moelle épinière. *C R Soc Biol (Paris)*, 3:76, 1851.
37. Sur plusieurs cas de cicatrisation de plaies faites à la moelle épinière, avec retour des fonctions perdues. *C R Soc Biol (Paris)*, 3:77, 1851.
38. Sur une nouvelle espèce de tournoiement. *C R Soc Biol (Paris)*, 3:79, 1851.
39. Influence d'une partie de la moelle épinière sur les capsules surrénales. *C R Soc Biol (Paris)*, 3:146, 1851.

40. Recherches expérimentales et observations cliniques sur le rôle de l'encéphale et particulièrement de la protubérance annulaire dans la respiration. (This work was reported in the thesis of J-B Coste, Paris, 1 August 1851.)
41. Experiments proving that life may be preserved in warm-blooded animals after the destruction of a considerable part of the spinal marrow. Med Exam (Philadelphia), 8:321, 1852.
42. On the reparative power of the spinal cord after complete division. Med Exam (Philadelphia), 8:379, 1852.
43. Researches on the reflex faculty. Med Exam (Philadelphia), 8:485, 1852.
44. Researches on the influence of the nervous system upon the functions of organic life. Med Exam (Philadelphia), 8:486, 1852.
45. On turning and rolling as phenomena produced by injuries of the nervous system. Med Exam (Philadelphia), 8:498, 1852.
46. On the relations existing between the organization of nerve tubes and their vital properties. Med Exam (Philadelphia), 8:563, 1852.
47. On a new fact relative to the physiology of the spinal cord. Boston Med Surg J, 47:334, 1852.
48. Cause of the stopping of the heart's movements, produced by an excitation of the medulla oblongata or the par vagum. Med Exam (Philadelphia), 9:141, 1853.
49. On a singular disturbance in the voluntary movements, apparently produced by an action of atmospheric air on the gray matter of the spinal cord, in birds. Med Exam (Philadelphia), 9:143, 1853.
50. Cause of loss of sensibility on one side of the body, and loss of voluntary movements on the other. Med Exam (Philadelphia), 9:288, 1853.
51. On the different degrees of excitability of the different parts of the sensitive nerve-fibres. Med Exam (Philadelphia), 9:291, 1853.
52. The auditive nerve is a nervous centre. Med Exam (Philadelphia), 9:491, 1853.
53. Expériences sur les résultats de la section d'une moitié latérale de la moelle épinière. C R Soc Biol (Paris), 5:151, 1853.
54. Des effets de la section des nerfs vagues sur la force du coeur. C R Soc Biol (Paris), 5:152, 1853.
55. Nouveau fait relatif à l'arrêt du coeur par la galvanisation du nerf vague. C R Soc Biol (Paris), 5:153, 1853.
56. Nouvelles preuves de l'entre-croisement des fibres sensitives dans la moelle épinière. C R Soc Biol (Paris), 5:154, 1853.
57. Sur une question de priorité relative au tournoiement. C R Soc Biol (Paris), 5:167, 1853.

58. Note sur la découverte de quelques-uns des effets de la galvanisation du nerf grand sympathique au cou. *Gaz Med (3rd Series)*, 9:22, 1854.
59. Sur les résultats de la section et de la galvanisation du nerf grand sympathique au cou. *C R Acad Sci*, 38:72, 1854.
60. Influence of the vagus nerves on the blood vessels of the lungs. *Virg Med Surg J*, 4:161, 1855.
61. Experimental and clinical researches on the physiology and pathology of the spinal cord and some other parts of the nervous centres. *Virg Med Surg J*, 4:177 and 283, 1855.
62. Recherches expérimentales sur la voie de transmission des impressions sensitives dans la moelle épinière. *C R Acad Sci*, 41:118, 1855; and in more detail in *Gaz Hebd Med*, 2:575 and 655, 1855.
63. Recherches sur la voie de transmission des impressions sensitives dans la moelle épinière. *C R Acad Sci*, 41:347, 1855; *Mem Soc Biol (Paris)*, 7:51, 1855.
64. Recherches expérimentales sur la distribution des fibres des racines postérieures dans la moelle épinière et sur la voie de transmission des impressions sensitives dans cet organe. *Mem Soc Biol (Paris)*, 7: 77, 1855; Recherches experimentales sur la voie de transmission des impressions sensitives dans la moelle épinière. *C R Acad Sci*, 41:477, 1855.
65. Recherches expérimentales sur les voies de transmission des impressions sensitives et sur des phénomènes singuliers qui succèdent à la section des racines des nerfs spinaux. *Mem Soc Biol (Paris)*, 7:331, 1855.
66. Lettre sur les propriétés et les fonctions de la moelle épinière. *Gaz Hop*, p. 468, 1855 [unverified].
67. Sur quelques caractères, non encore signalés, des mouvements réflexes chez les mammifères. *C R Soc Biol (Paris)*, 9:102, 1857.
68. Experimental researches on the spinal cord as a leader for sensibility and voluntary movements. *Proc R Soc Lond*, 8:591, 1857.
69. On the resemblence between the effects of the section of the sympathetic nerve in the neck and of a transverse section of a lateral half of the spinal cord. *Proc R Soc Lond*, 8:594, 1857.
70. Recherches expérimentales sur la transmission des impressions sensitives dans la moelle épinière. *Bull Acad Med (Paris)*, 23:7, 1857; Notes sur quelques points importants de la physiologie de la moelle épinière. *C R Acad Sci*, 45:146, 1857; Exposé critique des idées de M. Chauveau sur la physiologie de la moelle épinière, et faits nouveaux à l'appui des théories que j'ai proposées à l'égard de la transmission des impressions sensitives. *J Physiol (Paris)*, 1:177, 1858.

71. Recherches sur les causes de mort après l'ablation de la partie de la moelle allongée qui a été nommée point vital. *J Physiol (Paris)*, 1:217, 1858.
72. Note sur l'influence qu'une moitié latérale de la moelle épinière exerce, dans certains cas, sur la moitié correspondante de l'encéphale et de la face. *J Physiol (Paris)*, 1:241, 1858.
73. Sur la sensibilité tactile et sur un moyen de la mesurer dans l'anesthésie et l'hyperesthésie. *J Physiol (Paris)*, 1:344, 1858.
74. Recherches sur la physiologie et la pathologie de la protubérance annulaire. [In 3 parts.] *J Physiol (Paris)*, 1:523 and 755, 1858; *J Physiol (Paris)*, 2:121, 1859.
75. Expériences montrant que les cordons antérieurs de la moelle épinière servent à la transmission des impressions sensitives. *J Physiol (Paris)*, 1:809, 1858.
76. Physiologie du système nerveux. *J Prog Sci Med (Paris)*, 4:323, 1859.
77. Possibility of repair and of return of function after a partial or a complete division of the spinal cord in man and animals. *Lancet*, 1:96, 1859.
78. Expériences nouvelles sur la transmission des impressions sensitives par la moelle épinière. *J Physiol (Paris)*, 2:65, 1859.
79. Remarques sur le mode d'influence du système nerveux sur la nutrition. *J Physiol (Paris)*, 2:112, 1859.
80. Du rhythme dans le diaphragme et dans les muscles de la vie animale après leur séparation des centres nerveux. *J Physiol (Paris)*, 2:115, 1859.
81. Remarques sur l'ephidrose parotidienne. (Production de sueur par action réflexe.) *J Physiol (Paris)*, 2:449, 1859.
82. Recherches expérimentales sur la physiologie de la moelle allongée. *J Physiol (Paris)*, 3:151, 1860.
83. Sur l'indépendance des propriétés vitales des nerfs moteurs. *J Physiol (Paris)*, 3:160, 1860.
84. Sur une modification spéciale de la nutrition dans une partie limitée du corps sous l'influence d'irritations de l'encéphale ou de la moelle épinière, dans certains cas d'épilepsie. *J Physiol (Paris)*, 3:167, 1860.
85. Experimental researches on various questions concerning sensibility. *Proc R Soc Lond*, 10:510, 1860; Recherches expérimentales sur diverses questions relatives à la sensibilité. *J Physiol (Paris)*, 4:140, 1861.
86. Note sur les mouvements rotatoires. *J Physiol (Paris)*, 3:720, 1860.
87. *Course of lectures on the physiology and pathology of the central nervous system, delivered at the Royal College of Surgeons of England in May 1858.* Philadelphia: Collins, 1860; published originally in multiple parts in *Lancet*, 2:1, 27, 53, 109, 137, 165, 219, 245, 271, 295, 345, 367, 391, 415, 441, 467, 493, 519, 545, 571, 599, 625, and 651, 1858.

88. *Lectures on the diagnosis and treatment of the principal forms of paralysis of the lower extremities.* Philadelphia: Collins, 1861.
89. Note sur la production de symptomes cérébraux à la suite de certaines lésions du nerf auditif. *Gaz Hebd Med,* 8:56, 1861.
90. Lectures on the diagnosis and treatment of the various forms of paralytic, convulsive and mental affections, considered as effects of morbid alterations of the blood, or of the brain or other organs. [In several parts.] *Lancet,* 2:1, 29, 55, 79, 153, 199, 391, 415, 515, and 611, 1861.
91. Remarques sur le mémoire de Du Bois-Reymond sur l'hémicranie. *J Physiol (Paris),* 4:137, 1861.
92. Remarques sur la physiologie du cervelet à propos du travail précédent. *J Physiol (Paris),* 4:413, 1861; Remarques sur la physiologie du cervelet et du nerf auditif. *J Physiol (Paris),* 5:484, 1862.
93. Remarques sur quelques points de la physiologie de la moelle épinière et du cerveau. *J Physiol (Paris),* 4:584, 1861.
94. Remarks on a case of wound of the spinal cord. *Lancet,* 2:166, 1862.
95. Remarques sur l'action du nerf vague sur le coeur. *J Physiol (Paris),* 5:295, 1862.
96. Sur l'entre-croisement de quelques-unes des branches des nerfs trijumeau dans la protubérance annulaire. *J Physiol (Paris),* 5:307, 1862.
97. Première note sur l'existence de sang rouge dans les veines et sur l'influence du système nerveux sur la couleur du sang veineux. *J Physiol (Paris),* 5:566, 1862.
98. Note sur les fibres nerveuses des muscles. *J Physiol (Paris),* 5:574, 1862.
99. Recherches sur la transmission des impressions de tact, de chatouillement, de douleur, de température et de contraction (sens musculaire) dans la moelle épinière. [In 3 parts.] *J Physiol (Paris),* 6:124, 232, and 581, 1863.
100. Production d'ataxie musculaire par l'irritation superficielle d'une petite portion de la moelle épinière chez les oiseaux. *J Physiol (Paris),* 6:701, 1864.
101. Aesthésiomètre. In: *Dictionnaire Encyclopedique des Sciences Médicales.* (Vol. 2, p. 47). Paris: Asselin & Masson, 1865.
102. Lectures on the recent advances of our knowledge in the diagnosis and treatment of functional nervous affections. Lecture 1. General remarks on the causes, diagnosis, and treatment of functional nervous affections. [In several parts.] *Lancet,* 1:1, 85, 139, and 247, 1866.

103. *Lectures on the diagnosis and treatment of functional nervous affections.* New York: GP Putnam's Sons, 1868.
104. Note sur une altération spéciale de la sensibilité tactile dans certaines affections de la base de l'encéphale. *Arch Physiol Norm Pathol,* 1:461, 1868.
105. Nouvelles recherches sur le trajet des diverses espèces de conducteurs d'impressions sensitives dans la moelle épinière. [In several parts.] *Arch Physiol Norm Pathol,* 1:610 and 761, 1868; *Arch Physiol Norm Pathol,* 2:236 and 693, 1869.
106. Expériences sur l'influence de l'irritation des nerfs de la peau sur la température des membres. [With J-S Lombard.] *Arch Physiol Norm Pathol,* 1:688, 1868.
107. Lectures on the physiology and pathology of the nervous system; and on the treatment of organic nervous affections. Lecture 1. On spinal hemiplegia. [In several parts.] *Lancet,* 2:593, 659, 755, and 821, 1868.
108. Lectures on the physiology and pathology of the nervous system; and on the treatment of organic nervous affections. Lecture 2. On organic affections and injuries of the spinal cord, producing some of the symptoms of spinal hemiplegia. [In several parts.] *Lancet,* 1:1, 219, 703, and 873, 1869.
109. Faits démontrant que le cordon latéral de la moelle épinière ne sert pas à la respiration. *C R Soc Biol (Paris),* 21:64, 1869; *C R Soc Biol (Paris),* 24:18, 1872.
110. Sur une différence radicale entre la moelle épinière et les nerfs, quant au retour des fonctions perdues. *C R Soc Biol (Paris),* 21:65, 1869.
111. De l'influence du centre nerveux cérébro-rachidien sur les échanges entre le sang et les tissus. *C R Soc Biol (Paris),* 21:98, 1869.
112. Paralysie réflexe de l'abdomen après la section du nerf sciatique. *C R Soc Biol (Paris),* 21:111, 1869.
113. Influence sur la pupille, de parties de la moelle épinière, en arrière du centre cilio-spinal. *C R Soc Biol (Paris),* 21:121, 1869.
114. Influence de la section du nerf sciatique sur la sécrétion lactée. *C R Soc Biol (Paris),* 21:129 and 319, 1869.
115. Influence des nerfs cutanés du bras chez l'homme sur la circulation de la face. *C R Soc Biol (Paris),* 21:146, 1869.
116. Sur des altérations de nutrition au cou après la section du nerf sciatique. *C R Soc Biol (Paris),* 21:147, 1869.
117. La section des canaux semi-circulaires ne cause le tournoiement que parce qu'elle s'accompagne d'une irritation du nerf auditif. *C R Soc Biol (Paris),* 21:157, 1869.

118. De l'influence du système nerveux sur la nutrition. *C R Soc Biol (Paris)*, 21:239, 1869; *C R Soc Biol (Paris)*, 22:43, 1870.
119. Fait démontrant que l'absorption peut avoir lieu par action réflexe. *C R Soc Biol (Paris)*, 21:308, 1869.
120. Remarques à propos de l'observation précédente. [Un cas de tumeur de la moelle épinière.] *Arch Physiol Norm Pathol*, 2:296, 1869.
121. Sur l'augmentation d'énergie des mouvements respiratoires, du côté d'une section d'une moitié latérale de la moelle épinière. *Arch Physiol Norm Pathol*, 2:299, 1869.
122. Faits qui semblent montrer que les fibres nerveuses servant aux mouvements volontaires ne sont pas celles qui font contracter les muscles dans les convulsions. *Arch Physiol Norm Pathol*, 2:672, 1869.
123. Remarques sur une cause d'erreur dans l'appréciation des degrés de sensibilité dans les cas de maladie des centres nerveux et particulièrement des cordons postérieurs de la moelle épinière. *Arch Physiol Norm Pathol*, 2:761, 1869.
124. Faits démontrant qu'il existe trois espèces de syncope, caractérisées: l'une par l'arrêt du coeur, une seconde par l'arrêt de la respiration, sans asphyxie, et la troisième par l'arrêt de quelques-uns des échanges entre le sang et les tissus. *Arch Physiol Norm Pathol*, 2:767, 1869.
125. Lectures on the physiology and pathology of the nervous system; and on the treatment of organic nervous affections. Lecture 3. On hemiparaplegia. *Lancet*, 2:429 and 867, 1869.
126. Faits contraires à la théorie des centres trophiques de Waller. *C R Soc Biol (Paris)*, 22:5, 1870; *C R Soc Biol (Paris)*, 23:170 and 207, 1871.
127. Hypertrophie des capsules surrénales, causée par une lésion de la moelle épinière. *C R Soc Biol (Paris)*, 22:27, 1870.
128. Différences entre les deux moitiés du cerveau, montrant que le côté droit devient surtout un centre de nutrition et le gauche un centre de vie intellectuelle. *C R Soc Biol (Paris)*, 22:27 and 97, 1870; *C R Soc Biol (Paris)*, 23:96, 1871.
129. Remoter consequences of nerve-lesions. In: Holmes T, ed., *A system of surgery, theoretical and practical, in treatises by various authors*, 2nd edition. (Vol. 4, p. 184). London: Longmans, Green & Co., 1870.
130. Faits montrant que la sécrétion des plumes s'augmente en arrière et du côté d'une hémisection de la moelle épinière. *C R Soc Biol (Paris)*, 22:41, 1870.
131. Influence des parties inférieures de la moelle épinière sur les parties supérieures. *C R Soc Biol (Paris)*, 22:45, 1870.

132. Pointe sentie lorsqu'une seule des pointes de l'aesthésiomètre est sentie. *C R Soc Biol (Paris)*, 22:61, 1870.
133. Fait démontrant que le symptôme connu sous le nom de constriction en ceinture et qu'on croit dépendre toujours d'une affection de la moelle épinière, peut être causé par une irritation d'un nerf cutané. *C R Soc Biol (Paris)*, 22:87, 1870.
134. Une piqûre du poumon peut causer une occlusion partielle des paupières. *C R Soc Biol (Paris)*, 22:97, 1870.
135. Constance d'une congestion des capsules surrénales après une lésion considérable d'un côté de l'encéphale. *C R Soc Biol (Paris)*, 22:113, 1870.
136. Production d'hémorrhagie pulmonaire par certaines lésions cérébrales. *C R Soc Biol (Paris)*, 22:117, 1870.
137. Similarité des effets produits par la section d'une moitié latérale de la moelle épinière et par une irritation des nerfs dorsaux, sur les mouvements volontaires et sur la respiration. *C R Soc Biol (Paris)*, 22:140, 1870.
138. Tournoiement causé par l'irritation du ganglion thoracique. *C R Soc Biol (Paris)*, 22:141, 1870.
139. On the location in the spinal cord of a special set of motor nerves distinct from the voluntary motor. *Lancet*, 1:2, 1870.
140. Relations entre l'hypocondrie et une altération particulière des poils. *C R Soc Biol (Paris)*, 23:52, 1871.
141. Mouvements rotatoires dus à une lésion de la partie lombaire de la moelle épinière. *C R Soc Biol (Paris)*, 23:104, 1871.
142. Faits démontrant que la mort, dans les affections cérébrales, peut être due à ce qu'elles ont produit des lésions pulmonaires. *C R Soc Biol (Paris)*, 23:101, 1871.
143. Fait nouveau relatif à la sensibilité tactile. *C R Soc Biol (Paris)*, 23:105, 1871.
144. Hémorrhagie et gangrène de l'oreille, produites par des lésions du système nerveux. *C R Soc Biol (Paris)*, 23:119 and 126, 1871; *Gaz Hebd Med (2nd series)*, 6:184 and 201, 1869.
145. Arrêt de la respiration par action réflexe. *C R Soc Biol (Paris)*, 23:134, 138, and 156, 1871.
146. Eschare se montrant du côté opposé à celui d'une lésion de la moelle épinière. *C R Soc Biol (Paris)*, 23:146, 1871.
147. Altération de nutrition d'un centre nerveux due à une lésion lointaine dans un nerf. *C R Soc Biol (Paris)*, 23:171, 1871.

148. On the production of haemorrhage, anaemia, oedema, and emphysema in the lungs by injuries to the base of the brain. *Lancet*, 1:6, 1871.
149. Pneumonie double, causée par une action réflexe provenant de l'inflammation d'un seul nerf vague. *C R Soc Biol (Paris)*, 24:18, 1872.
150. Preuves que c'est par une irritation de fibres centripètes venant des racines du nerf spinal que l'insufflation pulmonaire arrêt la respiration. *C R Soc Biol (Paris)*, 24:22, 1872.
151. Faits nouveaux contre l'opinion que c'est par une action du nerf vague que se produisent les ecchymoses pulmonaires dans les lésions cérébrales. Etude comparative de l'action physiologique des deux nerfs pneumogastriques. *C R Soc Biol (Paris)*, 24:181, 1872.
152. Production immédiate d'emphysème pulmonaire, par la galvanisation du nerf vague. *C R Soc Biol (Paris)*, 24:181 and 187, 1872.
153. Sécrétion de mucus palpébral par la galvanisation du nerf trijumeau dans le crâne. *C R Soc Biol (Paris)*, 24:188, 1872.
154. La section du nerf sciatique peut causer de l'exophthalmie unilatérale. *C R Soc Biol (Paris)*, 24:194, 1872.
155. Atrophie du cerveau causée par une lésion de la moelle épinière et par la section du nerf grand sympathique cervical. *C R Soc Biol (Paris)*, 24:194 and 195, 1872.
156. Remarks on some interesting effects of injuries of nerves, as shown in three cases. *Arch Sci Pract Med (NY)*, 1:54, 1873.
157. On the sudden or rapid arrest of many normal or morbid phenomena. *Arch Sci Pract Med (NY)*, 1:87, 1873.
158. On the mechanism of production of symptoms of diseases of the brain. *Arch Sci Pract Med (NY)*, 1:117 and 251, 1873.
159. On kinds of hemiplegia hitherto unknown or very little known, and on their diagnosis with spinal, altern and cerebral hemiplegia. *Arch Sci Pract Med (NY)*, 1:134, 1873.
160. Leçons sur les nerfs vaso-moteurs, sur l'épilepsie et sur les actions réflexes normales et morbides. Paris, 1872.
161. On ecchymoses and other effusions of blood caused by a nervous influence. *Arch Sci Pract Med (NY)*, 1:148, 1873.
162. Brown-Séquard's Lectures. A course of six lectures delivered at the Lowell Institute, Boston, in February and March 1874. *The Tribune*, 9 April 1874, and *Tribune Extras* No. 15, 1874.
163. Effets de l'irritation du nerf grand sympathique obtenus, chez l'homme, par action réflexe. *C R Soc Biol (Paris)*, 27:131, 1875.
164. On localization of functions in the brain. *Boston Med Surg J*, 93:119, 1875.

165. Production des effets de la paralysie du nerf grand sympathique cervical par l'excitation de la surface du cerveau. *C R Soc Biol (Paris),* 27:353 and 372, 1875; *Arch Physiol Norm Pathol (2nd Series)* 2:854, 1875.
166. Atrophie de l'oeil du côté de la cautérisation du cerveau. *C R Soc Biol (Paris),* 27:354, 1875.
167. Des altérations qui surviennent dans la muqueuse de l'estomac, consécutivement aux lésions cérebrales. *Bull Soc Anat (Paris)* 50 (3rd Series), 10:597, 1875.
168. L'ataxie des mouvements après la piqûre du sinus rhomboidal de la moelle épinière, chez les oiseaux, est due à l'irritation de nerfs des méninges. *C R Soc Biol (Paris),* 27:393, 1875.
169. Sur la variété des effets paralytiques ou spasmodiques causés par l'irritation thermique du cerveau. *C R Soc Biol (Paris),* 27:146, 360, 372, and 376, 1875; *C R Soc Biol (Paris),* 28:8, 1876.
170. Sur l'apparition d'une paralysie du côté d'une lésion encéphalique. *C R Soc Biol (Paris),* 27:424, 1875; *C R Soc Biol (Paris),* 28:2 and 13, 1876; A lecture on the appearance of paralysis on the side of a lesion of the brain. [In several parts.] *Lancet,* 1:2, 79, and 159, 1876.
171. Où se font les entre-croisements des conducteurs des ordres de la volonté aux muscles? *C R Soc Biol (Paris),* 28:14, 1876.
172. Sur l'anesthésie du côté de la lésion encéphalique. *C R Soc Biol (Paris),* 28:24, 1876.
173. Sur les convulsions unilatérales du côté de la lésion encéphalique. *C R Soc Biol (Paris),* 28:38, 1876.
174. La volonté n'agit pas comme on l'admet quand elle produit des mouvements. *C R Soc Biol (Paris),* 28:40, 1876.
175. Introductory lecture to a course on the physiological pathology of the brain. *Lancet,* 2:75, 1876.
176. Lectures on the physiological pathology of the brain: delivered at the Royal College of Physicians of London, July 1876. [In several parts.] *Lancet,* 2:109, 143, 211, 245, 279, 315, 387, 419, 453, and 527, 1876; *Lancet,* 1:39, 77, 117, 155, 265, 339, 485, 599, 709, and 827, 1877; *Lancet,* 1:153 and 225, 1878.
177. Course of lectures delivered before the President and Fellows of the King and Queen's College of Physicians, November 1876: Anaesthesia as an effect of brain-disease. *Dublin J Med Sci,* 63:1, 1877; Anaesthesia and amaurosis as effects of brain-disease. *Dublin J Med Sci,* 63:113, 1877; Aphasia as an effect of brain-disease. *Dublin J Med Sci,* 63:209, 1877.

178. Introduction à une série de mémoires sur la physiologie et la pathologie des diverses parties de l'encéphale. *Arch Physiol Norm Pathol (2nd series)*, 4:409 and 655, 1877.
179. The localisation of the functions of the brain applied to the use of the trephine. *Lancet*, 2:107, 1877.
180. On convulsions and paralysis, considered as effects of lesions of the base of the brain. Two lectures given in Philadelphia on 15 and 16 February 1878 and published as a 32-page brochure.
181. Recherches démontrant la non-nécessité de l'entre-croisement des conducteurs servant aux mouvements volontaires à la base de l'encéphale, ou ailleurs. *C R Acad Sci*, 86:1113, 1878.
182. Remarques sur la perception des impressions sensitives. Communicated to the Société de Biologie at its meeting on 4 May 1878 [not cited in *C R Soc Biol (Paris)*, 1878].

B. Researches on Epilepsy

183. D'une affection convulsive qui survient chez les animaux ayant eu une moitié latérale de la moelle épinière coupée. *C R Soc Biol (Paris)*, 2:105, 1850.
184. D'une affection convulsive consécutive à la section transversale de la moelle épinière. *C R Soc Biol (Paris)*, 2:169, 1850.
185. Recherches expérimentales sur la production d'une affection convulsive, épileptiforme, à la suite de lésions de la moelle épinière. *C R Acad Sci*, 42:86, 1856; with more details in *Arch Gen Med (Paris)*, 7:143, 1856.
186. Researches on epilepsy. Its artificial production in animals and its etiology, nature and treatment in man. Boston: Clapp, 1857; Experimental and clinical researches applied to physiology and pathology. [In several parts.] *Boston Med Surg J*, 55:337, 377, 421, and 457, 1856–1857; *Boston Med Surg J*, 56:54, 112, 155, 174, 216, 271, 338, 433, and 473, 1857.
187. Note sur des faits nouveaux concernant l'épilepsie consécutive aux lésions de la moelle épinière. *J Physiol (Paris)*, 1:472, 1858.
188. De la transmission par hérédité chez les mammifères, et particulièrement chez les cochons d'inde, d'une affection épileptiforme, produite chez les parents par des lésions traumatique de la moelle épinière. *C R Soc Biol (Paris)*, 11:194, 1859; Hereditary transmission of an epileptiform affection accidentally produced. *Proc R Soc Lond*, 10:297, 1860.

189. Sur l'arrêt immédiat de convulsions violentes par l'influence de l'irritation de quelques nerfs sensitifs. *Arch Physiol Norm Pathol*, 1:157, 1868.
190. Note sur l'avortement d'attaques d'épilepsie par l'irritation de nerfs à action centripète. *Arch Physiol Norm Pathol*, 1:317, 1868.
191. Nouvelles recherches sur l'épilepsie due à certaines lésions de la moelle épinière et des nerfs rachidiens. *C R Soc Biol (Paris)*, 21:29, 65, 111, 140, 156, 158, 190, 222, and 294, 1869; *Arch Physiol Norm Pathol*, 2:211, 422, and 496, 1869.
192. Du lieu de passage, dans la moelle épinière, des conducteurs spéciaux qui font contracter les muscles dans les convulsions de l'épilepsie. *Arch Physiol Norm Pathol*, 2:775, 1869.
193. Remarques sur l'épilepsie causée par la section du nerf sciatique chez les cobayes. *Arch Physiol Norm Pathol*, 3:153, 1870.
194. Des relations qui existent entre la cessation de l'état morbide épileptogène, à la face et au cou, et le retour de la sensibilité à la patte, chez les cobayes ayant été soumis à la section du nerf sciatique. *Arch Physiol Norm Pathol*, 3:302, 1870.
195. Faits nouveaux concernant la physiologie de l'épilepsie. *C R Soc Biol (Paris)*, 22:9, 33, 45, 50, 59, 82, 91, 113, and 124, 1870; *Arch Physiol Norm Pathol*, 3:516, 1870.
196. Quelques faits nouveaux relatifs à l'épilepsie qu'on observe à la suite de diverse lésions du système nerveux, chez les cobayes. *Arch Physiol Norm Pathol*, 4:116, 1871; *C R Soc Biol (Paris)*, 23:95, 146, and 169, 1871; *C R Soc Biol (Paris)*, 24:1, 18, and 195, 1872.
197. Note sur un moyen de produire l'arrêt d'attaques d'épilepsie et des convulsions causées par la strychnine ou les pertes de sang. *Arch Physiol Norm Pathol*, 4:204, 1871.
198. Production d'épilepsie chez le pigeon. *C R Soc Biol (Paris)*, 23:145 and 155, 1871.
199. Différences remarquables entre les États-Unis et la France à l'égard de la production de l'épilepsie par la section du nerf sciatique. *C R Soc Biol (Paris)*, 23:52, 1871.
200. Convulsions épileptiformes ou mouvements rotatoires causés par les capsules surrénales. *C R Soc Biol (Paris)*, 23:188, 1871.
201. Étendue considérable de la zone épileptogène, dans un cas de lésion de la moelle cervicale. *C R Soc Biol (Paris)*, 23:169, 1871.
202. Faits montrant que la moelle épinière en arrière de l'origine du nerf sciatique n'a pas la puissance de produire l'épilepsie. *C R Soc Biol (Paris)*, 24:1, 1872.

203. Production d'épilepsie par une lésion du nerf grand sympathique dans l'abdomen. *C R Soc Biol (Paris)*, 24:17, 1872.
204. L'hypertrophie du coeur est un effet constant de l'épilepsie artificielle, après un certain temps. *C R Soc Biol (Paris)*, 24:195, 1872.

C. General Physiology, and Physiology of the Muscles, Heart, Blood, Skin and Viscera

205. Note sur la source de l'irritabilité musculaire. *NY Med Times*, p. 74, 1847 [unverified].
206. Sur l'état de l'irritabilité dans les muscles paralysés. *NY Med Times*, p. 83, 1847 [unverified].
207. Hybernation des tenrecs. *C R Soc Biol (Paris)*, 1:37, 1849.
208. Recherches sur la rigidité cadavérique et la putréfaction. *C R Soc Biol (Paris)*, 1:39, 1849.
209. Tremblement des cholériques après la mort. *C R Soc Biol (Paris)*, 1:81, 1849.
210. Du sang veineux comme excitateur de certains mouvements. *C R Soc Biol (Paris)*, 1:105, 1849.
211. Usages des poches anales des tortues. *C R Soc Biol (Paris)*, 1:132, 1849.
212. Contraction de la peau et mouvements vermiculaires de scrotum, sous l'influence de l'électro-magnétisme. *C R Soc Biol (Paris)*, 1:134, 1849; Nouvelles recherches sur les contractions de la peau produites par le galvanisme. *C R Soc Biol (Paris)*, 2:132, 1850.
213. Influence de l'électro-magnétisme et de la foudre sur la durée de la rigidité cadavérique. *C R Soc Biol (Paris)*, 1:138, 1849.
214. Sur la mort par la foudre et par l'électro-magnétisme. *C R Soc Biol (Paris)*, 1:154, 1849.
215. Le tissu cellulaire de la peau est contractile. *C R Soc Biol (Paris)*, 1:158, 1849; *C R Soc Biol (Paris)*, 2:133, 1850.
216. Mouvements rhythmiques des muscles respirateurs et locomoteurs après la mort. *C R Soc Biol (Paris)*, 1:158, 1849.
217. Des rapports qui existent entre l'irritabilité musculaire, la rigidité cadavérique et la putréfaction. *C R Soc Biol (Paris)*, 1:173, 1849.
218. Sur la coagulabilité du sang des batraciens en hiver. *C R Soc Biol (Paris)*, 1:194, 1849.
219. De l'influence du système nerveux, du galvanisme, du repos et de l'action sur la nutrition des muscles. *C R Soc Biol (Paris)*, 1:195, 1849.

220. Existence d'un mouvement rhythmique dans le jabot des oiseaux. *C R Soc Biol (Paris)*, 2:83, 1850.
221. Apparition de la rigidité cadavérique avant la cessation des battements du coeur. *C R Soc Biol (Paris)*, 2:194, 1850.
222. Sur la persistance de la vie dans les membres atteints de la rigidité qu'on appelle cadavérique. *C R Acad Sci*, 32:855, 1851.
223. Recherches sur le rétablissement de l'irritabilité musculaire chez un supplicié treize heures après la mort. *C R Acad Sci*, 32: 897, 1851; *Mem Soc Biol (Paris)*, 3:147, 1851.
224. Preuve nouvelle à l'appui de la doctrine de Haller relative à l'indépendance de l'irritabilité musculaire. *C R Soc Biol (Paris)*, 3:101, 1851.
225. Recherches sur le rétablissement de l'irritabilité musculaire chez un second supplicié, plus de quatorze heures après la mort. *C R Soc Biol (Paris)*, 3:103, 1851.
226. Sur l'irritabilité des muscles paralysés. *C R Soc Biol (Paris)*, 3:144, 1851.
227. Preuve de la contractilité du tissu cellulaire. *C R Soc Biol (Paris)*, 3:164, 1851.
228. On the nutrition of muscles during their contraction. *Med Exam (Philadelphia)*, 8:428, 1852.
229. On the source of the vital properties. *Med Exam (Philadelphia)*, 8:481, 1852.
230. On the use of defibrinated blood in transfusion. *Nelson's Northern Lancet (Am J Med Jurisprudence)*, 6:237, 1852/1853; On the maintenance of life in limbs separated from the body, by means of injection of blood. *NY Med Times*, 1:355, 1852.
230.* On the causes of torpidity in the tenrec, (*Erinaceus ecaudatus*, Linn.). *Med Exam (Philadelphia)*, 8:549, 1852 [omitted by Brown-Séquard; added by the present author]
231. On a singular case of animal graft. *Med Exam (Philadelphia)*, 8:560, 1852.
232. On muscular irritability in paralyzed limbs, and its semeiological value. *Med Exam (Philadelphia)*, 9:25, 1853.
232.* Influence of red blood on muscles and nerves deprived of their vital properties. *Med Exam (Philadelphia)*, 9:280, 1853 [omitted by Brown-Séquard; added by the present author]
233. Sur l'emploi du sang défibriné dans la transfusion. *Med Times Gaz (London)*, Febr. 1854, p. 237.

234. Laws of the dynamical actions in man and animals. *Med Exam (Philadelphia)*, 9:211, 1853; Lois relatives aux phénomènes dynamiques de l'économie animale. *J Physiol (Paris)*, 1:1, 1858.
235. On apparently spontaneous actions of the contractile tissues of the animal body. *Med Exam (Philadelphia)*, 9:491, 1853.
236. On the cause of the beatings of the heart. *Med Exam (Philadelphia)*, 9:504, 1853.
237. Expériences prouvant qu'un simple afflux de sang à la tête peut être suivi d'effets semblables à ceux de la section du nerf grand sympathique au cou. *C R Acad Sci*, 38:117, 1854.
238. Recherches expérimentales sur la faculté que possèdent certains éléments du sang de régénérer les propriétés vitales. *C R Acad Sci*, 41:628, 1855; Experimental researches on the faculty possessed by certain elements of the blood of regenerating the vital properties. *Lond Med Times Gaz*, 32:492, 1855.
239. Experimental researches on the influence of efforts of inspiration on the movements of the heart. *Proc R Soc Lond*, 8:596, 1857; Note sur l'association des efforts inspiratoires avec une diminution ou l'arrêt des mouvements du coeur. *J Physiol (Paris)*, 1:512, 1858.
240. Recherches expérimentales sur la physiologie et la pathologie des capsules surrénales. *Bull Acad Med (Paris)*, 21:1067, 1856; *C R Acad Sci*, 43: 422 and 542, 1856; *C R Acad Sci*, 44:246, 1857; *C R Acad Sci*, 45:1036, 1857; and with more detail in *Arch Gen Med (Paris)*, 8:385 and 572, 1856; Nouvelle recherches sur l'importance des fonctions des capsules surrénales. *J Physiol (Paris)*, 1:160, 1858.
241. On the influence of oxygen on the vital properties of the spinal cord, nerves, and muscles. *Proc R Soc Lond*, 8:598, 1857.
242. Recherches sur les lois de l'irritabilité musculaire, de la rigidité cadavérique et de la putréfaction. *C R Acad Sci*, 45:460, 1857; republished with more details as The Croonian Lecture – On the relations between muscular irritability, cadaveric rigidity, and putrefaction. *Proc R Soc Lond*, 11:204, 1861; republished with additions – Leçon Croonienne sur les relations entre l'irritabilité musculaire, la rigidité cadavérique et la putréfaction. *J Physiol (Paris)*, 4:266, 1861.
243. Recherches expérimentales sur les propriétés physiologiques et les usages du sang rouge et du sang noir, et de leurs principaux éléments gazeux, l'oxygène et l'acide carbonique. *C R Acad Sci*, 45:562 and 925, 1857; with more details in *J Physiol (Paris)*, 1:95, 352, and 729, 1858.
244. Expériences sur la transformation de l'amidon en glucose dans l'estomac. [With FG Smith.] *J Physiol (Paris)*, 1:158, 1858.

245. Note sur les modifications que subissent les globules circulaires du sang de mammifère, injecté dans le système circulatoire des oiseaux, et sur les altérations des globules ovales du sang d'oiseau, injecté dans le système circulatoire des mammifères. *J Physiol (Paris)*, 1:173, 1858.
246. Limites de la possibilité du retour spontané de la rigidité cadavérique après qu'on l'a fait disparaître par l'élongation des muscles. *J Physiol (Paris)*, 1:281, 1858.
247. Sur des faits qui semblent montrer que plusieurs kilogrammes de fibrine se forment et se transforment, chaque jour, dans le corps de l'homme et sur le siège de cette production et de cette transformation. *J Physiol (Paris)*, 1:298, 1858.
248. Recherches sur la possibilité de rappeler temporairement à la vie des individus mourant de maladie. *J Physiol (Paris)*, 1:666, 1858.
249. Note sur l'existence de contractions rhythmiques dans les conduits excréteurs des principales glandes. *J Physiol (Paris)*, 1:775, 1858.
250. Remarques sur la production des phénomènes consécutifs à la ligature de l'oesophage. *J Physiol (Paris)*, 1:799, 1858.
251. Expériences sur l'absorption de la graisse. *J Physiol (Paris)*, 1:808, 1858.
252. Recherches sur l'irritabilité musculaire. *J Physiol (Paris)*, 2:75, 1859.
253. Recherches expérimentales et cliniques sur quelques questions relatives à l'asphyxie. *J Physiol (Paris)*, 2:93, 1859.
254. Remarques sur l'éphidrose parotidienne. *J Physiol (Paris)*, 2:449, 1859.
255. On the importance of the application of physiology to the practice of medicine and surgery. *Dublin Q J Med Sci*, 39:421, 1865.
256. *Advice to Students. An address delivered at the opening of the medical lectures of Harvard University*. Cambridge: John Wilson & Son, 1867.
257. Importance de l'emploi de sang défibriné dans la transfusion. *C R Soc Biol (Paris)*, 21:71, 1869.
258. Cas de transfusion de sang d'oiseau rappelant à la vie un chien mourant d'hémorrhagie. *C R Soc Biol (Paris)*, 21:72, 1869.
259. Absence de tuberculose secondaire, malgré l'existence de ses causes ordinaires. *C R Soc Biol (Paris)*, 21:153, 1869; *C R Soc Biol (Paris)*, 22:61, 1870.
260. Expériences démontrant que les poils peuvent passer rapidement du noir au blanc chez l'homme. *Arch Physiol Norm Pathol*, 2:442, 1869.
261. De l'état syncopal causé par l'acide carbonique. *C R Soc Biol (Paris)*, 21:204, 1869.
262. Les irritations mécaniques des muscles sont plus puissantes que la galvanisation. *C R Soc Biol (Paris)*, 22:73, 1870.

263. Des congestions consécutives aux ligatures d'artères. *C R Soc Biol (Paris)*, 22:82, 1870; *Arch Physiol Norm Pathol*, 3:518, 1870.
264. Reproduction de lames des vertèbres chez le chien. *C R Soc Biol (Paris)*, 22:144, 1870.
265. Transmission par hérédité de nombre d'altérations accidentelles. *C R Soc Biol (Paris)*, 22:5, 16, 17, 59, 64, 96, and 124, 1870; *C R Soc Biol (Paris)*, 24:188, 1872; On the hereditary transmission of effects of certain injuries to the nervous system. *Lancet*, 1:7, 1875.
266. Modification de mères par leurs embyrons, d'après des faits observés chez le cobaye. *C R Soc Biol (Paris)*, 22:5, 1870.

D. Animal Heat

267. On the normal degree of the temperature of man. *Med Exam (Philadelphia)*, 8:554, 1852.
268. On the influence exerted upon the general temperature of the body by a change in the temperature of one of the extremities. *Med Exam (Philadelphia)*, 8:556, 1852.
269. On the increase of animal heat after injuries of the nervous system. *Med Exam (Philadelphia)*, 9:137, 1853.
270. De l'influence de l'asphyxie sur la chaleur animale. *C R Soc Biol (Paris)*, 8:89, 1856.
271. Sur la basse température de quelques palmipèdes longipennes. *J Physiol (Paris)*, 1:42, 1858.
272. Recherches expérimentales sur quelques-uns des effets du froid sur l'homme. [With M Tholozan.] *J Physiol (Paris)*, 1:497, 1858.
273. Remarques sur l'influence du froid appliqué à une petite partie du corps de l'homme. *J Physiol (Paris)*, 1:502, 1858.
274. Recherches sur l'influence des changements de climat sur la chaleur animale. *J Physiol (Paris)*, 2:549, 1859.
275. Se produit-il plus de chaleur dans le sang circulant dans les poumons lorsque l'air inspiré, de chaud et humide, devient froid et sec? *Arch Physiol Norm Pathol*, 2:19, 1869.

E. Physiology and Pathology of the Eye and of Vision

276. Recherches expérimentales concernant l'action de la lumière et celle d'un changement de température sur l'iris, dans les cinq classes d'animaux vertébrés. *C R Acad Sci*, 25:482 and 508, 1847.

277. Action de la lumière lunaire sur la pupille. *C R Soc Biol (Paris)*, 1:9, 1849.
278. Action de la chaleur et du froid sur l'iris. *C R Soc Biol (Paris)*, 1:40, 1849.
279. Explication d'un phénomène de visibilité. *C R Soc Biol (Paris)*, 1:90, 1849.
280. Diagnostic de la paralysie de la rétine. *C R Soc Biol (Paris)*, 1:91, 1849.
281. Le resserrement et la dilatation de la pupille produits par la chaleur et le froid sont-ils des effets purement physiques, ou résultent-ils d'une véritable contraction musculaire? *C R Soc Biol (Paris)*, 1:115, 1849.
282. De la prétendue nécessité d'une turgescence vasculaire de l'iris pour produire le resserrement de la pupille. *C R Soc Biol (Paris)*, 1:116, 1849.
283. On certain actions of cold, warmth and light upon the crystalline lens. *Med Exam (Philadelphia)*, 8:553, 1852.
284. Researches on the action of certain part of the solar spectrum upon the iris. *Proc R Soc Lond*, 8:233, 1856.
285. Recherches expérimentales sur l'influence excitatrice de la lumière, du froid et de la chaleur sur l'iris, dans les cinq classes d'animaux vertébrés. *J Physiol*, 2:281 and 451, 1859.
286. Production d'amaurose et d'exophthalmie par une lésion du corps restiforme ou de la moelle épinière. *C R Soc Biol (Paris)*, 23:125, 1871.
287. Recherches sur les communications de la rétine avec l'encéphale. *Arch Physiol Norm Pathol*, 4:261, 1871.

F. Diverse

288. Helminthes trouvés chez des lapins. *C R Soc Biol (Paris)*, 1:46, 1849.
289. Recherches sur une cause de mort qui existe dans un grand nombre d'empoisonnements. *C R Soc Biol (Paris)*, 1:102, 1849.
290. Recherches sur le mode d'action de la strychnine. *C R Soc Biol (Paris)*, 1:119, 1849.
291. Sur la disposition spéciale des faisceaux et des couches musculaires du coecum chez le lapin et le lièvre. *C R Soc Biol (Paris)*, 1:190, 1849.
292. De l'existence constante des cysticerques chez les lapins, et de l'accroissement simultané de ces parasites et des animaux qui les portent. *C R Soc Biol (Paris)*, 2:79, 1850.
293. Recherches expérimentales sur l'action convulsivante de certains poisons. [In collaboration with F-N Bonnefin and published in his thesis.] Paris, 29 August 1851.
294. De l'emploi du trépan dans les fractures du rachis. *C R Soc Biol (Paris)*, 3:6, 1851; Trephining in cases of fracture of the spine. *Lancet*, 1:477, 1863.

295. On the treatment of epilepsy. *Med Exam (Philadelphia)*, 9:205, 1853.
296. Sur le fusel-oil. *C R Soc Biol (Paris)*, 5:160, 1853.
297. On a new mode of treatment of functional dyspepsia, anaemia and chlorosis. *Arch Sci Pract Med (NY)*, 1:30, 1873.
298. On a rare cause of mistake in testing urine for albumen by the ordinary processes. *Arch Sci Pract Med (NY)*, 1:277, 1873.
299. Opium and the actual cautery in the treatment of cholera. *Arch Sci Pract Med (NY)*, 1:467, 1873.
300. Leçon sur l'emploi du cautère actuel, surtout dans les affections nerveuses. *Boston Med Surg J*, 93:?, 1875 [incorrect citation: could not be verified].
301. Feeding per rectum in nervous affections. *Lancet*, 1:144, 1878.

Part 2: 1878 to 1886

302. Recherches démontrant la non-nécessité de l'entrecroisement des conducteurs servant aux mouvements volontaires, à la base de l'encéphale ou ailleurs. *France Med*, 25:305, 1878.
303. Lectures on the physiological pathology of the brain. Lecture 3. On ptosis as an effect of brain disease. *Lancet*, 2:573 and 611, 1878.
304. Injection de lait dans les veines: son innocuité, son importance. *C R Soc Biol (Paris)*, 30:292, 1878.
305. Production d'hémorrhagies dans le péricarde et dans le foie, par une lésion du corps strié et prédominance du côté droit du cerveau quant à la puissance de produire des altérations de nutrition et des troubles vaso-moteurs. *C R Soc Biol (Paris)*, 30:371, 1878.
306. Doctrines relatives aux principales actions des centres nerveux. Leçon d'ouverture du cours de médecine au Collège de France, faite le 2 décembre. *Gaz Hebd Med (2nd Series)*, 15:805, 1878.
307. Lectures on the physiological pathology of the brain. Lecture 3. On paralysis of limbs as an effect of disease of the medulla oblongata. *Lancet*, 1:1, 1879; On paralysis of limbs as an effect of disease of the medulla oblongata and neighbouring parts. *Lancet*, 2:451 and 565, 1879.
308. Prolongation extraordinaire des principaux actes de la vie après la cessation de la respiration. *Arch Physiol Norm Pathol (2nd Series)*, 6:83, 1879.
309. Quelques faits relatifs au mécanisme de production des paralysies et des anesthésies d'origine encéphalique. *Arch Physiol Norm Pathol (2nd Series)*, 6:199, 1879.

310. Nouveaux faits démontrant que des changements de forme et d'autres altérations organiques, dépendant d'une cause accidentelle, peuvent être transmis par hérédité. *C R Soc Biol (Paris)*, 31:113 and 125, 1879.

311. Faits montrant que des lésions de diverses parties de l'encéphale peuvent déterminer l'inhibition des cellules nerveuses et d'autres éléments de la moelle épinière, servant aux mouvements réflexes. *C R Soc Biol (Paris)*, 31:129, 1879.

312. Transfert d'anesthésie et d'hyperesthésie, par l'influence d'une lésion organique. *C R Soc Biol (Paris)*, 31:131, 1879.

313. Paralysie de cause organique cérébrale transférée dans le côté opposé du corps par une seconde lésion organique du même côté que la première. *C R Soc Biol (Paris)*, 31:135, 1879.

314. Production d'hémorrhagie dans les méninges spinales, par influence nerveuse, à la suite d'une lésion encéphalique. *C R Soc Biol (Paris)*, 31:136, 1879.

315. Recherches montrant combien est variable la limite des parties de la base de l'encéphale qui déterminent soit une paralysie croisée, soit une paralysie directe. *C R Soc Biol (Paris)*, 31:136, 1879.

316. Faits montrant: 1, que la zone motrice d'une moitié de la surface cérébrale peut produire des mouvements du côté correspondant; 2, qu'une partie très minime du faisceau pédonculaire de la base de l'encéphale peut suffire pour la production des mouvements dans les membres des deux côtés du corps, sous l'influence de l'excitation de la zone motrice de l'une quelconque des deux moitiés du cerveau. *C R Soc Biol (Paris)*, 31:139 and 140, 1879.

317. Expériences donnant ce résultat, en apparence paradoxal, que l'extirpation d'une partie du cerveau plus étendue que la zone motrice détermine moins d'effet paralytique que l'extirpation de cette zone seulement. *C R Soc Biol (Paris)*, 31:141, 1879.

318. Faits nouveaux absolument contraires à la théorie des centres psychomoteurs. *C R Soc Biol (Paris)*, 31:152, 1879.

319. Inhibition des cellules motrices de la moelle épinière par une lésion de la protubérance annulaire, chez les chats. *C R Soc Biol (Paris)*, 31:153, 1879.

320. Faits montrant que la galvanisation de la surface de chaque hémisphère cérébral agit sur les muscles des membres du côté opposé par deux voies bien distinctes l'une de l'autre. *C R Soc Biol (Paris)*, 31:165, 1879.

321. Expériences montrant: 1, que l'excitation galvanique des parties considérées comme motrices à la base de l'encéphale produit plus

souvent des mouvements du côté correspondant que du côté opposé; 2, qu'une lésion d'un côté de la moelle épinière ou d'un des nerfs sciatiques peut produire l'inhibition des cellules motrices et sensitives du bulbe et de la protubérances. *C R Soc Biol (Paris)*, 31:200, 1879.

322. Une lésion d'un côté de la base de l'encéphale qui, chez l'homme, produit si rarement de la paralysie à la paroi abdominale, en produit toujours chez le lapin et le cobaye. *C R Soc Biol (Paris)*, 31:201, 1879.

323. Faits nouveaux relatifs à la mise en jeu ou à l'arrêt (inhibition) des propriétés motrices ou sensitives de diverses parties du centre cérébro-rachidien. *Arch Physiol Norm Pathol (2nd Series)*, 6:494, 1879.

324. Faits relatifs au côté où se perd le mouvement volontaire, dans les cas de lésion d'une moitié latérale de la base de l'encéphale. *Arch Physiol Norm Pathol (2nd Series)*, 6:498, 1879.

325. Côté où se produisent des mouvements de membres quand on irrite une des moitiés latérales de la base de l'encéphale. *Arch Physiol Norm Pathol (2nd Series)*, 6:499, 1879.

326. Expériences montrant: 1, Que la même lésion d'un centre nerveux peut déterminer un état paralytique avec perte du ton musculaire ou une contracture; 2, Qu'une irritation mécanique violente de l'encéphale peut produire de l'inhibition dans certaines parties de la moelle épinière et de la dynamogénie dans d'autres. *C R Soc Biol (Paris)*, 31:296, 1879.

327. Recherches montrant la puissance, la rapidité d'action et les variétés de certaines influences inhibitoires (influences d'arrêt) de l'encéphale sur lui-même ou sur la moelle épinière et de ce dernier centre sur lui-même ou sur l'encéphale. *C R Acad Sci*, 89:657, 1879.

328. Alimentation par lavements de pancréas et de viande. *Gaz Hebd Med (2nd Series)*, 16:732, 1879.

329. Recherches expérimentales sur une nouvelle propriété du système nerveux. *C R Acad Sci*, 89:889, 1879.

330. Inhibition de la faculté réflexe de la moelle épinière: arrêt de mouvements rythmiques du vagin, du rectum et du spincter vésical. *Gaz Hebd Med (2nd Series)*, 17:393, 1880.

331. Expériences montrant que l'anesthésie due à certaines lésions du centre cérébro-rachidien peut être remplacée par de l'hyperesthésie, sous l'influence d'une autre lésion de ce centre. *C R Acad Sci*, 90:750, 1880.

332. De l'accroissement de l'activité du coeur après qu'il a été soumis à une inhibition complète. *C R Soc Biol (Paris)*, 32:211, 1880; *Gaz Med (6th Series)*, 2:351, 1880; Preuves qu'il y a augmentation de force dans le coeur, pendant son inhibition. *Gaz Hebd Med (2nd Series)*, 17:429, 1880.

333. Sur l'inhibition (arrêt) des échanges entre les tissus et le sang. *C R Soc Biol (Paris)*, 32:238, 1880; *Gaz Med (6th Series)*, 2:374, 1880; *Gaz Hebd Med (2nd Series)*, 17:457, 1880.

334. Unilateral convulsions due to brain disease. *Br Med J*, 2:332, 1880.

335. The effects produced by various lesions of the base of the brain on the excitability of the so-called motor centres. *Br Med J*, 2:383, 1880.

336. Sur des modifications profondes produites rapidement par certaines irritations de la peau, dans les grandes fonctions organiques et animales, ainsi que dans les propriétés des tissus nerveux et musculaire. *C R Soc Biol (Paris)*, 32:335, 1880; *Gaz Med (6th Series)*, 2:621, 1880; *Gaz Hebd Med (2nd Series)*, 17:795, 1880.

337. Sur le rôle des nerfs cutanés et de la moelle épinière dans la production de l'anesthésie, de la stupeur et d'autres phénomènes, après des applications de chloroforme sur la peau. *C R Soc Biol (Paris)*, 32:356, 1880; *Gaz Med (6th Series)*, 2:637, 1880; Rôle des nerfs cutanés et de la moelle épinière dans la production des phénomènes observés après des applications de chloroforme sur la peau; lésions héréditaires de l'oeil. *Gaz Hebd Med (2nd Series)*, 17:780, 1880.

338. Transmission par hérédité de certaines altérations des yeux chez les cobayes. *C R Soc Biol (Paris)*, 32:358, 1880; *Gaz Med (6th Series)*, 2:638, 1880.

339. Nouvelles preuves que c'est à une irritation des nerfs cutanés que sont dus les effets inhibitoires et autres que produit le chloroforme appliqué sur la peau. *C R Soc Biol (Paris)*, 32:376, 1880; *Gaz Med (6th Series)*, 2:652, 1880; *Gaz Hebd Med (2nd Series)*, 17:812, 1880.

340. Nouveaux faits relatifs à l'action du chloroforme appliqué à la périphérie du système nerveux (peau et conduit auditif externe). *C R Soc Biol (Paris)*, 32:383, 1880; *Gaz Med (6th Series)*, 2:669, 1880; Effets produits par l'application du chloroforme dans le conduit auditif et sur la peau. *Gaz Hebd Med (2nd Series)*, 17:812, 1880.

341. Existence de mouvements rhythmiques dans les vaisseaux du coeur. *C R Soc Biol (Paris)*, 32:384, 1880; *Gaz Med (6th Series)*, 2:669, 1880; Battements des vaisseaux du coeur. *Gaz Hebd Med (2nd Series)*, 17:813, 1880.

342. Discussion on the influence of injuries and morbid conditions of the nervous system on nutrition. *Br Med J*, 2:384, 1880; Remarks on some of the physiological and pathological influences of the nervous system on nutrition. *Br Med J*, 2:915, 1880.

343. Faits nouveaux observés à la suite d'excitations de la base de l'encéphale. p. 87. Rapport sur l'École Pratique des Hautes Études, Paris, 1879–1880.

344. Preuves que la perte de connaissance dans l'épilepsie, l'apoplexie, la syncope soudaine et d'autres circonstances, ne dépend pas essentiellement d'une diminution de circulation dans les vaisseaux encéphaliques. p. 88. Rapport sur l'École Pratique des Hautes Études, Paris, 1879–1880.

345. Preuves que la physiologie de l'appareil moteur cérébro-spinal repose sur des faits expérimentaux mal interprétés. p. 88. Rapport sur l'École Pratique des Hautes Études, Paris, 1879–1880.

346. Nouvelles recherches sur l'action du chloroforme appliqué sur la peau. *C R Soc Biol (Paris)*, 33:1, 1881; *Gaz Med (6th Series)*, 3:31, 1881.

347. Recherches sur les effets d'application de chloroforme sur les muqueuses nasale, buccale, pharyngée et laryngée. *C R Soc Biol (Paris)*, 33:1, 1881; *Gaz Med (6th Series)*, 3:31, 1881.

348. Effets produits par le chloral liquide pur (anhydre) appliqué sur la peau. *C R Soc Biol (Paris)*, 33:2, 1881; *Gaz Med (6th Series)*, 3:32, 1881.

349. Faits montrant que certaines parties du système nerveux peuvent agir de façon à augmenter plus ou moins soudainement les propriétés d'autres parties de ce système. *C R Soc Biol (Paris)*, 33:16, 1881; *Gaz Med (6th Series)*, 3:56, 1881.

350. D'un état syncopal particulier causé par l'application de chloral anhydre sur la peau. *C R Soc Biol (Paris)*, 33:18, 1881; *Gaz Med (6th Series)*, 3:57, 1881.

351. Sur l'absence de putréfaction chez les animaux tués par le chloral anhydre, appliqué sur la peau. *C R Soc Biol (Paris)*, 33:18, 1881; *Gaz Med (6th Series)*, 3:57, 1881.

352. Recherches sur les effets de l'élongation du nerf sciatique chez des animaux ayant eu une hémisection de la moelle épinière. *Mem Soc Biol (Paris)*, 33:1, 1881; *Gaz Med (6th Series)*, 3:65, 1881.

353. Sur un nouveau procédé de recherche des modes d'action des poisons. *Gaz Hebd Med (2nd Series)*, 18:87, 1881; Sur un nouveau mode de recherche de l'action des poisons. *C R Soc Biol (Paris)*, 33:28, 1881; *Gaz Med (6th Series)*, 3:81, 1881.

354. Production d'anesthésie par le tiraillement du bulbe et de la moelle cervicale, en abaissant fortement la tête d'un animal. *C R Soc Biol (Paris)*, 33:29, 1881; *Gaz Med (6th Series)*, 3:81, 1881.
355. Nouveaux faits relatifs aux effets produits par le chloral anhydre et par le chloral hydraté, appliqués sur la peau. *C R Soc Biol (Paris)*, 33:30, 1881; *Gaz Med (6th Series)*, 3:81, 1881.
356. Influence de l'irritation mécanique du bulbe rachidien sur les poumons. *C R Soc Biol (Paris)*, 33:53, 1881; *Gaz Med (6th Series)*, 3:130, 1881.
357. Nouveaux faits relatifs à l'élongation du nerf sciatique. *C R Soc Biol (Paris)*, 33:54, 1881; *Gaz Med (6th Series)*, 3:130, 1881.
358. Existence de sensibilité aux excitations mécaniques, dans certains cas, à la surface du cerveau des mammifères. *C R Soc Biol (Paris)*, 33:171, 1881; *Gaz Med (6th Series)*, 3:304, 1881.
359. De l'inhibition et de la dynamogénie des nerfs et des muscles à la suite d'irritations lointaines dues à des poisons, au froid ou à des causes mécaniques. *C R Soc Biol (Paris)*, 33:194, 1881; *Gaz Med (6th Series)*, 3:358, 1881.
360. Faits montrant que le corps calleux est excitable et qu'il sert en partie à la transmission des excitations galvaniques des prétendus centres psycho-moteurs aux membres. *C R Soc Biol (Paris)*, 33:204, 1881; *Gaz Med (6th Series)*, 3:377, 1881.
361. Faits montrant que l'excitabilité des nerfs moteurs et l'irritabilité musculaire, loin d'avoir des relations constantes, peuvent varier en sens inverse l'une de l'autre. *C R Soc Biol (Paris)*, 33:206, 1881; *Gaz Med (6th Series)*, 3:377, 1881.
362. De l'influence dynamogénique de certaines excitations des nerfs moteurs. *C R Soc Biol (Paris)*, 33:208, 1881; *Gaz Med (6th Series)*, 3:391, 1881.
363. Des phénomènes unilatéraux, inhibitoires et dynamogéniques dus à une irritation des nerfs cutanés par le chloroforme. *C R Acad Sci*, 92:1517, 1881.
364. On certain physiological effects of stretching of the sciatic nerve. *Lancet*, 1:206, 1881.
365. Phénomènes d'inhibition et de dynamogénie. *Gaz Hebd Med (2nd Series)*, 18:380, 1881.
366. Experimental facts showing that the admitted views relating to paralysis of cerebral origin and to the physiology of the so-called motor tract in the brain must be rejected. *Lancet*, 2:254, 1881.

367. Des localisations dans les maladies de l'encéphale et de la moelle épinière, au point de vue du diagnostic. International Medical Congress: Abstracts, London, 1881 [unverified].
368. Faits nouveaux relatifs à la contracture d'origine encéphalique. *C R Soc Biol (Paris)*, 33:325, 1881; *Gaz Med (6th Series)*, 3:678, 1881.
369. Contracture post-hemiplégique supprimée par l'élongation du sciatique. *Gaz Hebd Med (2nd Series)*, 18:763, 1881.
370. Atrophie du tissu adipeux et d'autres tissus non musculaires dans l'hémiplégie de cause cérébrale. *Gaz Med (6th Series)*, 3:679, 1881.
371. Recherches sur une nouvelle propriété du système nerveux. *C R Acad Sci*, 93:885, 1881.
372. Recherches expérimentales montrant que des causes diverses, mais surtout des lésions de l'encéphale, et en particulier du cervelet, peuvent déterminer, après la mort, une contracture générale ou locale. *C R Acad Sci*, 93:1149, 1881.
373. Production excessive de force nerveuse et musculaire pendant une attaque d'extase. *C R Soc Biol (Paris)*, 34:23, 1882.
374. Nouvelles recherches sur l'apparition de contracture après la mort. *C R Soc Biol (Paris)*, 34:25, 1882.
375. Recherches ayant pour objet d'établir que les lésions encéphaliques unilatérales, si elles déterminent une hémiplégie complète ou considérable, produisent aussi de la parésie dans les autres membres, surtout dans l'inférieur. *C R Soc Biol (Paris)*, 34:28, 1882.
376. Régénération du nerf sciatique dans une longueur de douze centimètres, dans l'espace de dix semaines, chez un petit singe. *C R Soc Biol (Paris)*, 34:30, 1882.
377. Persistance de l'état normal de la nutrition dans un membre de singe paralysé par suite de l'ablation du nerf sciatique dans toute sa longueur. *C R Soc Biol (Paris)*, 34:31, 1882.
378. Recherches sur une influence spéciale du système nerveux, produisant l'arrêt des échanges entre le sang et les tissus. *C R Acad Sci*, 94:491, 1882.
379. Faits montrant que les mouvements produits par l'irritation des diverses parties de l'encéphale sont très différents de ceux qui devraient survenir d'après les doctrines admises à l'égard des appareils moteur et sensitif du système nerveux cérébro-spinal. *C R Soc Biol (Paris)*, 34:246, 1882.
380. Recherches relatives à la production des mouvements dans les membres, sous l'influence d'irritations de diverses parties de l'encéphale. *C R Soc Biol (Paris)*, 34:279, 1882.

381. Recherches expérimentales et cliniques sur l'inhibition et la dynamogénie. Application des connaissances fournies par ces recherches aux phénomènes principaux de l'hypnotisme, de l'extase et du transfert. [In several parts.] *Gaz Hebd Med (2nd Series)*, 19:35, 53, 75, 105, and 136, 1882.
382. Faits montrant combien sont variées et nombreuses les voies de communication entre les zones motrices de la surface cérébrale et les membres. *C R Soc Biol (Paris)*, 34:328, 1882.
383. Faits nouveaux établissant l'extrême fréquence de la transmission, par hérédité, d'états organiques morbides, produits accidentellement chez des ascendants. *C R Acad Sci*, 94:697, 1882.
384. Recherches sur l'un des principaux fondements des doctrines relatives au mécanisme de production des mouvements volontaires et des convulsions. *C R Acad Sci*, 94:1285, 1882.
385. Possibilité d'introduire un tube dans le larynx sans produire de douleur ou une réaction quelconque. *C R Acad Sci*, 95:553, 1882.
386. Nouvelles recherches sur la production d'une anesthésie complète au larynx. *C R Soc Biol (Paris)*, 34:649, 1882.
387. Production d'anesthésie générale sous l'influence de l'irritation de la muqueuse laryngée par de l'acide carbonique ou du chloroforme. *C R Soc Biol (Paris)*, 34:799, 1882.
388. Epilepsy (p. 444) and Spinal Irritation (p. 1499). In: Quain R, ed. *A dictionary of medicine*. New York: Appleton, 1883.
389. Nerve-lesions and their more immediate effects; and locomotor ataxia [in collaboration with J L Clarke]. In: Holmes T, Hulke JW, eds., *A system of surgery, theoretical and practical, in treatises by various authors*, 3rd edition (pp. 178 and 223). London: Longmans, Green & Co, 1883.
390. Remoter consequences of nerve-lesions; and Suture and stretching of nerves. In: Holmes T, Hulke JW, eds., *A system of surgery, theoretical and practical, in treatises by various authors*, 3rd edition (pp. 199 and 214). London: Longmans, Green & Co, 1883.
391. Production d'anesthésie surtout dans une des moitiés du corps par une irritation du larynx, après la section d'un des nerfs laryngés supérieurs. *C R Soc Biol (Paris)*, 34:816, 1882.
392. Recherches sur la production d'une anesthésie générale ou d'une anesthésie surtout unilatérale, sous l'influence d'une simple irritation périphérique. *C R Acad Sci*, 95:1369, 1882.
393. Sur la possibilité de produire par une irritation périphérique, soit une paralysie générale sans anesthésie, soit de l'anesthésie sans paralysie, suivant le lieu de l'irrition. *C R Soc Biol (Paris)*, 35:27, 1883.

394. Sur l'inhibition soudaine des activités et des fonctions de l'encéphale, avec arrêt des échanges entre les tissus et le sang, sous l'influence d'une piqûre du bulbe rachidien. C R Soc Biol (Paris), 35:87, 1883.
395. Production d'hyperesthésie sous l'influence d'une application du chloral anhydre dans le conduit auditif externe chez des mammifères. C R Soc Biol (Paris), 35:91, 1883.
396. Recherches sur le rôle de l'inhibition dans une espèce particulière de mort subite et à l'égard de la perte de connaissance dans l'épilepsie. C R Acad Sci, 96:417, 1883.
397. Paralysies directes et croisées par irritation de la protubérance. Gaz Hebd Med (2nd Series), 20:154, 1883.
398. Inhibition en général et spécialement production d'une anesthésie générale par une simple irritation de la muqueuse laryngée ou de ses nerfs sensitifs. p. 89. Rapport sur l'École Pratique des Hautes Études, Paris, 1882–1883.
399. L'anesthésie dans les affections organiques de l'encéphale se produit par un mécanisme semblable à celui de l'analgésie due à l'irritation de la muqueuse laryngée, c'est-à-dire par inhibition. p. 90. Rapport sur l'École Pratique des Hautes Études, Paris, 1882–1883.
400. Production d'une anesthésie presque générale sous l'influence d'une irritation galvanique intense d'un des nerfs laryngés supérieurs. C R Soc Biol (Paris), 35:156, 1883.
401. Sur l'apparition d'un état cataleptiforme après la mort. C R Soc Biol (Paris), 35:191, 1883.
402. Sur l'apparition, après la mort, d'un état cataleptiforme dû à certaines lésions du centre cérébro-spinal, chez les oiseaux. C R Soc Biol (Paris), 35:206, 1883.
403. Sur l'importance de l'emploi simultané de la morphine et de l'atropine dans la plupart des cas où l'on doit faire usage de l'une de ces substances. C R Soc Biol (Paris), 35:289, 1883.
404. Recherches expérimentales et cliniques sur le mode de production de l'anesthésie dans les affections organiques de l'encéphale. C R Soc Biol (Paris), 35:417 and 454, 1883.
405. De l'importance du rôle de l'inhibition en thérapeutique. C R Acad Sci, 96:617, 1883.
406. Recherches expérimentales et cliniques sur le mode de production de l'anesthésie dans les affections organiques de l'encéphale. C R Acad Sci, 96:1766, 1883.
407. Production d'inhibition et de dynamogénie dans le système nerveux et les tissus contractiles. 1. Faits relatifs à l'inhibition de la sensibilité

générale par une irritation du larynx ou de la peau du cou. 2. a) inhibition exercée par l'encéphale sur la moelle et vice versâ; b) inhibition de la contractilité, ou de l'excitabilité des nerfs moteurs; c) transfert d'états thermiques. p. 92. Rapport sur l'École Pratique des Hautes Études, Paris, 1883–1884.

408. Production d'une contracture immobilisant le corps et les membres, dans certains cas de mort subite, contracture qui persiste après la mort. *Nature*, 1884 [incorrect citation: unverified].

409. Dynamogénie. In: *Dictionnaire Encyclopédique des Sciences Médicales.* (Vol. 30, p. 756) Paris: Asselin & Masson, 1884.

410. Persistance de la parole, dans le chant, dans les rêves et dans le délire, chez des aphasiques. *C R Soc Biol (Paris)*, 36:256, 1884.

411. Existence de l'excitabilité motrice et de l'excitabilité inhibitoire dans les régions occipitales et sphénoïdales de l'écorce cérébrale. *C R Soc Biol (Paris)*, 36:301, 1884.

412. Faits montrant que toutes ou presque toutes les parties de l'encéphale, chez l'homme, peuvent déterminer certaines inhibitions. *C R Soc Biol (Paris)*, 36:320, 1884.

413. Inhibition de certaines puissances réflexes du bulbe rachidien et de la moelle épinière, sous l'influence d'irritations de diverses parties de l'encéphale. *C R Soc Biol (Paris)*, 36:350, 1884.

414. Du rôle de certaines influences dynamogéniques réflexes dans des cas de suture de nerfs récemment publiés. *C R Soc Biol (Paris)*, 36:423, 1884.

415. De la puissance inhibitrice et de la puissance convulsivante de l'acide carbonique. *C R Soc Biol (Paris)*, 36:556, 1884.

416. Causes des altérations de nutrition qui suivent la section du nerf sciatique et du nerf crural, chez les cobayes. *C R Soc Biol (Paris)*, 37:146, 1885.

417. Production d'épilepsie spinale par une lésion du cervelet. *C R Soc Biol (Paris)*, 37:149, 1885.

418. Inhibition de la sensibilité à la douleur dans le corps tout entier sous l'influence de l'irritation de la muqueuse laryngée par la cocaïne. *C R Soc Biol (Paris)*, 38:167, 1885.

419. Du rôle de l'arrêt des échanges entre le sang et les tissus, de la contracture et de l'inhibition à l'égard du degré d'énergie et de la durée des propriétés des nerfs et des muscles après la mort. *C R Soc Biol (Paris)*, 37:185, 1885.

420. Recherches sur l'augmentation de la tonicité musculaire et sur l'inhibition de la propriété essentielle des tissus contractiles. *C R Soc Biol (Paris)*, 37:206, 1885.

421. Étude des effets produits par les irritations cutanées pour servir à l'explication des influences thérapeutiques exercées par les contre-irritants. *C R Soc Biol (Paris)*, 37:209, 1885.

422. Exposé de quelques faits jetant un jour nouveau sur la nature de la rigidité cadavérique. *Mem Soc Biol (Paris)*, 37:55, 1885.

423. Nouveaux faits relatifs à la rigidité cadavérique. *C R Soc Biol (Paris)*, 37:249, 1885.

424. Remarques sur l'altération de sensibilité, connue sous le nom d'allochirie. *C R Soc Biol (Paris)*, 37:268, 1885.

425. Production de globules semblables à ceux du sang des mammifères, dans diverses parties du corps d'animaux de cette classe, lorsqu'on y injecte du sang d'oiseau, même longtemps après la mort. *C R Soc Biol (Paris)*, 37:287, 1885.

426. Sur une espèce d'anesthésie artificielle, sans sommeil et avec conservation parfaite de l'intelligence, des mouvements volontaires, des sens et de la sensibilité tactile. *C R Acad Sci,* 100:1366, 1885.

427. Nouveaux faits relatifs à la formation de globules sanguins quand on injecte du sang d'oiseau dans les vaisseaux d'un mammifère, après la mort. *C R Soc Biol (Paris)*, 37:307, 1885.

428. Recherches expérimentales paraissant montrer que les muscles atteints de rigidité cadavérique restent doués de vitalite jusqu'à l'apparition de la putréfaction. *C R Acad Sci,* 101:926, 1885.

429. Nouveaux faits relatifs à la formation de globules sanguins quand on injecte du sang d'oiseau dans les vaisseaux d'un mammifère, après la mort. *C R Soc Biol (Paris)*, 37:307, 1885. [Same citation as No. 427; erroneously cited twice by Brown-Séquard.]

430. Indication d'un mode nouveau de production de l'emphysème pulmonaire. *C R Soc Biol (Paris)*, 37:354, 1885.

431. Sur la puissance de formation de globules sanguins, dans le système vasculaire des mammifères, après la mort. *C R Soc Biol (Paris)*, 37:393, 1885.

432. Faits relatifs aux voies de communication entre le cerveau et les muscles. *C R Soc Biol (Paris)*, 38:75, 1886.

433. Prolongation exceptionnelle de certains actes réflexes de la moelle épinière, après la mort. *C R Soc Biol (Paris)*, 38:101, 1886.

434. Simples procédés pour la prévention, dans certaines circonstances, d'affections catarrhales ou d'inflammations de nombre d'organes ou des muqueuses nasale, bucco-pharyngée, laryngée, trachéale ou bronchiale. *C R Soc Biol (Paris)*, 38:109, 1886.

435. Sur une nouvelle espèce de paralysie, locale ou générale, avec ou sans altération des sens et de la sensibilité générale. *C R Soc Biol (Paris)*, 38:131, 1886.

Part 3: 1886 to 1894

436. Nouveaux faits relatifs à l'anesthésie liée aux lésions organiques de la moelle épinière. *C R Soc Biol (Paris)*, 38:386, 1886.
437. Recherches expérimentales montrant que la rigidité cadavérique n'est due ni entièrement, ni même en grande partie, à la coagulation des substances albumineuses des muscles. *C R Acad Sci*, 103:622, 1886; *Gaz Hop (Paris)*, 59:1034, 1886; Recherches expérimentales paraissant démontrer que la rigidité cadavérique dépend d'une contracture, c'est-à-dire d'un acte de vie des muscles, commençant ou se continuant après la mort générale. *France Med*, 33:1507, 1886.
438. Recherches expérimentales montrant combien sont variés et nombreux les effets purement dynamiques provenant d'influences exercées sur l'encéphale par les nerfs sensitifs et sur les nerfs moteurs par les centres nerveux. *C R Acad Sci*, 103:790, 1886.
439. Sur divers effets d'irritation de la partie antérieure du cou et, en particulier, la perte de la sensibilité et la mort subite. *C R Acad Sci*, 104:951, 1887.
440. Fait nouveau à l'appui de la théorie d'après laquelle l'anesthésie, dans les cas de lésion partielle de la moelle épinière, dépend non d'une section de conducteurs, mais d'une inhibition. *C R Soc Biol (Paris)*, 39:238, 1887.
441. Sur l'existence dans chacun des hémisphères cérébraux de deux séries de fibres capables d'agir sur les deux moitiés du corps, soit pour y produire des mouvements, soit pour déterminer des phénomènes inhibitoires. *C R Soc Biol (Paris)*, 39:261, 1887.
442. Sur divers effets d'irritation de la partie antérieure du cou et, en particulier, la perte de la sensibilité et la mort subite. *Gaz Med (7th Series)*, 4:182, 1887; *Gaz Hop (Paris)*, 60:370, 1887; *Wien Med Bl*, 10:495, 1887.
443. Faits montrant que c'est parce que le bulbe rachidien est le principal foyer d'inhibition de la respiration qu'il semble être le principal centre des mouvements respiratoires. *C R Soc Biol (Paris)*, 39:293, 1887.
444. Dualité du cerveau et de la moelle épinière, d'après des faits montrant que l'anesthésie, l'hyperesthésie, la paralysie et des états variés

d'hypothermie et d'hyperthermie, dus à des lésions organiques du centre cérébro-spinal, peuvent être transférés d'un côté à l'autre du corps. *C R Acad Sci*, 105:646, 1887.

445. Recherches sur des mouvements de contraction et de ralâchement, en apparences spontanés, qui se produisent dans les muscles, après la mort, tant que dure la rigidité cadavérique. *C R Acad Sci*, 105:556, 1887; *France Med*, 34:1497, 1887.

446. Influence de la position de la tête sur les propriétés des prétendus centres moteurs et sur les manifestations morbides de cerveaux lésés. *C R Soc Biol (Paris)*, 39:607, 1887.

447. Recherches sur les deux principaux fondements des doctrines reçues à l'égard de la dualité cérébrales dans les mouvements volontaires. *C R Acad Sci*, 105:840, 1887.

448. Recherches sur l'importance, surtout pour les phtisiques, d'un air non vicié par des exhalaisons pulmonaires. [With A d'Arsonval.] *C R Acad Sci*, 105:1056, 1887.

449. Démonstration de la puissance toxique des exhalaisons pulmonaires provenant de l'homme et du chien. [With A d'Arsonval.] *C R Soc Biol (Paris)*, 39:814, 1887.

450. Discours aux funérailles de M. Vulpian. *C R Soc Biol (Paris)*, 39:321, 1887.

451. Funérailles de M. Vulpian. Discours prononcé, au nom de la Société de Biologie. *Arch Physiol Norm Pathol (3rd Series)*, 9:353, 1887.

452. Nouvelles recherches sur les phénomènes produits par un agent toxique très puissant qui sort sans cesse des poumons de l'homme et des mammifères, avec l'air expiré. [With A d'Arsonval.] *C R Acad Sci*, 106:165, 1888.

453. Nouvelles recherches démontrant que les poumons sécrètent un poison extrêmement violent qui en sort avec l'air expiré. [With A d'Arsonval.] *C R Soc Biol (Paris)*, 40:33, 1888.

454. Nouvelles remarques à l'égard du poison pulmonaire. [With A d'Arsonval.] *C R Soc Biol (Paris)*, 40:54, 1888.

455. Toxicité de l'air expire—nouvelles recherches. [With A d'Arsonval.] *C R Soc Biol (Paris)*, 40:90, 1888.

456. Remarques sur la valeur des faits qui nous ont servi à démontrer la toxicité de l'air expiré. [With A d'Arsonval.] *C R Soc Biol (Paris)*, 40:99, 1888.

457. Resemblances entre l'action toxique de certaines ptomaines et celle du poison pulmonaire. [With A d'Arsonval.] *C R Soc Biol (Paris)*, 40:108, 1888.

458. Description d'un appareil permettant de faire respirer à plusieurs animaux de l'air libre et pur quant à ses proportions d'oxygène et d'acide carbonique, mais contenant des quantités considérables du poison de l'air expiré. [With A d'Arsonval.] *C R Soc Biol (Paris)*, 40:110, 1888.
459. Sur quelques points importants relatifs à la durée de la survie des lapins après l'injection sous-cutanée du liquide contenant le poison de l'air expiré. [With A d'Arsonval.] *C R Soc Biol (Paris)*, 40:151, 1888.
460. Recherches démontrant que l'air expiré par l'homme et les mammifères, à l'état de santé, contient un agent toxique très puissant. [With A d'Arsonval.] *C R Acad Sci*, 106:106, 1888.
461. Remarques au sujet de la ventilation des lieux habités. [With A d'Arsonval.] *C R Soc Biol (Paris)*, 40:172, 1888.
462. Explication du retour, quelquefois si rapide, de la sensibilité et du mouvement volontaire, après la suture des bouts d'un nerf coupé. *C R Soc Biol (Paris)*, 40:245, 1888.
463. Notions nouvelles de physiologie générale des centres nerveux, pour servir à la pathogénie de la paralysie et de l'anesthésie. *C R Soc Biol (Paris)*, 40:276, 1888.
464. Notions nouvelles de physiologie générale des centres nerveux, pour servir à la pathogénie de la paralysie et de l'anesthésie. Seconde communication. *C R Soc Biol (Paris)*, 40:290, 1888.
465. Coexistence d'inexcitabilité de la zone excito-motrice du cerveau avec persistance des fonctions motrices de ce centre nerveux et aussi avec production d'attaques épileptiformes violentes. *C R Soc Biol (Paris)*, 40:354, 1888.
466. Note sur des phénomènes importants observés chez un chien après la section d'une moitié latérale du bulbe rachidien. *C R Soc Biol (Paris)*, 40:407, 1888.
467. Les nerfs moteurs perdent-ils leur excitabilité avant les muscles, lorsqu'ils sont privés de circulation sanguine? *C R Soc Biol (Paris)*, 40:694, 1888.
468. Recherches expérimentales montrant que, sous l'influence de la gravitation, les centres appelés moteurs et les autres parties d'une moitié de l'encéphale peuvent déterminer des mouvements dans chacune des moitiés du corps. *C R Acad Sci*, 106:1577, 1888; *France Med*, 35:817, 1888.
469. Champ d'action de l'inhibition en physiologie, en pathogénie et en thérapeutique. *Arch Physiol Norm Pathol (5th Series)*, 1:1, 1889.
470. Recherches cliniques et expérimentales sur les entre-croisements des conducteurs servant aux mouvements volontaires. *Arch Physiol Norm Pathol (5th Series)*, 1:219, 1889.

471. Le sommeil normal, comme le sommeil hypnotique, est le résultat d'une inhibition de l'activité intellectuelle. *Arch Physiol Norm Pathol (5th Series),* 1:333, 1889.

472. De la cause du rythme respiratoire, d'aprés un fait découvert par M. Charles Rouget. *Arch Physiol Norm Pathol (5th Series),* 1:336, 1889.

473. Quelques mots sur la decouverte de l'inhibition. *Arch Physiol Norm Pathol (5th Series),* 1:337, 1889.

474. Recherches sur la localisation des conducteurs des impressions sensitives dans les diverses parties de l'encéphale, et sur la pathogénie des anesthésies de cause encéphalique. *Arch Physiol Norm Pathol (5th Series),* 1:484, 1889.

475. Nouvelles recherches démontrant que la toxicité de l'air expiré ne dépend pas de l'acide carbonique. [With A d'Arsonval.] *C R Acad Sci,* 108:267, 1889.

476. Remarques sur l'association entre l'effort inspiratoire et l'inhibition du coeur. *Arch Physiol Norm Pathol (5th Series),* 1:610, 1889.

477. Expériences montrant combien est grande la dissémination des voies motrices dans le bulbe rachidien. *Arch Physiol Norm Pathol (5th Series),* 1:606, 1889.

478. Recherches montrant que la mort par inhalation du poison que contient l'air expiré n'est pas activée par les émanations de vapeurs provenant de l'urine et des matières fécales des animaux soumis à cette inhalation. [With A d'Arsonval.] *C R Acad Sci,* 108:1294, 1889.

479. Inhibition. In: *Dictionnaire Encyclopédique des Sciences Médicales* (Vol 16, 4th Series; p. 1). Paris: Masson and Asselin & Houzeau, 1889.

480. Des effets produits chez l'homme par des injections sous-cutanées d'un liquide retiré des testicules frais de cobaye et de chien. *C R Soc Biol (Paris),* 41:415, 1889.

481. Seconde note sur les effets produits chez l'homme par des injections sous-cutanées d'un liquide retiré des testicules frais de cobaye et de chien. *C R Soc Biol (Paris),* 41:420, 1889.

482. Troisième note sur les effets des injections sous-cutanées de liquide testiculaire. *C R Soc Biol (Paris),* 41:430, 1889.

483. Remarques à l'occasion du travail de M. Variot, sur les injections de liquide testiculaire chez l'homme. *C R Soc Biol (Paris),* 41:454, 1889.

484. Note on the effects produced on man by subcutaneous injections of a liquid obtained from the testicles of animals. *Lancet,* 2:105, 1889.

485. Expérience démontrant la puissance dynamogénique chez l'homme d'un liquide extrait de testicules d'animaux. *Arch Physiol Norm Pathol (5th Series),* 1:651, 1889.

486. Des contractions et des élongations en apparences spontanées des muscles atteints de la rigidité cadavérique. *Arch Physiol Norm Pathol (5th Series)*, 1:675, 1889.

487. Du rôle physiologique et thérapeutique d'un suc extrait de testicules d'animaux, d'aprés nombre de faits observés chez l'homme. *Arch Physiol Norm Pathol (5th Series)*, 1:739, 1889.

488. Sur des actions inconnues ou à peine connues des muscles aprés la mort. *Arch Physiol Norm Pathol (5th Series)*, 1:726, 1889.

489. De quelques règles générales relatives à l'inhibition. *Arch Physiol Norm Pathol (5th Series)*, 1:751, 1889.

490. Preuves de l'insignifiance d'une expérience célèbre de MM. Victor Horsley et Beevor sur les centres appelés moteurs. *Arch Physiol Norm Pathol (5th Series)*, 2:199, 1890.

491. Nouveaux faits relatifs à l'injection sous-cutanée, chez l'homme, d'un liquide extrait de testicules de mammifères. *Arch Physiol Norm Pathol (5th Series)*, 2:201, 1890.

492. Influence du système nerveux pour retarder la putréfaction. *C R Soc Biol (Paris)*, 42:2, 1890.

493. Recherches sur les mouvements rythmés des ailes et du thorax chez les oiseaux décapités ou ayant subi d'autres lésions des centres nerveux. *Arch Physiol Norm Pathol (5th Series)*, 2:371, 1890.

494. Théorie des mouvements involontaires coordonnés, des membres et du tronc chez l'homme et les animaux. *Arch Physiol Norm Pathol (5th Series)*, 2:411, 1890.

495. Exposé de faits nouveaux à l'égard de l'influence sur les centres nerveux d'un liquide extrait de testicules d'animaux. *Arch Physiol Norm Pathol (5th Series)*, 2:443, 1890.

496. Remarques sur les effets produits sur la femme par des injections sous-cutanées d'un liquide retiré d'ovaires d'animaux. *Arch Physiol Norm Pathol (5th Series)*, 2:456, 1890.

497. Recherches sur l'existence d'une période intermédiaire à l'irritabilité musculaire et à la rigidité cadavérique. *Arch Physiol Norm Pathol (5th Series)*, 2:628, 1890.

498. Nouveaux faits relatifs à l'influence sur les centres nerveux de l'homme d'un liquide extrait de testicules d'animaux. *Arch Physiol Norm Pathol (5th Series)*, 2:641, 1890.

499. Quelques mots sur les recherches de M. Nicaise sur la physiologie de la trachée et des bronches. *Arch Physiol Norm Pathol (5th Series)*, 2:657, 1890.

500. Influence du système nerveux pour retarder la putréfaction. *Gaz Med (7th Series)*, 7:28, 1890.

501. Du rajeunissement. *Scalpel (Liége)*, 48:8, 1890–1891 [Unverified].
502. Nombreux cas de vivisection pratiquée sur le cerveau de l'homme; leur verdict contre la doctrine des centres psycho-moteurs. *Arch Physiol Norm Pathol (5th Series)*, 2:762, 1890.
503. Have we two brains or one? *Forum*, 9:627, 1890.
504. Remarques sur un ouvrage du Dr. Bateman sur l'aphasie. *C R Soc Biol (Paris)*, 42:537, 1890.
505. Nouvelles remarques sur le liquide testiculaire. *C R Soc Biol (Paris)*, 41:717, 1890.
506. De la perte de connaissance dans l'épilepsie après l'ablation du ganglion cervical supérieur du nerf grand sympathique, des deux côtés, chez l'homme et chez le cobaye. *Arch Physiol Norm Pathol (5th Series)*, 3:216, 1891.
507. Exposé de faits nouveaux montrant la puissance du liquide testiculaire contre l'affaiblissement dû à certaines maladies et en particulier la tuberculose pulmonaire. *Arch Physiol Norm Pathol (5th Series)*, 3:224, 1891.
508. Remarques sur la spermine et le liquide testiculaire. *Arch Physiol Norm Patho (5th Series)*, 3:401, 1891.
509. Quelques mots sur un réflexe nouveau, décrit par les Drs. Onanoff et C-H Hughes. *Arch Physiol Norm Pathol (5th Series)*, 3:403, 1891.
510. De l'injection des extraits liquides provenant des glandes et des tissus de l'organisme comme méthode thérapeutique. [With A d'Arsonval.] *C R Soc Biol (Paris)*, 43:248, 1891.
511. Additions à une note sur l'injection des extraits liquides de divers organes, comme méthode thérapeutique. [With A d'Arsonval.] *C R Soc Biol (Paris)*, 43:265, 1891.
512. Remarques à propos de l'emploi du liquide testiculaire. *C R Soc Biol (Paris)*, 43:318, 1891.
513. Remarques à l'occasion du fait de guérison d'ataxie locomotrice, communiqué par M. Depoux. *C R Soc Biol (Paris)*, 43:404, 1891.
514. Recherches sur les extraits liquides retirés des glandes et d'autres parties de l'organisme et sur leur emploi, en injections sous-cutanées, comme méthode thérapeutique. [With A d'Arsonval.] *Arch Physiol Norm Pathol (5th Series)*, 3:491, 1891.
515. Rejet de l'emploi de tous les antiseptiques autres que la glycérine et l'acide carbonique pour la préparation des extraits organiques destinés aux injections thérapeutiques sous-cutanées. [With A d'Arsonval.] *C R Soc Biol (Paris)*, 43:535, 1891.

516. Préparation des extraits liquides provenant des différents organes de l'économie animale destinés aux injections sous-cutanées therapeutiques. [With A d'Arsonval.] *Arch Physiol Norm Pathol (5th Series)*, 3:593, 1891.

517. Recherches sur l'inhibition de la sensibilité aux causes de douleur sous l'influence d'une irritation de la muqueuse laryngée par de l'acide carbonique. *Arch Physiol Norm Pathol (5th Series)*, 3:645, 1891.

518. Innocuité de l'injection dans le sang d'extraits liquides du pancréas, du foie, du cerveau et de quelques autres organes. [With A d'Arsonval.] *C R Soc Biol (Paris)*, 43:722, 1891.

519. Faits montrant combien est grande et variée l'influence du système nerveux sur la nutrition et les sécrétions: influence curative du liquide testiculaire dans un grand nombre d'affections locales ou générales, organiques ou fonctionnelles. *Arch Physiol Norm Pathol (5th Series)*, 3:747, 1891.

520. Recherches sur la production d'une analgésie générale par des irritations traumatiques ou mécaniques de la peau du cou, de la trachée ou du larynx par la faradisation ou par l'application de chloroforme ou de cocaïne au larynx. *Arch Physiol Norm Pathol (5th Series)*, 3:773, 1891.

521. Sur une inhibition dont les chirurgiens pourraient tirer profit si elle se produit chez l'homme comme chez le chien et le singe. Les plaies par incision ou par brûlure, après une irritation du larynx ou de ses nerfs sensitifs, peuvent conserver de l'analgésie pendant plusieurs jours et même deux semaines ou plus longtemps. *Arch Physiol Norm Pathol (5th Series)*, 3:805, 1891.

522. Mort par arrêt des échanges entre le sang et les tissus sous l'influence d'une irritation de la muqueuse laryngée. *Arch Physiol Norm Pathol (5th Series)*, 3:818, 1891.

523. Faits établissant que la vie locale peut durer bien plus longtemps qu'on ne croit dans la moelle épinière, les nerfs et les muscles, après la mort générale, chez des mammifères. *Arch Physiol Norm Pathol (5th Series)*, 4:119, 1892.

524. Injection dans le sang d'extraits liquides du pancréas, du foie, du cerveau et de quelques autres organes. [With A d'Arsonval.] *Arch Physiol Norm Pathol (5th Series)*, 4:148, 1892.

525. Nouveaux modes de préparation du liquide testiculaire pour les injections sous-cutanées. [With A d'Arsonval.] *Arch Physiol Norm Pathol (5th Series)*, 4:164, 1892.

526. Localisation prétendue de fonctions diverses dans les centres nerveux et surtout dans certaines parties des organes auditifs. *Arch Physiol Norm Pathol (5th Series)*, 4:366, 1892.

527. Traitement de nombreux états morbides par des injections sous-cutanées du liquide testiculaire. *Bull Med (Paris)*, 6:965, 1892 [unverified].

528. Effets physiologiques d'un liquide extrait des glandes sexuelles et surtout des testicules. *C R Acad Sci*, 114:1237, 1892.

529. Effets produits sur de nombreux états morbides par des injections sous-cutanées d'un extrait liquide retiré des testicules. *C R Acad Sci*, 114:1318, 1892; *Gaz Hop (Paris)*, 65:645, 1892.

530. Influence de l'extrait aqueux de capsules surrénales sur les cobayes presque mourants à la suite de l'ablation de ces organes. *C R Soc Biol (Paris)*, 44:410, 1892.

531. Suc testiculaire: remarques sur la communication de MM. Nourry et Michel. *C R Soc Biol (Paris)*, 44:508, 1892.

532. Influence curative du liquide testiculaire dans l'ataxie locomotrice. *C R Soc Biol (Paris)*, 44:505, 1892.

533. Influence dynamogénique du liquide testiculaire chez des animaux que l'on va faire mourir par hémorragie. *C R Soc Biol (Paris)*, 44:607, 1892.

534. Des douleurs et des congestions causées par les injections de liquide testiculaire et d'un moyen très simple de ne pas les produire. [With A d'Arsonval.] *Arch Physiol Norm Pathol (5th Series)*, 4:599, 1892.

535. Note sur le traitement du cancer et du choléra par le liquide testiculaire. *C R Acad Sci*, 115:375, 1892.

536. Note sur quelques faits nouveaux relatifs à la physiologie de l'épilepsie. *C R Acad Sci*, 115:394, 1892.

537. Effets physiologiques d'un liquide extrait des glandes sexuelles et surtout des testicules. *Gaz Med (8th Series)*, 1:399, 1892.

538. Des injections sous-cutanées ou intra-veineuses d'extraits liquides de nombre d'organes, comme méthode thérapeutique. [With A d'Arsonval.] *C R Acad Sci*, 114:1399, 1892; *Nice Med*, 16:129, 1891–1892.

539. Hérédité d'une affection due à une cause accidentelle: faits et arguments contre les explications et les critiques de Weismann. *Arch Physiol Norm Pathol (5th Series)*, 4:686, 1892.

540. Sur la durée du travail de production des mouvements involontaires, coodonnés. *Arch Physiol Norm Pathol (5th Series)*, 4:703, 1892.

541. Importance de l'analgésie due à une irritation laryngienne dans l'étude expérimentale de la puissance motrice des diverses parties de l'encéphale. *Arch Physiol Norm Pathol (5th Series)*, 4:725, 1892.

542. Remarques sur l'influence du liquide testiculaire dans plusieurs cas nouveaux d'ataxie locomotrice et dans un cas de paraplégie de cause organique. *C R Soc Biol (Paris)*, 44:551, 1892.

543. Remarques sur le traitement de l'ataxie locomotrice par de liquide testiculaire, à propos du cas de M. Depoux. *C R Soc Biol (Paris)*, 44:796, 1892.

544. Sur l'emploi du liquide testiculaire pour augmenter la vigueur du foetus dans le sein maternel, d'après un fait du Dr. Kahn. *C R Soc Biol (Paris)*, 44:797, 1892.

545. Remarques sur l'emploi du liquide testiculaire par plus de douze cents médecins et en particulier sur l'influence favorable exercée par ce liquide dans vingt et un cas de cancer et dans quelques autres affections. [With A d'Arsonval.] *C R Soc Biol (Paris)*, 44:815, 1892.

546. Résultats thérapeutiques des injections de liquide testiculaire. [With A d'Arsonval.] *L'Union Médicale (3rd Series)*, 54:638, 1892.

547. Questions relatives à la physiologie de l'encéphale. *Arch Physiol Norm Pathol (5th Series)*, 5:409, 1893.

548. Quelques règles relatives à l'emploi du liquide testiculaire. *C R Soc Biol (Paris)*, 45:35, 1893.

549. Remarques sur l'innocuité du liquide testiculaire. *C R Soc Biol (Paris)*, 45:307, 1893.

550. Note sur les conclusions physiologiques et cliniques qui ressortent de certaines expériences dans lesquelles l'ataxie locomotrice ou la paralysie, dues à des lésions de la moelle épinière, ont été guéries ou améliorées par des injections de liquide testiculaire. *C R Soc Biol (Paris)*, 45:365, 1893.

551. Influence heureuse de la transfusion de sang normal après l'extirpation des capsules surrénales chez le cobaye. *C R Soc Biol (Paris)*, 45:448, 1893.

552. Faits cliniques et expérimentaux contre l'opinion que le centre respiratoire se trouve uniquement ou principalement dans le bulbe rachidien. *Arch Physiol Norm Pathol (5th Series)*, 5:131, 1893.

553. Effets physiologiques et thérapeutiques d'un liquide extrait de la glande sexuelle mâle. [With A d'Arsonval.] *Gaz Hop (Paris)*, 66:488, 1893.

554. Régles relatives a l'emploi du liquide testiculaire. [With A d'Arsonval.] *Arch Physiol Norm Pathol (5th Series)*, 5:192, 1893.

555. Remarques sur les recherches de MM Gad et Marinesco, sur le centre respiratoire. *Arch Physiol Norm Pathol (5th Series)*, 5:194, 1893.

556. Des transmissions dans la moelle épinière d'après les dégénérescences secondaires. *Arch Physiol Norm Pathol (5th Series)*, 5:197, 1893.

557. La dilatation de la pupille est-elle une phénomène d'inhibition ou l'effet d'une contraction musculaire. *Arch Physiol Norm Pathol (5th Series)*, 5:198, 1893.

558. Nouvelles remarques sur les injections sous-cutanées ou intra-veineuses d'extraits liquides de nombre d'organes, comme méthode therapeutique. [With A d'Arsonval.] *Arch Physiol Norm Pathol (5th Series)*, 5:200, 1893.

559. Remarques sur la valeur des fondements des doctrines relatives au siège de la puissance motrice volontaire dans les centres nerveux. *Arch Physiol Norm Pathol (5th Series)*, 5:203, 1893.

560. Quelques mots sur les progrès de nos connaissances à l'égard des actions physiologiques et thérapeutiques du liquide orchitique (testiculaire) *Arch Physiol Norm Pathol (5th Series)*, 5:205, 1893.

561. Remarques sur une série de faits nouveaux. *Arch Physiol Norm Pathol (5th Series)*, 5:208, 1893.

562. Importance de la sécrétion interne des reins démontrée par les phénomènes de l'anurie et de l'urémie. *Arch Physiol Norm Pathol (5th Series)*, 5:778, 1893.

563. Faits tendant à montrer que le retour de la sensibilité et du mouvement après la suture des nerfs est dû à une dynamogénie remplaçant de l'inhibition. *Bull Acad Med Paris (3rd Series)*, 29:582, 1893.

564. Remarques à l'égard des cas d'ataxie, chez l'homme et chez le chien, communiqués par M. Depoux et M. Mégnin. *C R Soc Biol (Paris)*, 45:520, 1893.

565. Note additionnelle à propos de la communication de M. Depoux, sur un cas de quérison d'ataxie locomotrice. *C R Soc Biol (Paris)*, 45:527, 1893.

566. Traitement de l'acromégalie par certains liquides organiques. *C R Soc Biol (Paris)*, 45:527, 1893.

567. On a new therapeutic method consisting in the use of organic liquids extracted from glands and other organs. *Br Med J*, 1:1145 and 1212, 1893.

568. Nutrition et cicatrisation après la section du nerf sciatique très haut, et amputation de la cuisse. *C R Soc Biol (Paris)*, 45:688, 1893.

569. Effets physiologiques et thérapeutiques d'un liquide extrait de la glande sexuelle mâle. [With A d'Arsonval.] *C R Acad Sci*, 116:856, 1893.

570. Quelques faits relatifs à certaines puissances antiseptiques du liquide orchitique préparé au Collège de France. *Arch Physiol Norm Pathol (5th Series)*, 5:797, 1893.

571. Remarques sur un travail de M. d'Arsonval. *C R Acad Sci,* 116:1532, 1893.
572. Nouvelles recherches démontrant que la toxicité de l'air expiré dépend d'un poison provenant des poumons et non de l'acide carbonique. [With A d'Arsonval.] *Arch Physiol Norm Pathol (5th Series),* 6:113, 1894.
573. Remarques sur la durée des propriétés des muscles et des nerfs après la mort. *Arch Physiol Norm Pathol (5th Series),* 6:188, 1894.
574. Remarques à propos des recherches du Dr. F. W. Mott sur les effets de la section d'une moitié latérale de la moelle épinière. *Arch Physiol Norm Pathol (5th Series),* 6:195, 1894.
575. Remarques sur les variétés extrêmes des manifestations paralytiques dans des cas de lésions de la base de l'encéphale et sur les conclusions qui en ressortent. *Arch Physiol Norm Pathol (5th Series),* 6:204, 1894.
576. Remarques sur une série de faits intéressants. *Arch Physiol Norm Pathol (5th Series),* 6:213 and 496, 1894.
577. Faits nouveaux montrant que la conductibilité nerveuse est absolument distincte de l'irritabilité. *Arch Physiol Norm Pathol (5th Series),* 6:752, 1894.

Glossary

A NUMBER OF TECHNICAL medical or physiological terms have been used in this text. Although they have generally been defined at first use, readers without a medical background may nevertheless find it useful to have these definitions gathered in a single place for their convenience. They are listed here alphabetically.

Acetylcholine. A neurotransmitter in both the central and peripheral nervous systems, it is released by certain nerves at their terminations to excite the neurons or effector organs (such as muscle) with which they connect. For example, the vagus nerve releases acetylcholine at its terminations in the heart, leading to slowing of the heart rate. Similarly, motor nerves release acetylcholine where they terminate on muscle fibers.

Adrenal glands. Endocrine glands that lie close to the kidneys and consist of an outer part, the cortex, and an inner part, the medulla.

Adrenaline. *See* Epinephrine.

Afferent or sensory nerves. Nerves that carry impulses toward the central nervous system.

Analgesia. Loss or absence of pain perception.

Anesthesia. Loss or absence of sensation (including but not limited to pain).

Anatomy. 1: The form and structure of a body and the interrelationship of its parts. 2: The study of such form and structure. 3: Dissection of the body.

Anterior. In or toward the front of.

Autonomic nervous system. Portion of the nervous system, with both central and peripheral components, that is present in vertebrates and enables the body to adapt to its environment. For example, it regulates the force and frequency of the heart beats, the blood pressure, respiration, the body temperature, and the functions of various organs of the body as well as bladder, bowel, and sexual function. It is divided into the sympathetic and parasympathetic systems, which are controlled by a portion of the brain called the hypothalamus, and the balance in activity of the two systems—which have opposing effects—governs behavior depending on the environment and emotion. Both systems operate continuously, but the sympathetic system plays a major role in stressful situations, whereas the parasympathetic system is dominant at other times. Thus, in response to fear or anger, for example, the sympathetic system causes the heart to beat faster and with greater strength; blood flow to the skin is reduced (being diverted to the muscles, in case the animal needs to fight or run away), the blood pressure is increased, the hair may stand on end (so the animal appears larger and more frightening), the pupils dilate, the airways widen to allow for greater airflow in the lungs, the concentration of sugar in the blood is increased, and so on.

Axon. *See* Neuron.

Brainstem. Part of the brain that connects with the spinal cord and is—in turn—connected with the cerebral hemispheres. It consists of the midbrain, pons, and medulla. In some usages, it also includes the hypothalamus (q.v.), thalamus (a relay point for nerve traffic to and from the cerebral cortex), and other diencephalic structures (i.e., structures that are interposed between the cerebral hemispheres and the midbrain).

Brown-Séquard syndrome. The symptoms and signs that result from a lateral hemisection or other lesion of the lateral half of the spinal cord. It is characterized by hyperesthesia (increased sensitivity to touch) and weakness below the level of the lesion, such as in the lower limb, on the ipsilateral (transected) side, and a loss of pain (analgesia) and temperature appreciation on the opposite (contralateral) side.

Central nervous system. The brain and spinal cord.

Cerebellum. The "little brain," a part of the brain that lies at the back of the head between the cerebral hemispheres and brainstem. It is concerned with the coordination of movement and with the preservation of balance. It also has less clearly defined cognitive functions and a role in motor learning. In humans, it consists of two lateral hemispheres or lobes and a midline portion (the vermis). It is connected with the spinal cord and with other parts of the brain.

Cerebral cortex. The outer (gray) layer of the cerebral hemispheres, consisting mainly of neurons.

Cerebral hemispheres. The two halves of the brain that are most evident in humans when the skull is opened. They are in continuity with the midbrain and hindbrain, and thus with the spinal cord.

Cholinergic. Related to acetylcholine. When used with reference to nerve fibers, it indicates that the fibers release the neurotransmitter acetylcholine.

Commissure. A band of nerve fibers that crosses the midline and connects corresponding parts of the central nervous system on the two sides.

Contralateral. The opposite side to.

Cutaneous. Of or relating to the skin.

Defibrinated blood. Blood from which the protein fibrin has been removed to prevent clotting. Brown-Séquard achieved this by mechanical agitation; blood was whipped while it clotted and the fibrin threads were then removed and washed to free blood cells trapped among them. The fluid that remained was defibrinated blood.

Dendrite. *See* Neuron.

Dermatome. The skin region innervated mainly by a single spinal sensory nerve and nerve root, the sensory fibers thereby passing to a single segment of the spinal cord.

Efferent nerves. Nerves that carry impulses from the central nervous system to the muscles or other effector structures.

Elixir of life. Derogatory term used for an agent supposedly capable of making an old person permanently young again.

Elixir vitae. *See* Elixir of life.

Endocrine gland. Gland that passes its secretions directly into the blood, rather than through a duct.

Epilepsy. A disorder characterized by recurrent seizures.

Epinephrine. Adrenaline; a hormone secreted in the adrenal medulla and a chemical neurotransmitter released by certain neurons in the central nervous system. It leads to constriction of some blood vessels and dilatation of others (primarily in muscles), an increase in blood pressure, an increase in heart rate and output, a dilatation of the airways, and an increase in the blood level of glucose—the so-called "fight or flight" reaction to stress.

Excitation. The process of activating a cell or cells.

Externat **and** *internat.* French medical students were divided into externs and interns after initial training based upon competitive examinations (*concours*). Interns were paid, but externs received little compensation in the mid-nineteenth century. Typically, each medical service was directed by a senior physician and included an intern and three or four externs. Interns were in charge of patients, monitored their treatment, accompanied their chief on morning rounds, assisted during surgery, took call at night, and undertook autopsies. The externs were responsible for minor surgical tasks and for maintaining medical records.

Extrapyramidal pathways. Descending motor pathways that do not traverse the medullary pyramids.

Fibrin. An insoluble protein that is the main constituent of a blood clot.

Funiculus. Subdivision of the spinal cord containing longitudinally oriented bundles of nerve fibers. The anterior funiculus is situated between the anterior fissure and the anterior roots, the lateral funiculus between the anterior and posterior roots, and the posterior funiculus between the posterior roots and the posterior median sulcus.

Gerontology. The science of ageing.

Glial cells. Cells other than neurons in the central nervous system. They produce the myelin (insulating fatty sheath) surrounding axons, help to protect neurons, provide a suitable environment for neurons to function, aid in their development, and seem to modulate neuronal behavior.

Goiter. An enlarged thyroid gland.

Gyri. (sing. Gyrus). The convolutions or folds seen on the surface of the cerebral hemispheres and cerebellum.

Hormones. Chemical substances released into the blood to influence the function of other parts of the body. The term is customarily restricted to substances that have more specific functions than simply subserving the general metabolic requirements of the body.

Humoral. Chemical.

Hyperesthesia. Increased sensitivity to touch, sometimes painful.

Hyperalgesia. Increased sensitivity to painful stimuli.

Hypoesthesia. Reduction in sensitivity of the skin to sensory stimuli.

Hypothalamus. A part of the brain that controls autonomic function such as temperature, as well as appetite, fluid intake, sleep, sexual activity, and the release of various hormones as summarized in footnote A, Chapter 13. *See also* Brainstem.

Hypothyroidism. Underactivity of the thyroid gland.

Inhibition. The suppression or blocking of activation or functioning; the opposite of excitation.

Interneuron. A nerve cell in the central nervous system that connects one cell with another.

Ipsilateral. The same side as.

Lateral. 1: to the side of. 2: Away from the midline.

Law of Bell-Magendie. The principle that the anterior and posterior roots have different functions (the anterior roots being motor and the posterior roots sensory).

Level, motor. The lowest level of the spinal cord with normal motor function after disease or injury of the spinal cord.

Level, neurological. The lowest level of the spinal cord with normal function.

Level, sensory. The lowest level of the spinal cord below which sensory function is abnormal after disease or injury of the spinal cord.

Locomotor ataxia. A form of tertiary neurosyphilis. It may not manifest for years after the initial infection and is characterized by sensory deficits, spontaneous stabbing pains, and impaired coordination of movement, especially in the legs, so that the gait becomes unsteady (ataxic).

Medulla, medulla oblongata. The portion of the brainstem that is in continuity with the spinal cord and contains neurons regulating such bodily functions as the heart rate, blood pressure, respiration, swallowing, and the state of arousal, as well as fibers passing between the brain and spinal cord.

Medullary pyramids. The region of the medulla containing the descending corticospinal tract. At the bottom of the medulla, some of these fibers cross from one side to the other in the decussation of the pyramids.

Motor nerves. *See* Efferent nerves.

Motor neurons. Nerve cells in the spinal cord that innervate muscles.

Myxedema. (Br., myxedoema). Syn. for hypothyroidism.

Myotome. The muscles supplied by a single segmental spinal nerve and root, and thus by a specific level of the spinal cord.

Nerve roots. Connection between the spinal nerves and the spinal cord. The spinal nerves arise at each segmental level of the spinal cord by an anterior root (predominantly motor) and a posterior root (predominantly sensory).

Nerve impulse. The transient self-propagating electrochemical events that occur along nerve fibers and constitute the message that is being transmitted.

Neurasthenia. A disorder described by the American neurologist George Beard in 1869, and supposedly characterized by nonspecific symptoms such as fatigue, lassitude, headache, anxiety, depression, aches and pains, disturbed sleep, and diverse other complaints. It is doubtful that it exists as a distinct diagnostic entity.

Neurology. The study of the nervous system in health and disease.

Neuron. A nerve cell, a cell that is excitable and able to transmit electrical impulses. A neuron typically consists of a cell body (*perikaryon*), a single elongated *axon* or nerve fiber that transmits impulses away from the cell body to other neurons or an effector structure such as muscle, and a number of small branches or *dendrites* that receive impulses from other neurons and transmit them toward the cell body.

Neurotransmitter. Chemical that is released from vesicles in the axonal terminals on one neuron to influence the activity of another. Neurotransmitters act on receptors that may be excitatory or inhibitory. *See* Synapse for further details.

Norepinephrine. Noradrenaline; a chemical neurotransmitter released by the adrenal medulla and at the termination of most sympathetic nerves and by certain neurons (noradrenergic neurons) in the central nervous system. It leads to constriction of some blood vessels and dilatation of others (primarily in muscles); increases the blood pressure, heart rate, and cardiac output; dilates the airways; and increases the blood level of glucose. Such changes constitute the so-called "fight or flight" reaction to stress.

Nuclei, in the central nervous system. Aggregates or compact collections of neurons, which appear gray within the white matter of the brain. The brain looks white where it consists primarily of nerve fibers rather than the cell bodies of neurons.

Nucleus tractus solitarius. Nucleus in the medulla that receives taste, cardiovascular, respiratory, and gastrointestinal inputs, and mediates the gag, cough, and various cardiovascular and respiratory reflexes, as well as reflexes affecting motility and secretion within the gastrointestinal tract.

Opotherapy. The administration for medical purposes of tissues derived from the body.

Organotherapy. The administration for medical purposes of tissues derived from the body.

Parasympathetic nervous system. *See* Autonomic nervous system.

Peripheral nervous system. The nerves that run from the central nervous system to other parts of the body, such as the muscles, skin, bodily organs, and sensory organs.

Physiology. The functional processes of living organisms, or the study of these functions and processes.

Posterior. 1: Behind or at the back of a structure. 2: Toward the back surface of the body.

Posterior columns, of spinal cord. Ascending fibers in the posterior funiculi at the back of the spinal cord, which conduct certain sensory information to the brain.

Professeur libre. Teacher without an official academic position.

Pyramids. *See* Medullary pyramids.

Pyramidal fibers or pathways. Fibers or pathways that traverse the medullary pyramids.

Reflex. 1: The process by which a stimulus generates an automatic, nonvolitional response, as when a muscle contracts when it is stretched by a tap with a tendon hammer (stretch reflex), a blink occurs when the cornea of the eye is touched with a wisp of cotton wool (corneal reflex), or retching occurs when the back of the throat is touched (gag reflex). 2: an involuntary or automatic reaction of the body to a specific stimulus. The simplest reflexes, such as the stretch reflex, involve an afferent (sensory) neuron whose axon conveys information to the central nervous system and an efferent (motor) neuron whose axon goes to an effector structure such as a muscle. There is a single synaptic connection between the two neurons (that is, the reflex is monosynaptic). Other reflexes involve one or more intermediate neurons between the afferent and efferent arcs in the spinal cord. For the more complex reflexes, the afferent or efferent loop may involve a number of neurons at different levels of the central nervous system. This arrangement permits the reflex to be modified, allows for a variety of responses, and permits more coordinated complex responses.

Roots. *See* Nerve roots.

Scratch reflex. Response to a cutaneous stimulus characterized by an involuntary scratching movements that usually relieves the itch. Scratch reflexes are components of normal grooming behavior but—especially after certain lesions of the spinal cord—are elicited by a variety of innocuous or inappropriate mechanical stimuli, such as rubbing the skin.

Sensory receptor. A cell or nerve ending that is specialized to respond to stimuli from the external or internal environment of an organism.

Spinal cord. The cylindrical portion of the central nervous system that extends down from the brain, within the bony vertebral column or backbone. It connects with the peripheral nervous system through the nerve roots and spinal nerves.

Spinal shock. The sudden but temporary loss of spinal cord activity (that is, of neural function) below the level of an acute injury to the spinal cord.

Stretch reflex. The reflex contraction of a muscle in response to its sudden stretch. The involved reflex involves receptors and afferent fibers that convey information to the spinal cord concerning the state of stretch of the muscle, and efferent fibers that pass from the motor neurons in the spinal cord back to the muscle to activate its contraction.

Sympathetic nervous system. *See* Autonomic nervous system.

Synapse. The junction between one neuron and another, or between an axon and muscle (or other) cell. A small gap, the *synaptic cleft*, separates the two interconnecting structures. The electrical impulse traveling down the axon of the presynaptic neuron leads to the release of vesicles containing a neurotransmitter that excites receptors on the postsynaptic membrane of the second cell.

Testicle. Or testis, the organ that produces sperms in male animals.

Testosterone. A steroid hormone manufactured in the testicles and, to a lesser extent, in the ovaries.

Tissue. A group of cells with a similar structure and function.

Vasomotor nerves. Nerves that supply the blood vessels, controlling their caliber.

Vasomotor reflexes. Reflexes that affect the circulation—and specifically the regional distribution of blood—as a result of internal or external stimuli.

Vestibular apparatus. Structures within the inner ear that provide information concerning the position of the body in space. Vestibular derangements lead to vertigo, imbalance, and related complaints.

White matter. Of brain or spinal cord, the part that is composed mainly of nerve fibers (rather than nerve cells).

Index

Page numbers followed by *f* indicate figures; those followed by *n* indicate footnotes.

Académie des Sciences, ix, 3, 4, 51, 53, 69, 85n, 88, 88n, 91, 97, 107, 137n, 151, 164, 199, 200, 201n, 227, 222, 277, 291
Academy of Natural Sciences of Philadelphia, 107
Acland, Henry, 202
Aconite, for dysentery, 124, 124n
Acquired epilepsy, inheritance of, 192–193
Addison, Thomas, 90–91, 90n, 93, 211, 246, 257n
Addison's disease, 90–91, 90n, 93, 211, 246
Adenauer, Konrad, 252
Adolescents, masturbation and, 241
Adrenal cortex, 235n
Adrenal glands, vii, 7, 52, 67, 85n, 89–93, 211, 235n, 245, 246–247, 253–254, 256, 256n, 285, 287, 335
    Addison's disease, 90–91, 90n, 93, 211, 246
    adrenaline, 67, 90, 93, 253, 254n, 335,337
    animal extracts from, 211, 246, 256
    blood pressure increase and, 253–254, 256n
    Brown-Séquard, C. E., on, 91–93, 246–247
    kidney and, 67, 89–90, 92
    Vulpian's work on, 85n
Adrenaline, 67, 90, 93, 253–254, 254n, 268, 335, 337

Adrenocorticotrophic hormone, 235n
Afferent nerves, 32–33, 33f, 35–36, 67, 73, 159–160, 160f, 184–186, 217, 218f
Agassiz, Louis, 132n, 134, 137, 137n, 141–144, 146–148, 205
Aging. *See also* Rejuvenation
    delaying/counteracting of, 7, 205–207, 238–253, 249n, 251n
    gerontology, 237, 253, 286
Agoraphobia, 88
Air toxicity, 197, 271–272
Aldosterone, 90, 235n
Alexander the Great, 183
Althaus, Julius, 106, 106n
Altitude sickness, 163n
America. *See also specific city or institution*
    Brown-Séquard C. E., in, 81–85,121–134, 144–146
    Civil War in, 75n, 116, 121–126, 125n, 146, 264
    clinical practice in New York, 145–146
    first move to, 55–57
    music halls in, xii, 205, 206
    response to animal extract research, 240–242
American Academy of Arts and Sciences, 132, 132n

344 Index

American Academy of Neurology, 125n
American Medical Association, 82, 85, 131, 251, 254
American Neurological Association, 125n
American Philosophical Society, 107, 132, 132n
American Physiological Society, 8, 8n
Amputation, 116, 122–124, 124n, 125n, 189–191, 275
 as epilepsy treatment, 192
 experimental epilepsy and, 189–191
Amyotrophic lateral sclerosis, Charcot and, 76n
Anastomosis, of blood vessels, 275–278, 278n
Anderson, John, 143
Anemia, 90–91
 "anemic" concept, of sleep, 262
 pernicious, 91, 257n
Anesthesia, 122, 335
 animal vivisection without, 40, 40n, 45–46, 140
 introduction of, 45–46
 measurement of, 111
 as sensory loss, 213–214
 Snow, John, and 59n
Aneurysm, 76n, 222, 222n
Angiotensin, 235n
Animal extracts, 5, 197–198, 205–211, 238–248,
 from adrenal glands, 211, 246, 256
 American response to, 240–242
 bone tissue, 245
 brain tissue, 245
 "elixir of life," 7, 206, 210, 239–240, 337
 kidney, 245
 muscle tissue, 245
 ovaries, 242, 242n, 257
 pancreas, 245
 Pasteur and, 202, 221–224
 pituitary gland, 245
 procedure for preparing, 242
 Schiff's work with, 244n
 spleen, 245
 testicles, 7, 30, 122, 205–211, 238–248, 248n, 252
 from thyroid, 245–246, 256
 treatment of disease and rejuvenation, 238–248, 258
Animal heat (temperature), 310
Animal research, 6, 8n, 45–46, 83, 140, 192–193. *See also* Antivivisection; Vivisection
 Galen and, 35
 vivisection without anesthesia, 40, 40n, 45–46, 140
Anticoagulants, 123n
Antidiuretic hormone, 235n
Antigens, 123n
Antineuralgic Pills, Brown-Séquard's, 124, 124n
Antiseptic technique, 108, 201, 203–204
 germ theory of disease, 112n, 184n, 201
 tetanus and, 122, 122n
Antivivisection, ix, 6, 40n, 45–46, 138–140, 140n, 172n, 204, 210–211, 240, 244n, 287 *See also* Vivisection
 Cobbe, Frances Power, 139
 Kingsford, Anna, 140, 140n
Aphasia, 167, 167n, 168n
 Brown-Séquard, C. E., on aphasia/ hemispheric functions, 168–170
Archives de Médecine Expérimentale et d'Anatomie Pathologique, 221n
Archives de Physiologie Normale et Pathologique, 137n, 221, 221n
Archives of Scientific and Practical Medicine, 144–145, 198
Arnott, James, 112
d'Arsonval, Jacques Arsène, 198–199, 201, 209, 211, 221, 223n, 224, 225, 227
Aseptic technique, 92, 122, 201
 germ theory of disease, 112n, 184n, 201
Atherton, Gertrude, 249n
Athletic performance, enhancement of, 247
Atrial natriuretic factor, 236n
Atropine, diarrhea and, 124
Auget, Antoine Jean Baptiste Robert, Baron de Montyon, 88, 88n
Autonomic nervous system, 37, 66–68, 72, 336–337. *See also* Vasomotor nerves

Awards
　Baly medal, to Brown-Séquard,
　　C. E., 201
　to Brown-Séquard, C. E., 86, 107,
　　163–164, 163n, 199, 201–202
　Montyon Prize, awarded to
　　Bernard, Claude, 50
Axon, 157–158, 158f

Babinski, Joseph, 209–210, 209n, 274
Babinski sign, 209n, 274
Baillière, 145
Balance, sense of, 261–262
Baly medal, from Royal College of
　　Physicians of London, 201
Bárány, Robert, 262
Bartholinus, Caspar, 89
Bartholow, Roberts, 171
Bayliss, William, 250n
Bed sores, 74–76, 78
Bell, Alexander Graham, 204
Bell, Charles, 38–40, 38n, 86
Belladonna, 124, 124n
Bence Jones, Henry, 108
Bence Jones protein, 108
Bentley, Edwin, 124, 124n
Berdoe, Edward, 210
Berger, Hans, 188, 188n
Bernard, Claude, 31, 39n, 46, 50, 52, 53n,
　　65–66, 68–72, 85, 88–89, 130, 130n,
　　150–151, 197–199, 221n
　on Brown-Séquard, C. E., 137n, 151
　concept of internal secretions and, 237
　funeral of, 150–151
　Montyon Prize awarded to, 50
　President of Société de Biologie, 201
　as rival of Brown-Séquard, C. E., 27, 52,
　　65, 83, 127, 150
Bernard, Tristan, 7
Bert, Paul, 163, 163n, 199–200, 201n
Berthelot, Marcelin, 151, 151n
Berthold, Arnold Adolph, 237
Bipolar disease, Brown-Séquard and, 100,
　　133–134, 197, 283–284
Bismarck, Otto von, 141
Blood,
　irrigation of tissues by, 48–49, 84, 97, 123,
　　199, 261, 264, 275–278, 286
　research on control of circulation, 5,
　　70–72, 306–310
　transfusion, 91, 123–124, 123n
Bois-Reymond, Emil du, 69n, 77, 298
Boissier, 4
Bonaparte, the Emperor Napoleon III, 54,
　　55, 137, 138, 141, 151, 211n
Bonnefin, Frederic, 30
Bordeu, Théophile de, 236
Borell, Merriley, 257
Boston, 5, 56, 57, 58, 59, 89, 126–133, 134,
　　137, 141, 142, 143, 145, 146, 147,
　　148, 150
Boston Society of Natural History, 173
Bouchard, Charles, 201n, 201n, 209, 222, 227
Bouley, Henri, 85n
Bowditch, Henry Pickering, 8, 8n, 129–131
Bowman, William, 98–99, 201–202
Bradykinin, 72
Brain, *See also specific topics.*
　anatomy of brain function, 165–177, 168f
　Broca, Pierre Paul, and language,
　　167–69, 168f
　Brown-Séquard, C. E., on aphasia/
　　hemispheric functions, 168–170
　Brown-Séquard, C. E., on functional
　　localization, 173–176, 197
　composition of, 32–33, 33f, 35, 157–158
　duality of, 157, 177–179
　equipotentiality of two hemispheres,
　　178–179
　focal v. diffuse disturbances in, 112
　functional connectivity of, 176–177
　functional localization in, 149, 165–177
　and heart and lung function, 203, 269n,
　　267–271
　inhibitory activities of, 111, 162–165, 263
　tumors, 112, 159n, 171, 172, 268
　Wernicke, Carl, and language,
　　167–168, 168f
Brazil, emperor of, 146, 146n, 201–202, 201n
De Brazza, Pierre Paul François Camille
　　Savorgnan, 200–201
Breathing (ventilation), 269–271, 269n

Bright, Richard, 90, 90n
Brinkley, John, 251, 251n
British Association for the Advancement of Science, 138–140
British East India Company, 15–16
British Medical Council, 202
British Medical Journal, Brown-Séquard, C. E., and, 138, 246–247
Broca, Pierre Paul, 56, 83, 86, 102, 167–169, 168f
Broca's area, 167–169, 168f
Bromides, 109, 122, 187
Brooks, Preston "Bully," 146
Brown, Augusta, 242
Brown, Charles Edward, Captain, 18
Brown, Graham, 190, 191
Browne, J. Crichton, 208n
Browning, Robert, 139
Brown-Séquard, Charles Edouard. *See also individual topics*
  on adrenal glands, *see* Adrenal glands.
  Charcot and, 137, 137n, 163, 208–209, 221n. *See also* Charcot, Jean-Martin.
  daily life, as Paris professor, 220–226
  doctoral thesis and, 31–32, 41–42
  early days as physician-scientist, 46–55
  early years in Mauritius, 11–12, 17–19, 19n
  in England, 98–116, 121
  experiments on self, 29–30, 62, 84, 205, 221, 225, 238–239, 248, 248n, 257–258, 264–266
  eye and vision research, 310–311
  French citizenship and home, 148–152
  at Harvard, 126–133
  hero of Mauritius cholera epidemic, 59–62, 81, 107, 266
  legacy of, 5, 237, 253–258, 284–288
  as medical student, 20, 27–32
  mother's death, 30
  on organ extracts, *see* Organ extracts.
  publications, 151, 261, 291–333
  on sensation, *see* Sensory pathway.
  on slavery, 81, 84, 121
  terminal illness and death, 226–228
  work published to 1878, 292–304
  work published from 1878 to 1886, 312–323
  work published from 1886 to 1894, 323–333
Brown-Séquard, Edouard (son), 89, 100, 127, 133–134, 283
Brown-Séquard, Charlotte Ellen (first daughter), 108
Brown-Séquard, Charlotte (second daughter), 147–150, 221, 225–227
Brown-Séquard, Ellen (first wife), 58, 59–61, 84, 89, 99, 100–101, 116, 121, 127
Brown-Séquard, Ellen Grace (granddaughter), 227
Brown-Séquard, Emma (third wife), 4, 148–150, 198–199, 221–223, 225–227
Brown-Séquard, Maria Rebecca (second wife), 142, 145–147
Brown-Séquard's Antineuralgic Pills, 124, 124n
Brown-Séquard syndrome, 5, 48–49f, 87, 213–220, 215f
Brukhonenko, Sergei Sergeevich, 278n
Bucknill, J. C., 208n
Byron, George Gordon, 183

Caloric test, 261–262
Cambridge University, 201
Cannabis, for diarrhea, 124, 124n
Carbon dioxide, 56, 186, 263, 270, 271–272, 272n
Carbon monoxide, 272n
Cardiopulmonary bypass, viii, 275, 277
Carlisle, Maria Rebecca (second wife), 142, 145–147
Carpenter, William Benjamin, 112
Carrel, Alexis, 278n
Carroll, Lewis, 77
Carter, Brudenell, 208, 208n
Casserius, Iulius, 89
Cell body, 157–158, 158f
Cellular therapy, 252
Cerebellum, 34f, 35, 157, 336, 338
Cerebrospinal fluid, 39n
Cervantes, Miguel de, 77
Chandler, Edward, 104
Chandler, Harry, 251

Chandler sisters (Johanna and Louisa), 104–105, 106
Chaplin, Charles, 252
Charcot, Jean-Martin, 31, 76, 76n, 87, 130, 137, 137n, 141, 144, 163–164, 190, 201n, 202–204, 207n, 208–209, 221n, 222, 272–273
Charlotte (queen of England), 103–104
Charrin, Albert, 221
Chloroform, 46, 55, 59n, 172
Cholecystokinin, 236n
Cholera, 54–55, 59–62, 59n, 81, 107, 266
Churchill, Winston, 6, 252
Cinematography, 5n
Circadian rhythms, 235n
Circulation, 5, 65–73, 159, 166n, 244n, 286, 306–310. *See also* Vasomotor nerves
Circumcision, for masturbation, 241
Civil War, American, 75n,116, 121–126, 125n, 146, 264
Cleveland, Grover, 125n
Cobbe, Frances Power, 139
Collège de France, ix, 3, 4, 5, 26–27, 39, 66, 88, 130n, 137n, 150–151, 151n, 197–199, 207n, 221, 221n, 222, 223, 223n, 227
Complex partial seizures, 188, 188n
Comroe, Julius, 262
Congress of Italian Naturalists, inhibition and, 161n
Considérant, Victor, 51
Convulsive syncope, 186n, 188–189
Corning, James, and vagal nerve stimulation, 188
Crimean War, 103n
Croonian Lecture, 112, 263
Crossed aphasia, 167–169, 167n, 168n
Cushing, Harvey, 252, 252n
Cussons, Andrea, testicular extracts and, 248
Czermak, Johann, 88

Dakin, Emma (third wife), 4, 148–150, 198–199, 221–223, 225–227
d'Alcantara, Dom Pedro (emperor of Brazil), 146, 146n, 201–202, 201n
Daly, César, 51, 52

Dareste, Gabriel Madeleine Camille, 151, 151n
Darwin, Charles, 13, 16, 77, 112n, 113, 142, 192, 207n
Darwin, Erasmus, 77
Dastre, Albert, 221, 221n
Daudet, Alphonse, 146
Dax, Gustav, 167n
Dax, Marc, 167, 167n
Debussy, Claude, 77
Decompression sickness, 163n
Decubitus ulcers. *See* Bed sores
Defibrination, 123, 123n, 276
de Gaulle, Charles, 252
Dejerine, Joseph Jules, 207, 207n
De Maupassant, Guy, 183
Dendrite, 157–158, 158f, 179, 337, 339–340
Denny-Brown, Derek, 214–216, 215f
D'Epinay, Prosper, 4, 5n
Deprez, Marcel, 223, 223n
Descartes, René, 36
Diabetes, 146n, 221n, 251, 255–256
Diarrhea, treatment of, 61, 124
Dickens, Charles, 183
Dissecting room hazards, 28–29
Dodo bird, 12
Donders, Franciscus, 201, 201n, 262
Donnelly, John, 139, 139n
Dostoyevsky, Fyodor, 183
Doyle, Conan, 250
The Duality of Mind (Wigan), 177
Dublin, Ireland, 18, 101, 107, 148,150
Du Bois-Reymond, 69n, 77
Dufresne, Guillaume, 13
Dumontpallier, Alphonse, 4, 207
Dunbar, Newell, 241–242
Dupuy, Eugene, 4, 225
Dutch East India Company, 13
Dynamometer, for power measurement, 111, 266
Dysentery, 91,124, 163, 201

Ears, water irrigation of, 261–262
École Pratique, 28–29, 53, 53n
Edinburgh University, 38n, 256n
Edinger-Westphal nucleus, 88

Efferent nerves, 32–34, 33f, 36, 67, 159, 160–161, 160f, 184, 190–191, 337, 341
Efron, R., 187
Eiffel, Gustav, 222
Electroencephalogram (EEG), 188, 188n
Eliot, George, 276–277
"Elixir of life", of Brown-Séquard, xii, 7, 206, 206n, 210, 239–242
Elliott, T. R., 254, 254n
Ems dispatch, 141
Endocrine/hormonal system, 5, 8, 89, 235–237, 236n, 249n, 252–256, 285, 286, 288. *See also specific gland/hormone*
  adrenal glands, vii, 7, 52, 67, 85n, 89–93, 211, 235n, 245, 246–247, 253–254, 256, 256n, 285, 287, 335
  adrenaline, 67, 90, 93, 253, 254n, 335, 337
  Schäfer on, 93, 256, 256n
Endocrine Society, founding of, 256
Endocrinology, journal, 256
England, 98–116, 121. *See also* London
Enteric nervous system, 66
Epigenetics, 192–193
Epilepsy, 183–193. *See also* Seizures
  bromide treatment for, 109, 187
  Brown-Séquard, C. E., experimental model of, 189–193
  Brown-Séquard, C. E., publications on, 304–306
  Brown-Séquard, C. E., treatment recommendations for, 186–188
  centric v. eccentric, 184
  convulsive syncope v., 186n, 188–189
  explanations for, 184–186
  hemispherectomy for, 179
  inheritance of acquired, 192–193
  lice infestations and, 191
  post-traumatic, 125
  reflex, 185–186, 185n, 192. *See also* Scratch reflex
  spinal, 189–193
Epinephrine, 67, 90, 93, 253–254, 254n, 268, 335, 337
Equipotentiality, of two cerebral hemispheres, 177–179
Erb, Wilhelm Heinrich, 190, 190n

Erb's palsy, 190n
Erectile dysfunction, 237
Ergot, 78
Esmarch, 202
Estrogens, 242n
Ether, 59n
Eugenics, 112n
Eustachius, Bartholomaeus, 89–90, 89n
Evans, Herbert McLean, 255, 255n
Expired air, toxicity of, 197, 271–272
Explosives, Berthelot, Marcelin, and 151n
Externat, 25–26, 337–338
Extrapyramidal system, 274
Eyes, vision and, 310–311

Fanton-Cameron, 208, 208n
Federal Radio Commission, 251
Feltus, Henry, 18, 57, 130
Fernández, Domingos, and Mauritius, 13
Ferrier, David, 170–173, 172n, 188, 203, 207, 208n
"Fight or flight" response, 66–67
Fillmore, Millard, 54
Fingerprint classification system, 112n
Flaubert, Gustave, 183
Fletcher, Ellen (first wife), 58, 59–61, 84, 89, 99, 100–101, 116, 121,127
Flourens, Pierre, 97, 166, 166n, 170, 270
Follicle-stimulating hormone, 235n
Forster, F. M., 187
Fouquier, Pierre-Eloy, 32
Fourcroy, Antoine François, Comte de, 24, 24n
Fourier, François Marie Charles, 51
Fourierism, 51, 55, 61
France. *See also specific province/city, institution, or topic.*
  Brown-Séquard, C. E., citizenship and home in, 138, 148–152, 220–226
  Franco-Prussian War, 141–142, 151n
  Mauritius's cultural link to, 13–17
  medical training in, 25–29
François-Franck, Charles-Emile, 221, 221n
François I (king of France), 150
Franco-Prussian War, 65n, 140–142, 143, 151n

Freud, Sigmund, 249
Frey-Gottesman, Lucja, 266–267, 266n
Fritsch, Gustav Theodor, 170, 171, 188
Functional localization in brain, 149, 165–177
   Brown-Séquard, C. E., v., 173–177, 197
   Ferrier and Goltz confrontation, 171–172, 172n

Galen of Pergamon, 35, 77, 183–184
Gall, Josef, 165–166
Galton, Francis, 112, 112n, 285
Galvanism, 69n
Galvin, Jim "Pud," 247
Gambetta, Léon, 141
Garfield, James, 203
Gastrin, 236n
George III (king), 35, 104
Germ theory of disease, 112n, 184n, 201
Gerontology, 237, 253, 286
Ghrelin, 236n
Gilles de la Tourette, Georges, 209, 209n
Girardin, Saint-Marc, 65–66, 65n
Glycogen, 39n, 237
Godlee, Rickman, 171
Goltz, Friedrich, 171–172, 202–203
Gonads, 7, 30, 205–211, 238–248, 248n, 253
   grafting/transplantation of animal/human, 249–252
   injection of animal, 7, 30, 205–211, 236–248, 248n
   ovaries, 236, 242, 242n, 249–250, 257, 342
   testicles, 7, 30, 122, 205–211, 238–248, 248n, 252, 253
   testosterone, 238n, 248, 248n, 252, 253, 342
   vasectomy, 249–250
Goubaux, Armand-Charles, 85n
Graham, Sylvester, 240
Gratiolet, 92
Grooming behavior, in animals, 191, 193
Gros-Caillou Hospital, 60
Gull, William, 91, 91n, 202
Gulstonian Lectures, 113
Gunshot wounds, 121, 124–126, 125n
Guttman, Ludwig, 126

Guyon, Jean Casimir Félix, 222, 222n, 285
Guy's Hospital, London, 90n, 91n, 109

Haldane, John Scott, 272, 272n
Hall, Marshall, 36–37, 36n, 41, 42, 184, 187
Hamilton, David, rejuvenation and, 248–249
Hammond, William A., 122, 122n, 208, 262
Hardy, William, 90
Harley, George, 92
Harrower, Henry, 256
Hart, Ernest, 211
Harvard College, 126–134
Harvey, William, 89
Hashimoto's thyroiditis, 243n
Heart, vagal nerve stimulation and, 254, 269
Heart, Weber brothers and, 161, 161n
Heart-lung machine, 277–278, 278n
Hemispherectomy, 179
Henle, Friedrich Gustav, 184n
Henle, Jakob, 67
Heredity, transmission of acquired characteristics, 139
Heubel, Emil, 263
Hibernation, viii, 262
Hippocrates, 77, 183
Hitzig, Eduard, 170–171, 188
Hodgkin, Thomas, 91, 91n
Holmes, Gordon, 115
Holmes, Oliver Wendell, 126–127, 126n, 143
Holmgren, I., 257
Homosexuality, 249
Honors
   Baly Medal to Brown-Séquard, C. E., 201
   Brown-Séquard, C. E., 86, 107, 163–164, 163n, 199, 201–202
Hormone, 90. *See also* Endocrine/hormonal system
Hormone replacement therapy, viii, 5, 7–8, 148, 203–211, 237, 254, 258, 285, 286
Horsley, Victor, 115n, 190, 207, 244, 245, 254n
Hospital
   Bellevue Hospital Medical College, 122n
   Gros-Caillou Hospital, Paris, 60

350 Index

Hospital (cont.)
   Guy's Hospital, London, 90n, 91n, 109
   Hospital for Diseases of the Nervous System, London, 106, 106n
   London Galvanic Hospital, Cavendish Square, 105–106
   Maida Vale Hospital, London, 106n
   Massachusetts General Hospital, Boston, 126
   Maudsley Hospital, London, 212n
   Middlesex Hospital, London, 38n
   National Hospital for the Paralysed and Epileptic, London, 102–116, 131, 208, 208n
   Philadelphia Orthopaedic Hospital and Infirmary for Nervous Diseases, 125n
   Turner's Lane General Hospital, Philadelphia, 125, 125n
   University of Pennsylvania Hospital, 125n
Hugo, Victor, 140
Hunter, John, 202, 237
Hunter, William, 38
Huot, Marie, 140, 140n
Huxley, Aldous, 250
Huxley, Thomas Henry, 98, 113, 115, 115n, 138, 139, 149, 171, 202, 207n
   Brown-Séquard, C. E., supported by, 139–140, 149
Hyperesthesia, 46–48, 47f, 48f, 87, 111, 212, 213, 214, 217, 226, 336, 338
Hypocretins, 235n
Hypothalamus, 66, 67, 235n, 236n, 263, 269, 336, 338
Hypothyroidism, 91n, 243–245, 243n, 246–247, 253, 256, 338
"Hysterical epilepsy", 109

Inhibition, 161–165
Inhibition theory of sleep, 263
Institut de France, 4, 51, 52, 86, 199, 200
Institut Pasteur, 224
Insulin, 255–256
Internat, 25–26, 337–338
International Medical Congress, 3, 131
International Medical Congress, London (1881), 171–172, 172n, 176, 202

Irrigation. *See also* Perfusion experiments.
   by blood, 48–49, 84, 97, 123,199, 261, 264, 275–278, 286
   with water, of ears, 261–262
Isabella (queen of Spain), 140

Jackson, Hughlings, 114, 116, 149, 159n, 168, 170, 178, 188, 207, 208n
Jacobin Club, 14, 24n
Jefferson, Thomas, 15, 77
Jefferson Medical College of Philadelphia, 201
Jenner, William, 201n, 202
Journal de la Physiologie de l'Homme et des Animaux, 97–98, 112
Journal de la Physiologie Expérimentale et Pathologique (Magendie), 39–40
Journal of Physiology, 137n
Julius Caesar, 183

Keen, William W., 125, 125n
Kellogg, John Preston, 240
Kennedy, John F., 90n
KFKB radio station, Kansas, 251n
Kidney, 171
   adrenal glands and, 67, 89–90, 92, 335
   Bowman's capsule, 99
   cholera and, 54
   extracts of, 245
   formation of renin in, 235n
   Henle and, 184n
   hormonal function and, 235, 235n
   reflex paraplegia and diseased, 101–102, 126, 273
Kingsford, Anna, 140, 140n
Koch, Robert, 184
Kocher, Theodore, 244
Konstantinov, I. E., 278n

Laborde, Jean Baptiste Vincent, 277n
Laboulaye, Edouard, 151
Lancet, Brown-Séquard and, 7, 99,100, 104, 105, 113, 116,149, 208n, 241
Language production, 167–170, 168f
La Phalange, 51

Larrey, Dominique Jean, 53n
Larrey, Félix-Hippolyte, 53–54
Laryngoscope, 88
Larynx, closure of, epilepsy and, 184, 186–187
Latta, Thomas, 55
Laudanum, 61, 62
Laurence, John Zachariah, 106, 108
Laurence-Moon-Biedl syndrome, 106
Laverdant, Gabriel Desiré, 61
Lavigerie, Charles, 146
Law of Bell-Magendie, 40
Legallois, Julien Jean César, 269, 269n
Legion of Honor, chevalier of, 199
Lenin, Vladimir, 183
Leopold (prince of Hohenzollern Sigmaringen), 140–141
Leptin, 236n
Lice infestations, epileptiform seizures and, 191, 193
Ligatures, for epilepsy, 186
Limbic system, 218f
Lincoln, Abraham, 116
Lippincott, publisher, 144, 145
Lister, Joseph, 108, 112, 112n, 202, 204
Littré, 31
Liver, 39n, 66, 92, 98n, 236–237, 236n, 245
  consumption of, for pernicious anemia, 257n
Lobb, Harry, 105
Locock, Charles, 109, 187
Loewy, Maurice, 3, 4n
London, England, 5, 5n, 38, 38n, 40n, 51n, 59, 68n, 87, 90, 93, 98–116, 146, 148–149, 150, 153n, 163–164, 163, 228. *See also* Hospitals *and specific institutions*
  Brown-Séquard, C. E., success in, 98–102
  Cavendish Square, 105–106, 115–116, 149
  cholera outbreak (1854), 54, 59n
  International Medical Congress, 171–172, 172n, 176, 202
  King's College, 98, 172, 172n
  London Neurological Society, 208n
  Royal College of Physicians of London, 112, 201, 250
  Royal Society of London, ix, 37, 68n, 87, 99, 107, 112, 113, 113n, 138, 171, 184, 212–213, 263
  University College, 38n, 93, 98, 250n, 254n, 256
London Neurological Society, 208n
Longet, M., 86
Lowell Institute, Boston, 147
Luteinizing hormone, 235n
Lymphatic fluid, 250n

MacArthur, Douglas, 124n
Magendie, François, 27, 39–40, 39n, 50, 66, 88, 90, 127, 139, 151, 198, 244n
Mahé de La Bourdonnais, Bertrand François, 14, 14n
Mahler, Gustav, 77
Maida Vale Hospital, London, 106n
Mann, Thomas, 252
Marey, Etienne-Jules, 5, 5n, 198–199, 221–222
Martin-Magron, 41, 50, 92, 102
Mascarenhas, Pedro de, 13
Massachusetts General Hospital, Boston, 126
Masturbation, 109, 209, 238, 240–241
Maudsley Hospital, London, 212n
Maugham, Somerset, 252
Mauritius, 11–17
  cholera epidemic, 59–62, 81, 107, 266
  colonial history of, 13–16
  population diversity, 16–17
  Slavery Abolition Bill and, 16–17, 16n
  sugar industry in, 16–17
  visitors to Paris from, 225
Medical College of Virginia, 82–85
Medulla, 34f, 35, 159, 166n, 217, 218f, 267, 268–271, 273–274
  epilepsy and, 185
Medulla, adrenal, 89–90, 92–93,
Melatonin, 235n
Mendelssohn, Felix, 184n
Microtome, 68n
Middlesex Hospital Medical School, 38n
Migraine, 77–78
Mill, John Stuart, 113

Minot, George, Nobel Prize and, 257
Mitchell, Silas Weir, 75, 75n, 125,125n, 132, 132n, 208, 277
Molière, Jean-Baptiste Poquelin, 183
Monet, Claude, 77
Monkey-gland operations, 250
Montefiore, Moses, 91n
Montparnasse, cemetery of, 4, 227
Montyon Prize, 50, 88, 88n, 97
Morath, Max, 206n
Morehouse, George R., 125, 125n
Motilin, 236n
Mott, Frederick, 212–213, 215f, 216
Motta Maia, Cláudio Velho de, 201n
Murphy, William, Nobel Prize and, 257
Murray, George Redmayne, 244
Muscle tissue,
    Brown-Séquard, C. E., research on, 306–310
    as extract, 245
    reciprocal innervation, 164n
    stretch reflex, 160–161, 160f, 190–191
Museum of Comparative Zoology, 143
Musicogenic epilepsy, 185n
Myasthenia gravis, 190n
Myxoedema. *See* Hypothyroidism

Napoleonic code, 16, 227
National Hospital for the Paralysed and Epileptic, London, 102–116, 131, 208, 208n
Nativel, Marie-Jeanne Geneviève Elisabeth, 18
Naussau, Maurice van, 13
Nervous system. *See also* Brain *and specific topics.*
    autonomic, 37, 66–68, 72, 336–337.
        See also Vasomotor nerves
    Brown-Séquard, C. E., publications on, to 1878, 292–304, 304–306
    Brown-Séquard, C. E., publications, 1878 to 1886, 312–323
    Brown-Séquard, C. E., publications, 1886 to 1894, 323–333
    Central nervous system, 32–33, 68n, 112, 157, 162–165, 177–179, 269n
    heart regulated by, 68–72

Neurasthenia, 251, 251n
Neuron, 32–33, 33f
Neurotransmitters, 158, 188, 217, 218, 236, 253, 254n, 263, 340
Newborns, Legallois' study of, 269n
New York, 3, 5, 18, 56, 57, 85, 97, 109, 115, 116,122n, 128, 132n, 134, 141, 142, 143,144, 145, 147, 148, 150, 159–160, 241
    clinical practice in, 145–146
Nice, Provence, 4, 6, 224–226, 228
Niehans, Paul, 252
Nietzsche, Friedrich, 77
Nightingale, Florence, 103, 103n
Nobel, Alfred, 131, 183
Nobel laureate,
    Bárány, 262
    Carrel, 278n
    Kocher, 244
    Landsteiner, 123n
    Minot, 257
    Murphy, 257
    Pavlov, 263n
    Pregl, 247
    Sherrington, 79, 164n, 165
    Whipple, 257
    Yeats, 249
Nodier, Charles, 11, 11n
Noradrenaline. *See* Norepinephrine
Norepinephrine, 67, 90, 217, 340
Nystagmus, 261–262

Oberon, Merle, 252
Ocean exploration, 163n
Oliver, George, 93, 256n
Opium extract, 124, 124n
Opotherapy, 236. *See* Organ extracts.
Organ extracts, 5, 197–198, 205–211, 238–248
    from adrenal glands, 211, 246, 256
    American response to, 240–242
    bone tissue, 245
    brain tissue, 245
    elixir of life, 7, 206, 210, 239–240, 337
    kidney, 245
    muscle tissue, 245

ovaries, 242, 242n, 249–250, 257
pancreas, 245
Pasteur and, 202, 221–224
pituitary gland, 245
procedure for preparing, 242–243
Schiff's work with, 244n
spleen, 245
from testicles, 7, 30, 122, 205–211, 238–248, 248n, 252
from thyroid, 244–245, 247, 256
treatment of disease and rejuvenation, 238–248, 258
Organotherapy, 5, 6, 7, 236–237, 254, 256. See also Organ extracts.
athletic performance and, 247
as hypothyroidism treatment, 244–245, 247
recapturing youth with, 7, 206–207, 206n, 210, 239–241, 255
Organ transplantation, 278n
Ovaries, 236, 242, 242n, 249–250, 257
Oxford University, England, 100, 207n
Oxytocin, 235n

Paget, James, 50–51, 51n, 75, 87, 97, 99, 100, 106, 108, 112, 202, 203
Pancoast, 202
Pancreas, 66, 236n, 245, 255–256
Paraplegia, 74, 78, 101,126
Parasympathetic system, 66–67, 72, 336
Paris, 3, 5, 6, 11, 20, 45, 54, 57, 59, 60, 65, 70, 83, 84, 87, 88, 89, 100, 102, 107, 108, 126, 130, 131,137–155, 166, 167, 197, 204. See also specific institutions and topics.
and the Collège de France, 197–228
Faculty of Medicine, 11, 20, 23–27, 29, 31, 53n, 85, 92, 148, 205, 222
first half of nineteenth century, 12
Franco-Prussian War, 65, 140–142, 151n
Mauritius and, 14–16
medical student in, 23–32, 81, 133
Treaty of, 16
visitors from Mauritius, 225
Paris Commune, 141–142

Paris Faculty of Medicine, 11, 20, 23–27, 29, 31, 53n, 85, 92, 148, 205, 222
Pasteur, Louis, 6, 140n
mourning death of Brown-Séquard, C. E., 226
on testicular extracts, 202, 221–224
Pavlov, Ivan Petrovich, 263, 263n
Perfusion experiments, 48–49, 84, 97, 123,199, 261, 264, 275–278, 286
Pernicious anemia, 257n
Phalange, 51
Phenobarbital, 109, 187
Phenytoin, 109, 187
Philadelphia, 56, 56n, 69, 70, 107, 125, 125n, 130, 132–133, 144
Brown-Séquard, C. E., father born in, 18
Jefferson Medical College of, 125n, 201
Philadelphia College of Pharmacy, 56n
Philadelphia Orthopaedic Hospital and Infirmary for Nervous Diseases, 125n
Philippeaux, 92
Photogenic epilepsy, 185n
Phrenology, 149, 165–166
Piastre, 18–19, 19n
Pineal gland, 235n
Pituitary gland, 235, 235n, 245, 252n
Pius XII (pope), 252
Plato, 77
Pliny the Elder, 236
Port Louis, Mauritius, 14, 16, 19–20, 19n, 60
American traders in, 15
Post-traumatic epilepsy, 125
Potassium bromide, 122
Pregl, Fritz, 247
Prix Lacaze, 199, 277
Prix Lallemand, 163, 163n
Prolactin, 235n
Prussia, Franco-Prussian War, 65, 141–142, 151n
Pulmonary edema, 267–269
Putnam's, publisher, 145
Pyramidotomy, 273–274

Quain, Richard, 149, 149n

Radcliffe, Charles Bland, 109, 116,149

Radcliffe College, 144
Ramskill, Jabez Spence, 106, 109
Rayer, Pierre, 31, 50, 52, 69, 97, 201, 272
Reflexes, 36–37, 110, 160–161, 160f, 184, 341. *See also* Scratch reflex.
Reflex epilepsy, 185–186, 185n, 192. *See also* Scratch reflex.
Reflex paraplegia, 101–102, 272–273
Reid, George, 108
Rejuvenation. *See also* Aging, 7, 205–207, 238–253, 249n, 251n
Rejuvenation (*cont.*)
  1875 experiments, 148
  1889 experiments, 205–211
  organ extracts and, 238–248, 248–253, 249n, 251n, 258
Renan, Ernest, 223, 223n
Renier, Leon, 151
Renin, 235n
Respiration, 123n, 159, 166, 189, 256n, 264, 267–272, 269n
Reverdin, J.L., 244
Richmond, Virginia, 5, 62, 81–85
Rigor mortis, 112–113, 263–264, 275–278
Riolan, Jean, 89
Robin, Charles, 31, 52, 87–88, 98, 199
Rolleston, H. D., 89
Romanes, George John, 207, 207n
Royal College of Physicians of London, 112, 201, 250
Royal College of Surgeons of England, 98, 107
Royal Commission of Enquiry on Vivisection, 139
Royal Society of Arts and Sciences of Mauritius, 107
Royal Society of London, ix, 37, 68n, 87, 99, 107, 112, 113, 113n, 138, 171, 184, 212–213, 263
  Philosophical Club of, 113, 113n

Salivary glands, 71–72
Sanderson, John Burdon, 98, 202, 272n
Sayers, Dorothy L., 251
Schäfer, Edward, 93, 256, 256n
Schiff, Moritz, 92, 208, 244, 244n

Schiller, Joseph, 137, 137n
School of Natural History, 143
Scratch reflex, 161, 191–193, 341
Sechenov, Ivan, 161–162, 162n
Secretin, 236n, 256
Seguin, Edward Constant, 144, 144n
Seizures, 124–125, 125n, 170, 185n. *See also* Epilepsy
  complex partial, 188, 188n
  convulsive syncope, 186n, 188–189
  generalized v. partial, 183
  inheritance of, 192–193
  epileptiform, lice infestations and, 191, 193
Sensory deficits, quantification of, 110–111
Sensory pathways, 29, 32–42, 33f, 42f, 46–48, 47f, 48f, 49f, 53, 85–87, 88, 89, 98, 201, 211–220, 212f, 215f, 218f, 244, 285, 286, 287
  Brown-Séquard, C. E., doctoral thesis on, 31–32, 41–42
Septicemia, 28
Séquard, Henriette Perrine Charlotte (mother), 11, 18–20, 30, 31, 32, 58, 81
Séquard, Pierre Paul (maternal grandfather), 18
Sexual behavior
  homosexuality, 249
  masturbation, 109, 210, 238, 239, 240–241
Sexual rejuvenation, 7, 205–207, 238–253, 249n, 251n
Shaw, George Bernard, 278
Sherrington, Charles Scott, 79, 164–165, 164n, 190, 191
Shock, 123n
Sibson, Francis, 112
Skin, 41n
  Brown-Séquard, C. E., research on, 306–310
Slavery. *See also* Colonialism
  Brazil's abolition of, 146, 146n
  Britain's Slavery Abolition Bill, 16–17, 16n
  Brown-Séquard, C. E., disapproval of, 84, 121
  Lincoln's emancipation proclamation, 116
Sleep
  Brown-Séquard, C. E., studies in, 262–263

hormones involved in regulating, 235n
neurasthenia, 251n
vascular concepts of basis of, 262
Snow, John, 59, 59n
Socialist ideals, of Brown-Séquard C. E., 51, 55, 61, 284
Société d'Anthropologie, 102, 107, 167
Société de Biologie, 4, 52–53, 68, 70, 85, 86, 87, 107, 168, 201, 205, 219, 227, 238, 240, 249n, 255, 292
Société Philomathique, 107
Space exploration, 163n
Speech (language), 167–170, 168f
　Broca and, 167–169, 168f
　Brown-Séquard, C. E., on aphasia, 168–170
　right v. left hemisphere and, 178–179
Sphygmograph, 198
Spigelius, 89
Spinal cord injuries, American Civil War and, 124–126, 125n
Spinal epilepsy, 189–193. See also Epilepsy
Spinal sensory pathways, See Sensory pathways.
Spinal shock, 36–37, 36n, 41, 42
Spleen, 245
"Split brain" surgical procedure, 179
Spurzheim, Johann Gaspar, 165
Stanford, Leland, 146, 146n
Stanford University, 146n
Stanley, Leo, 251
Starling, Ernest, 90, 250, 250n
Startle response, 73
Steinach, Eugen, 249, 249n, 252
Stevenson, Robert Louis, 177
Stilling, Benedikt, 68, 68n
Stramonium, 124, 124n
Stretch reflex, 35–37, 101, 110, 111, 160–161, 160f, 184, 190–191, 274, 341
Struthers, John, 108
Sumner, Charles, 146–147
Swanson, Gloria, 252
Sympathetic nerves/system, 66–73, 77, 78, 145, 221n, 254, 262, 266, 269, 336, 340, 341
Synapse, 36, 157–158, 158f, 159, 254, 341–342

Taylor, Zachary, 54
Tennyson, Alfred, 139
Testicles, 238n
　grafting/transplantation of animal/human, 242–243, 249–257
　injection of animal, 7, 30, 122, 205–211, 236–237, 238–248, 248n, 252
Testosterone, 238n, 248, 248n, 252
Tetanus, 122, 122n
Thalamus, 218f
Tholozan, Joseph Désiré, 72–73
Thompson, Henry, 211, 211n
Thyroid
　animal extracts, 245–246, 256
　hypothyroidism and, 91n, 243–245, 243n, 244n, 246–247, 253, 256, 338
Thyroid-releasing hormone, 235n
Thyroid replacement therapy, 243n
Todd, R. Bentley, 98, 98n
Tourette, Georges Gilles de la, 209, 209n
Transfusion, blood, 91, 123–124, 123n
Treaty of Paris, 16
Trichinosis, 51n
Trousseau, Armand, 25, 26, 31, 52, 87, 131
Turner's Lane General Hospital, 125, 125n

University College London, 38n, 93, 98, 250n, 254n, 256
University of Bern, 244n
University of Cambridge, 201
University of Geneva, 149, 244n
University of Pennsylvania Hospital, 125n

Vagus nerve, 161, 187–188, 201
Van Gogh, Vincent, 77, 183
Vasectomy, and rejuvenation, 249–250
Vasomotor nerves,
　discovery of, 58, 65, 67–72, 77, 78, 199, 221n
Vasomotor reflexes, 72–73, 221n
Vasomotor theory of epilepsy, 185–186, 186n
Vasomotor theory of migraine, 77–78
Vatican Academy of Science, 252
Vesey, W. T., 90
Vicq d'Azyr, Felix, 23, 23

Victoria (queen of England), 38n, 51n, 59n, 90n, 99, 102–103, 109, 112n, 166, 201
  International Medical Congress, 171–172
Victoria and Albert Museum, 139n
Virchow, 202
Viscera, Brown-Séquard, C. E., work on, 306–310
Vitamin B_{12}, 257n
Vitamin E, 255n
Vivisection, without anesthesia, 40, 40n, 45–46, 140
Vivisection Act, 172n
Volkmann, 202, 271
Von Langenbeck, Bernard, 203, 203n
Voronoff, Serge, 250–251, 252
Vulpian, Edmé-Félix Alfred, 85, 85n, 92, 137, 137n, 141, 148, 163, 166n, 190, 199, 200, 208, 213, 221n, 276, 291

Wakley, Thomas, 37n, 99, 100, 149
Walker, Alexander, 37–38, 38n
Wall, Patrick, 216, 216n
Waller, Augustus Volney, 70, 138, 138n
Warwyck, Wybrandt van, 13
Waterhouse, W. D., 4, 208
Watteville, Armand de, 208, 208n

Weber, Eduard Friedrich, 161, 161n
Weber, Ernst Heinrich, 110, 110n, 161, 161n
Webster, Daniel, 58n
Wernicke, Carl, 167–168, 168f
Wernicke's area, 168, 168f
Westphal, Carl Friedrich Otto, 88
Whipple, George, Nobel Prize and, 257
Whytt, Robert, 35–36
Wigan, Arthur, 177
Wilberforce, Samuel, 115, 115n
Wilhelm II (emperor of Germany/king of Prussia), 202n
Wilks, Samuel, 109
Willis, Thomas, 36, 68, 68n, 77
Wire, Alderman David, 104–105
Woakes, Edward, 78
Wood, George B., 56, 56n
Word recognition, 167–168, 168f
Wren, Christopher, 68n

Yale, Elihu, 103
Yeats, William Butler, 249
Yeo, Gerald, 172, 172n

Zoth, Oskar, 247

hormones involved in regulating, 235n
neurasthenia, 251n
vascular concepts of basis of, 262
Snow, John, 59, 59n
Socialist ideals, of Brown-Séquard C. E., 51, 55, 61, 284
Société d'Anthropologie, 102, 107, 167
Société de Biologie, 4, 52–53, 68, 70, 85, 86, 87, 107, 168, 201, 205, 219, 227, 238, 240, 249n, 255, 292
Société Philomathique, 107
Space exploration, 163n
Speech (language), 167–170, 168f
  Broca and, 167–169, 168f
  Brown-Séquard, C. E., on aphasia, 168–170
  right v. left hemisphere and, 178–179
Sphygmograph, 198
Spigelius, 89
Spinal cord injuries, American Civil War and, 124–126, 125n
Spinal epilepsy, 189–193. *See also* Epilepsy
Spinal sensory pathways, *See* Sensory pathways.
Spinal shock, 36–37, 36n, 41, 42
Spleen, 245
"Split brain" surgical procedure, 179
Spurzheim, Johann Gaspar, 165
Stanford, Leland, 146, 146n
Stanford University, 146n
Stanley, Leo, 251
Starling, Ernest, 90, 250, 250n
Startle response, 73
Steinach, Eugen, 249, 249n, 252
Stevenson, Robert Louis, 177
Stilling, Benedikt, 68, 68n
Stramonium, 124, 124n
Stretch reflex, 35–37, 101, 110, 111, 160–161, 160f, 184, 190–191, 274, 341
Struthers, John, 108
Sumner, Charles, 146–147
Swanson, Gloria, 252
Sympathetic nerves/system, 66 73, 77, 78, 145, 221n, 254, 262, 266, 269, 336, 340, 341
Synapse, 36, 157–158, 158f, 159, 254, 341–342

Taylor, Zachary, 54
Tennyson, Alfred, 139
Testicles, 238n
  grafting/transplantation of animal/human, 242–243, 249–257
  injection of animal, 7, 30, 122, 205–211, 236–237, 238–248, 248n, 252
Testosterone, 238n, 248, 248n, 252
Tetanus, 122, 122n
Thalamus, 218f
Tholozan, Joseph Désiré, 72–73
Thompson, Henry, 211, 211n
Thyroid
  animal extracts, 245–246, 256
  hypothyroidism and, 91n, 243–245, 243n, 244n, 246–247, 253, 256, 338
Thyroid-releasing hormone, 235n
Thyroid replacement therapy, 243n
Todd, R. Bentley, 98, 98n
Tourette, Georges Gilles de la, 209, 209n
Transfusion, blood, 91, 123–124, 123n
Treaty of Paris, 16
Trichinosis, 51n
Trousseau, Armand, 25, 26, 31, 52, 87, 131
Turner's Lane General Hospital, 125, 125n

University College London, 38n, 93, 98, 250n, 254n, 256
University of Bern, 244n
University of Cambridge, 201
University of Geneva, 149, 244n
University of Pennsylvania Hospital, 125n

Vagus nerve, 161, 187–188, 201
Van Gogh, Vincent, 77, 183
  Vasectomy, and rejuvenation, 249–250
Vasomotor nerves,
  discovery of, 58, 65, 67–72, 77, 78, 199, 221n
Vasomotor reflexes, 72–73, 221n
Vasomotor theory of epilepsy, 185–186, 186n
Vasomotor theory of migraine, 77–78
Vatican Academy of Science, 252
Vesey, W. T., 90
Vicq d'Azyr, Felix, 23, 23

Index

Victoria (queen of England), 38n, 51n, 59n, 90n, 99, 102–103, 109, 112n, 166, 201
  International Medical Congress, 171–172
Victoria and Albert Museum, 139n
Virchow, 202
Viscera, Brown-Séquard, C. E., work on, 306–310
Vitamin B_{12}, 257n
Vitamin E, 255n
Vivisection, without anesthesia, 40, 40n, 45–46, 140
Vivisection Act, 172n
Volkmann, 202, 271
Von Langenbeck, Bernard, 203, 203n
Voronoff, Serge, 250–251, 252
Vulpian, Edmé-Félix Alfred, 85, 85n, 92, 137, 137n, 141, 148, 163, 166n, 190, 199, 200, 208, 213, 221n, 276, 291

Wakley, Thomas, 37n, 99, 100, 149
Walker, Alexander, 37–38, 38n
Wall, Patrick, 216, 216n
Waller, Augustus Volney, 70, 138, 138n
Warwyck, Wybrandt van, 13
Waterhouse, W. D., 4, 208
Watteville, Armand de, 208, 208n

Weber, Eduard Friedrich, 161, 161n
Weber, Ernst Heinrich, 110, 110n, 161, 161n
Webster, Daniel, 58n
Wernicke, Carl, 167–168, 168f
Wernicke's area, 168, 168f
Westphal, Carl Friedrich Otto, 88
Whipple, George, Nobel Prize and, 257
Whytt, Robert, 35–36
Wigan, Arthur, 177
Wilberforce, Samuel, 115, 115n
Wilhelm II (emperor of Germany/king of Prussia), 202n
Wilks, Samuel, 109
Willis, Thomas, 36, 68, 68n, 77
Wire, Alderman David, 104–105
Woakes, Edward, 78
Wood, George B., 56, 56n
Word recognition, 167–168, 168f
Wren, Christopher, 68n

Yale, Elihu, 103
Yeats, William Butler, 249
Yeo, Gerald, 172, 172n

Zoth, Oskar, 247